Burnout

Burnout
The Emotional Experience of Political Defeat

Hannah Proctor

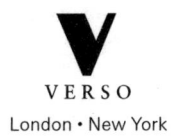

V
VERSO
London • New York

First published by Verso 2024
© Hannah Proctor 2024

All rights reserved

The moral rights of the author have been asserted

1 3 5 7 9 10 8 6 4 2

Verso
UK: 6 Meard Street, London W1F 0EG
US: 388 Atlantic Avenue, Brooklyn, NY 11217
versobooks.com

Verso is the imprint of New Left Books

ISBN-13: 978-1-83976-605-3
ISBN-13: 978-1-83976-607-7 (US EBK)
ISBN-13: 978-1-83976-606-0 (UK EBK)

British Library Cataloguing in Publication Data
A catalogue record for this book is available from the British Library

Library of Congress Cataloging-in-Publication Data

Names: Proctor, Hannah, author.
Title: Burnout : the emotional experience of political defeat / Hannah Proctor.
Description: London ; New York : Verso, 2024. | Includes bibliographical references and index.
Identifiers: LCCN 2023046427 (print) | LCCN 2023046428 (ebook) | ISBN 9781839766053 (paperback : alk. paper) | ISBN 9781839766077 (ebook)
Subjects: LCSH: Political participation--Psychological aspects. | Political activists--Psychology. | Struggle. | Distress (Psychology) | Defeat (Psychology)
Classification: LCC JF799 .P745 2024 (print) | LCC JF799 (ebook) | DDC 323/.042019--dc23/eng/20231201
LC record available at https://lccn.loc.gov/2023046427
LC ebook record available at https://lccn.loc.gov/2023046428

Typeset in Minion by Biblichor Ltd
Printed and bound by CPI Group (UK) Ltd, Croydon CR0 4YY

You who will emerge again from the flood
In which we have gone under
Think
When you speak of our faults
Of the dark times
Which you have escaped.

For we went, changing countries more often than our shoes
Through the wars of the classes, despairing
When there was injustice only, and no indignation.

And yet we know:
Hatred, even of meanness
Makes you ugly.
Anger, even at injustice
Makes your voice hoarse. Oh, we
Who wanted to prepare the land for friendliness
Could not ourselves be friendly.

You, however, when the time comes
When mankind is a helper unto mankind
Think on us
With forbearance.[1]

– Bertolt Brecht, 'To Those Born After' (1939)

Contents

Introduction   1

Part I. Historical Symptoms: Past Attachments   29

   1. Melancholia   31
   2. Nostalgia   42
   3. Depression   62

Part II. Survival Pending Revolution: Patient Urgency   87

   4. Burnout   89
   5. Exhaustion   103
   6. Bitterness   130

Part III. Concepts Transformed: Anti-Adaptive Healing   159

   7. Trauma   161
   8. Mourning   186

Afterword   203
Acknowledgements   215
Notes   219
Index   253

Introduction

*for every revolutionary   must at last will his own destruction
rooted as he is in the past he sets out to destroy*[1]
                                                    – Diane di Prima

Change is hard. Living under capitalism can be physically damaging and mentally draining; the harms it inflicts are unevenly distributed. Overturning prevailing social and economic conditions is necessary and urgent. But change is hard.

It's hard to change. People shaped by the societies they have grown up in transform in the process of trying to change them. Breaking with habitual rhythms to organise collectively, forging solidarity with others against a common enemy or gathering in the streets to fight injustice can alter lives forever, but struggles don't always continue. When movements are crushed, strategies fail, solidarity crumbles, energies wane, people turn on one another or groups reproduce the oppressive dynamics of the structures they are fighting, the dejection incurred can be as psychologically profound as the elation that preceded it. Trying to reform let alone overturn the existing state of things can inflict its own mental wounds, especially when movements end in defeat or retreat.

Burnout considers emotional experiences of political defeat, disillusionment and depletion in historical perspective, with chapters structured around eight concepts: melancholia, nostalgia, depression, burnout, exhaustion, bitterness, trauma and mourning. Confronting the psychological toll of political struggle, the book asks how activists, organisers and revolutionaries in various left-wing groups, parties and liberation movements have worked through the emotional impacts of their political experiences, whether collectively or in isolation. Analysing the psychic aftermath of cycles of struggle, the emotional fallout of defeated movements, the ongoing strain of day-to-day organising 'spade work', and the corrosive interpersonal tensions that emerge in radical political groups,

Burnout responds to the psychological challenges of sustaining momentum over long periods. By examining historical examples of defeat and attempts to overcome them, I hope to provide resources for working through difficult emotional experiences that arise in social movements, asking how to keep fighting against oppressive and exploitative social conditions even when victory seems remote. I also insist on the possibility, indeed the necessity, of acknowledging the magnitude of psychological questions in left-wing political movements, an acknowledgement that need not reduce social problems to individual ones in the process.

In *Enduring Time* Lisa Baraitser declares her interest in exploring 'the slowness of chronic time, rather than the time of rupture; the durational drag of staying alongside others, rather than the time of transgression; the elongated time of incremental change, rather than the time of breakthrough or revolution.'[2] In *Burnout*, I intend to substitute Baraitser's 'rather thans' for 'ands'. Instead of swapping an account of the epic for an account of the mundane – the big for the small, the political for the personal, the historical for the experiential, the exceptional for the quotidian – I take for granted that these seemingly distant poles are always entangled. By asking how people have tried to address psychological distress in the process of attempting to transform their shared social conditions through struggle, I explore how political defeats, disappointments and retreats have shaped people, who have shaped history in turn.

Revolutionary selfhood

Revolutionary left-wing traditions stereotypically equate an emphasis on individual psychology with an affirmation of bourgeois individualism. The image of the ideal revolutionary subject propagated by many revolutionaries historically is someone who relinquishes their personal life for the sake of the collective. Such a rhetoric of revolutionary selflessness is expressed in the documentary *Red Army/PLFP: Declaration of World War* (1971), which follows the activities of militants in the revolutionary socialist group Popular Front for the Liberation of Palestine (PFLP) and members of the Japanese Red Army who, following the defeats of the Japanese student movements of 1968, had travelled to Lebanon to fight in solidarity with the Palestinian cause. The film includes an interview with PFLP member Leila Khaled, whose image circulated widely following her involvement in the TWA 840 plane hijacking in 1969. She explains why, despite her recent fame, she rejects being called a hero:

> We do not talk of ourselves as individuals . . . revolution is always born of people, for people, and because it is for general humanity that is why being among the whole makes the individual pretty insignificant . . . we are never heroes . . . we are simply doing our duty, and I like to insist that we dedicate ourselves to revolution and that our lives are for revolution.³

Khaled underwent plastic surgery in 1970 to make her face less recognisable, in order to participate anonymously in further militant actions but also to evade her status as a revolutionary icon. She endured the painful procedures without anaesthetic, a decision she framed in her autobiography in terms of her revolutionary commitment: 'I have a cause higher and nobler than my own, a cause to which all private interests and concerns must be subordinated.'⁴ Khaled claimed that as a Palestinian woman, she was often accused of displaying too much emotion, and she admitted to feeling deep emotions about her losses – losses of home, community, present and future – yet she insisted that the fight for Palestinian liberation was guided by reason, not passion. The self must be renounced in favour of the collective; emotions must be channelled into political action.

In *Memoirs of a Revolutionary*, first published in French in 1951, Victor Serge likewise says of his role before, during and after the October Revolution of 1917: 'Individual existences were of no interest to me— particularly my own.'⁵ In a similar vein to Khaled, he frequently describes the self-sacrifice and anonymity demanded by a life dedicated to revolution:

> All we lived for was activity integrated into history; we were interchangeable . . . None of us had, in the bourgeois sense of the word, any personal existence: we changed our names, our postings, and our work at the Party's need . . . When I say *we*, I have in mind the typical international or Russian militant comrade.⁶

Yet the mental breakdown experienced by Serge's wife, Liuba Russakova, which unfolded in the paranoid context of the Stalinist purges, during which even the psychiatric clinics and sanatoria were full of police spies, indicates that this vision of ideal revolutionary dedication was strained by actual historical experiences. The same can be said for the many stories of despair, suicide and anguish documented in Serge's notebooks, which cover his last years in exile in Mexico in the 1940s after he fled first the Stalinist Terror and then Nazi-occupied France. Courageous commitment to a collective cause could not insulate individuals from forms of psychological torment or distress, which in turn impeded their capacity to participate in continued militancy.

Forgoing personal concerns for the sake of the greater good may be urgent, but completely suppressing individual desires, needs and difficulties does not necessarily advance collective political causes. Black Panther Party co-founder Huey P. Newton's 1973 memoir *Revolutionary Suicide* opens with an anecdote involving a piece of psychological research. While Newton was held in solitary confinement in the California Men's Colony in San Luis Obispo and banned from receiving reading material, a copy of the May 1970 issue of the magazine *Ebony* was pushed under his cell door. In it he read an article by Lacy Banks discussing research findings made by Dr Herbert Hendin, who had conducted a comparative study showing that suicide rates among black people in the US had doubled in the past ten to fifteen years, far surpassing the suicide rate for white people. The article reminded Newton of an argument made by Emile Durkheim in 1897 that linked the desire to commit suicide to people's economic circumstances. Hendin's research describes something Newton labels 'reactionary suicide': suicides that resulted from existing social conditions, a phenomenon Newton links to a metaphorical 'spiritual death' among black people in the US.[7] Rather than endure these deathly conditions, he concludes it would be better to fight them, even if doing so could be a dangerous and potentially fatal endeavour. Contemplating the high suicide rates among young black people led Newton to develop the concept of 'revolutionary suicide': total commitment to a transformative cause.

Newton's revolutionary suicide is not a death wish but expresses the desire to live in a less deathly world, while recognising, more explicitly than Khaled or Serge, the possibility of getting crushed in the process. The philosophy of revolutionary suicide accepts that the individual revolutionary may not live to see the liveable world they are fighting to create. In the book's epilogue Newton reflects on his comrades 'in the asylum, penitentiary, or grave', saluting those who continue to give up the 'I' for the sake of the 'we': 'By giving all to the present we reject fear, despair and defeat.'[8] The *Ebony* article Newton cited, which explains that Hendin's research focused on black men and women in New York City, also links the high suicide rate to social and economic factors: police violence, unemployment, cramped housing, inaccessible mental health care, hunger. Newton proposed militancy – individuals in the present abandoning their personal lives for the sake of the collective future – as the cure for reactionary suicide, whereas Banks discusses suicide prevention centres, counselling services and the 'rising corps' of black psychiatrists.[9] Could an attentiveness to psychic life accompany or enhance militancy without embracing mainstream psychiatric practices that encourage adaptation to existing norms and disconnect individual despair from social conditions? Newton's criticisms of Eldridge Cleaver for embracing violent rhetoric and 'defect[ing] from the community' by neglecting the Panthers' survival programmes that aimed to 'serve the people' – grocery giveaways, free medical clinics, community ambulances, breakfast clubs, prison bussing programmes, sickle cell anaemia screenings and so on – suggest an alternative to reactionary suicide in periods when the struggle is in abeyance.[10] Survival pending revolution is a form of resistance, not retreat. Fighting the oppressor by refusing their terms entails 'psychological warfare'.[11] Newton suggests that questions about the psychic life of revolutionaries and activists demand a dialectical response: in the absence of imminent revolution, it is necessary to build structures of support in the meantime.

Both Khaled and Newton invoke Ernesto 'Che' Guevara as a model revolutionary. In 1965, four years after the assassination of the independence leader and first Prime Minister of Democratic Republic of the Congo (DRC), Patrice Lumumba, Guevara travelled under an alias from Havana to Congo to lead a force of around 200 mostly Afro-Cuban soldiers to fight alongside the Marxist Simba movement against the Belgian colonialists. In the epilogue to *Congo Diary*, in which Guevara reflects on the many difficulties and errors he encountered, including the low morale and poor training among Congolese rebels, Guevara outlines an image of the ideal revolutionary subject capable of fighting in such a conflict, an image that reiterates the need for emotional toughness and a revocation of personal attachments:

> We must confirm what characteristics are required of a militant, so that he [sic] can overcome the violent traumas of a reality which he must confront . . . Revolutionary militants who go off to participate in a similar experience must begin without dreams, having abandoned everything that used to constitute their lives and exertions. The only ones who must go are those with a revolutionary strength of mind much greater than the average – even the average in a revolutionary country – with practical experience gained in struggle, with a high level of political development, and with strong discipline.[12]

This steeliness and self-sacrifice, he argues, could only be achieved in a small proportion of revolutionaries and would require trained revolutionary cadres and political education. This abstract image of the ideal militant is, however, quickly undercut by the severe self-criticisms that immediately follow in Guevara's text, based on his assessments of his own concrete experiences and behaviour.

Guevara admits to his own flaws: while able to endure a poor diet and worn-out shoes, he withdrew too often from the group to read. He also bemoans his failure to convince soldiers to look beyond the 'dark fog of the present' to contemplate the brighter future, and he castigates himself for his 'bitter and damaging' emotional outbursts. He speculates these could be 'due to some innate aspect of my character', implying that he assumes that the individual psyche is resistant to change. He concludes sourly, confessing: 'I didn't overcome subjectivity in the end.' 'These psychological considerations,' he writes, 'might appear out of place in the analysis of a struggle that is virtually continental in scale', and yet, reflecting on the problems he encountered in Congo alongside his own personal failures, he is compelled to admit their significance.[13]

That psychological considerations have a place in political struggles with totalising ambitions, that psychic transformation cannot always keep pace with political goals, that even the most politically committed individuals have contradictory psychic lives that can impede or complicate their political activities, is the subject of this book. Newton cites George Jackson's prison letters, which in turn cite Ho Chi Minh: 'Calamity has hardened me and turned my mind to steel,' while a more ambiguous line by Guevara forms an epigraph to a chapter in Khaled's autobiography, which captures the contradictory relationship between political struggle and psychic life that I have wrestled with while writing this book: 'We must grow tough, but without ever losing our tenderness.'[14]

Embers of hope

The question of how past experiences shape the present is central to both the individual lives of revolutionaries and to revolutionary history. As a left-wing historian, I am often tempted to cite past instances of revolutionary rupture as evidence that nothing about the present is inevitable, that things could be otherwise. I have previously produced arguments like this almost by rote. I have been moved by many texts that excavate hopeful moments from revolutionary history to stir politically sympathetic readers in the quiescent present, but when writing about political disillusionment and exhaustion, I found this rhetorical gesture insufficient. However seductive and politically consoling I find this mode of argumentation, experiences of political burnout necessitate contending with hopeful moments in the past that cannot be severed from individuals' subsequent experiences of despair.

Looking back on the 2020 George Floyd uprisings from the distance of a year, Tobi Haslett claimed that it would not be 'pat or naive or triumphalist to say that people were changed by the rebellion'. He describes watching footage of a crowd in Philadelphia shoving one police car into another, and slashing tyres and lighting fires, while outnumbered cops looked on helplessly. Watching the same footage again months later he 'cried hard': 'In an instant it brought back the floating feeling, the roaring weightlessness, of spring.' Haslett introduces the phenomenological rush of the uprising from the perspective of a later moment. The vivid immediacy of the streets is filtered through memory, narrated from the tear-streaked aftermath of defeat:

> I remembered the elation cut with fear, the shards of unreality and lakes of psychic calm – times when the knowledge rippled invisibly through the sprinting, shouting crowd that the young people of the city had outpaced the armed police. I remembered the first day of the uprising, the sense of being released from the grip of quarantine into the city's three-dimensionality. Here were buildings and swarms of people, thickly present in the stabbing sun.

The subjective transformations instigated by such experiences outlive the return of routine, but living through the reinstatement of the status quo is emotionally transformative in its own right: tears wept at the possibility of such a ruptural moment, tears wept because the crack in the social order has closed up again. This book is concerned with relations between floating feelings of freedom and hard tears that follow. I attempt to think through the psychological experiences that accompany defeat, emerge from political antagonism or arise from exhaustion without forgetting subjective shifts associated with prefigurative moments that glimpse the possibility of breaking (with) the present state of things.

'Graffiti for Two' (2014), co-written by Alaa Abd El-Fattah and Ahmed Douma, which intersperses prose by the former with poetry by the latter, articulates the relation between hope and despair as a relation between the past and the present, questioning the political utility of arguments that seek to access the former from the position of the latter. The text was written while both authors were political prisoners in Tora Prison in Egypt. It was published on 25 January 2014, the third anniversary of the outbreak of the revolution that overthrew the Mubarak regime. El-Fattah had been arrested in November 2013 and charged with organising protests against the reactivation of a law from the British colonial era, a law recently deployed to quash protest following Mohamed Morsi's ouster from the presidency in summer 2013. Composed while both Douma and El-Fattah were being held in solitary confinement, and based on ideas they developed by shouting to each other through the peepholes in their cells during the night, 'Graffiti for Two' was scribbled in pencil on scraps of paper that were smuggled out and later assembled into a full text.

Against those who would characterise despair as a form of treason and a betrayal of the hopeful revolution, the authors insist that denying despair's reality is both psychologically corrosive and politically counter-productive. They link the denial of despair in the present to an overly romanticised image of past hope, which in the Egyptian context took the form of an attachment to the mythic eighteen revolutionary days of rebellion in Tahir Square in January 2011. They reject the rhetoric of remaining mentally free in prison and do not find solace in retaining ideas and commitments despite being crushed. The denial of despair can be a refusal to speak frankly about hopeless or difficult conditions in the present:

> People say, 'You can't kill an idea.' But they say nothing about the usefulness of immortal ideas unheard in the noise of gunfire. Why are we afraid to admit weakness? To admit that we are human, that the APC's crush us and prisons desolate us and bullets scar our thoughts and our dreams. That we are humans suffering defeats, let down by our bodies, made weak by the whisperings of our selves, burned by our dreams and paralyzed by our nightmares. Humans looking to love for support against despair.[15]

Their essay captures the intertwinement of individual memory and revolutionary history central to this book, a relationship of the present to the past that is both individual and collective, micro and macro, in a manner that is not metaphorical but experiential. El-Fattah describes lying in his cell, his hopes overwhelmed by despair, his dreams overtaken by nightmares. He contemplates his parents' militancy in the 1970s and his own memories of Tahir Square in 2011 but remains wary of nostalgia. Singing old revolutionary songs 'is heritage, not resistance', while clinging to the mythic image of the square leads to neglect of revolutionary activity in the present: 'We strayed from the straight path of the revolution when we built shrines to our wounds.' To retain the revolutionary dream, 'a dream not bound by prison walls or surrounded by the edges of a square or limited by the borders of a homeland', it is necessary to contend with the pasts of both hope (the experience of the square) and despair (the experience of the cell).[16]

The psychic transformations brought about by the passage from hope to despair, from rupture to repression (or the return of routine) are encapsulated in a line from Raymond Williams' autobiographical novel *Border Country*: 'The end of the strike had changed Morgan.'[17] Morgan, a Labour Party activist and National Union of Railwaymen branch secretary, had organised a blockade of the railway during the miners' lockout in the UK general strike of 1926. His friend Harry 'recovered quickly' after the strike and resumed his former routines, working as a signalman in their Welsh village, but Morgan cannot get over it so fast.

Morgan is not crushed by the failure of the strike alone but by what its failure reveals to him about 'the real nature of society'. Fighting for a common goal has achieved nothing. The fusion of Morgan's political ideals with the practical experience of solidarity had once been energising; now it seems like a sham: 'His life had been centred on the idea of common improvement. The strike had raised this to an extraordinary practical vividness. Then, suddenly, a different reality had closed in.' He finds himself confronted by 'a grey, solid world of power and compromise'. Everything that had seemed meaningful and vibrant now seems to have been for nothing. It suddenly appears naive to have ever believed anything could have been otherwise. The possibility that had felt concrete when engaged in struggle with others has retreated to the realm of abstract fantasy:

> It was not only that the compromise angered him: not only that he was sickened by the collapse into mutual blame. It was that suddenly the world of power and compromise seemed real, the world of hope and ideas no more than a gloss, a mark in the margin.

Morgan is horrified that many strikers do not seem to have been changed either by the strike or by its end but have simply accepted that things will continue as before. Hope for a different future, for the kind of future that just days before had seemed within reach, now appears fanciful and absurd. After the strike, Morgan experiences a profound disorientation, 'a change in the whole structure of his life'. He watches as people scurry back to resume their social roles, retreating to pursue their personal interests: 'To see this happening was a deep loss of faith, a slow and shocking cancellation of the future.'[18]

Former firebrand Morgan moves away from the village to become an entrepreneur, making money from a preserves business while Harry remains true to his principles. I'm not so concerned with Morgan's specific trajectory and loss of faith as with the many possible outcomes suggested by the sentence, 'The end of the strike had changed Morgan.' How are people transformed by their political engagements and disappointments? How have people in different moments and movements narrated, made sense of, or attempted to recover from such experiences? Both the strike and its defeat change Morgan: his sense of self, his understanding of society, his relationship to other people, his attitude to what might come next. Likewise, the hope of the square and the despair of the cell both figure as part of the subjective transformation described by El-Fattah and Douma. Is it possible to survive defeat without feeling as though the future has been cancelled? What are the psychological consequences of trying to transform the world and glimpsing the possibility of an alternative reality but failing to achieve it? And do those psychological experiences have material implications?

Patient urgency

Dismissing psychological questions as bourgeois individualism detrimental to collective causes was typical on the Old Left, while people on the New Left, though often sceptical of therapy and steeped in the rhetoric of revolutionary self-sacrifice, were more likely to view subjectivity as a site of political transformation. In the sixties and seventies, radical psychiatry theories permeated New Left discourses in Western Europe and the US. Society was understood as sick, insanity framed as a rational response to a crazy world. Psychiatry was attacked for violently forcing labels of 'madness' onto people who failed to conform to social norms. In the words of members of the US-based Radical Therapist collective that formed in 1970:

Psychology and psychiatry are simply another expression of an oppressive society, we have to see our work not so much as reform of a profession but as one part of a whole socialist movement. We see mental hospitalization as coming from the same established power that drops bombs over Hanoi . . . We see more and more people who are misfits in society – outraged women and gays, 'psychotics', high-school drop outs, Vietnam veterans – all people whose lives are in contradiction to the system.[19]

Psychiatric hospitals were understood as one oppressive institution among many that needed to be abolished altogether or at least radically reworked. Asylums were often rhetorically treated as a metonym for the oppressive society that built them. Anti-psychiatrists lambasted the brutality of asylums, engaged in movements of deinstitutionalisation and developed less coercive alternative spaces, which in turn became magnets for people engaged in social movements and the counterculture. Black, women's and gay movements of the period also attacked mainstream psychiatry and campaigned against pathologising practices, while 'mad liberation', mental patients' unions and the survivors' movement, which saw psychiatric hospital patients organise against the psychiatric establishment, emerged alongside them.[20]

Around the time I first started thinking about the problem of activist burnout in historical perspective, I encountered a pamphlet produced in 1978 by a group called Red Therapy. Red Therapy was a self-organised, leaderless, radical therapy group that grew out of small informal meetings in London in autumn 1973; its members were involved in various political organisations and movements, including the women's liberation movement, the libertarian communist group East London Big Flame, and the Troops Out movement (an Irish republican organisation based in Britain that opposed the actions of the British army in Northern Ireland). In the words of their collaboratively written pamphlet, Red Therapy consisted of 'revolutionaries carrying on anti-authoritarian traditions that sprang for us in the student/workers/women's movements of the late '60s'.[21]

Before describing the eclectic practices they developed together, the pamphlet rehearses familiar left-wing arguments about the social causes of mental illness, echoing many other psychopolitical publications from this period. The pamphlet declares, for instance, that the 'conditions of life within contemporary capitalism lead to all kinds of unhappiness'.[22] The group criticises therapeutic methods and medical institutions, characterising psychoanalysis as patriarchal and psychiatric hospitals as carceral. Red Therapy's pamphlet nonetheless resists the hostility towards therapy exhibited by many socialists and communists who still viewed it as a form of bourgeois self-indulgence.[23] Instead, Red Therapy insisted that psychological issues were not merely individual but also structural and that therapy was not just about making life more bearable, but could foster processes of self-actualisation that would nourish political movements in turn. They perceived that self-transformation and social transformation were interlinked.

Though animated by theoretical concerns commonplace on the left in the seventies and outfitted with a predictable if eclectic bibliography (R. D. Laing, Herbert Marcuse and Wilhelm Reich, alongside feminist and spiritual titles and practical guides to psychotherapeutic techniques), the pamphlet is distinguished by the authors' suggestion that their original impetus for initiating a therapy group arose from difficulties they had experienced within their own political milieus. A participant in the Troops Out movement reflected on the fractious and resentful atmosphere that had developed in their meetings, where the tensions were so intense that they impeded the group's attempts to organise. Red Therapy also attempted to address the emotional issues that arose when its members had attempted to create alternative forms of living:

> We wanted to work together politically in non-hierarchical ways, find some kind of sexual freedom and non-oppressive relationships between men and women and adults and children. I think we found it was ALL HARDER THAN WE THOUGHT – that we couldn't somehow will ourselves liberated and wake-up the next morning feeling wonderfully collective, non-jealous, confident, non-competitive etc. We couldn't suddenly change the patterns of a lifetime which we had been forced to conform to in this society. The changes had to take place at a deeper level than just intellectual and political understanding. We had to go back into our pasts, unlearn our conditioning, break out of the blocks that had been instilled into us since childhood.[24]

The collective's therapeutic practices did not just respond to the strain of attempting to survive under capitalism but also confronted the difficulties associated with breaking with sexual and familial conventions.

Red Therapy's attempt to grapple with the frustrations of psychological experiences that arose within politicised social contexts, their acknowledgement of desires that pulled against their intellectual positions, their attempt to respond to the subjective impact of a historical moment characterised by dissipating political energies and splintering movements, their experiments with an eclectic array of radical therapeutic methods, and their insistence that psychological change demanded a patience that seemed to contradict their urgent revolutionary goals, open up questions worth exploring further, questions that could potentially also be a source of sustenance and inspiration for those committed to political change today. I use the concept of 'patient urgency' to capture the asynchronicity that Red Therapy discerned between social and psychic transformation. They found that they could not change their desires or behaviours overnight so as to live according to their political principles. This feeling of being out of sync or feeling psychic lag is also evident in many of the historical examples discussed in this book.

The political, then, is not only personal but also interpersonal. Red Therapy not only helped people to work through interpersonal tensions they encountered in other organisations but the group itself split into a women's and a men's group in response to difficult dynamics in the original mixed group. Gail Lewis, who was active in the Brixton Black Women's Group and later trained as a psychotherapist, has discussed finding the feminist analytic categories available in the seventies insufficient for contending with ambivalent feelings towards others and incapable of making sense of racial tensions, including those that arose in the women's liberation movement. She describes a confrontation over the legacies of imperialism that erupted between black and white feminists at the Women's Liberation Conference in 1978 as a wrenching moment of painful interpersonal conflict, proposing that such clashes cannot be made sense of solely as intellectual disagreements but demand a reckoning with the psychic: 'I want to understand how there can be such explosions, and I want to understand them psychically, affectively and emotionally, not only structurally, because I think politics needs an emotional understanding too.'[25] A desire to understand the origins and trace the fallouts of such explosions also provided the impetus for writing this book.

In his trenchant critique of the antipsychiatry movement and its legacies, *Psychopolitics* (1982), Peter Sedgwick points out that small-scale initiatives like Red Therapy, though capable of addressing 'the more moderate end of emotional miseries' and 'everyday problem[s] of conflict' were not equipped for helping people experiencing more extreme forms of psychological distress, such as psychosis, and could not provide a meaningful alternative to the infrastructures of a state-funded health-care system.[26] In this book, I am also primarily if not exclusively concerned with modest miseries and do not attempt to address the politics of mental health or the provision of mental health care in toto. Instead, I have attempted to show how efforts to ameliorate miseries of different magnitudes might enable people to overcome burnout to participate in movements for larger scale social transformations, including the transformation of health care. Rather than retreating from politics, many former members of Red Therapy continued their interest in politically committed psychotherapy, moving on from sessions among themselves to engage in community-based clinical projects. Joanna Ryan and Marie Maguire, for example, were both involved with the Battersea Action and Counselling Centre in the late 1970s, a community psychotherapy organisation in a shopfront in southwest London that offered 'drop-in' mental health services to local working-class people, using techniques grounded in an alertness to the psychological impact of social and economic conditions.[27]

Looking back on the early years of the women's liberation movement from the perspective of the late 1980s, British socialist feminist Sheila Rowbotham offered a generous reading of the shift from public to psychic questions pursued by many feminists in Britain (including those involved in Red Therapy, though she doesn't discuss that group specifically), arguing that they were responding to distressing experiences that arose within the movement, rather than retreating from it. Rowbotham emphasises the messiness and heterogeneity of unfolding social movements, declaring it unsurprising that many women withdrew or turned against one another in the process of attempting to live according to their newly identified political ideals: 'There are severe psychological costs in both pitting yourself against existing forms of relationship and dissolving aspects of identity.' She identifies frustrations with the pace of change as a major source of disillusionment, but also suggests that confronting this issue motivated people to explore their psychic lives in more depth, leading to a reappraisal of the movement's earlier rejection of therapy:

> The turn to therapy and psychoanalysis as a means of comprehending the complexity of sexual desire and identity in the family made it easier to understand why it was more difficult to change need, fantasy, habit and desire than we had imagined.[28]

The interest in therapy that emerged from the women's movement in Britain (and on the British left more broadly), Rowbotham suggests, was not symptomatic of an individualistic turn, as many accounts of the aftermath of the liberation movements that erupted in the sixties claim. Instead, it arose as part of an attempt to navigate the psychic lag encountered through organising. It was all harder – and slower – than they thought.

Jacqueline Rose made a similar point in a 1982 interview in *m/f*, a journal that provided a forum for theoretical debates about psychoanalysis and feminist politics. Querying the framing of a question from an interviewer who described Jacques Lacan as advancing a 'materialist theory of the subject', Rose claimed that rather than turning to psychoanalysis due to its compatibility with Marxism, feminists in the seventies had been drawn to it due to their 'dissatisfaction with certain accounts of the social'. Contesting Terry Eagleton's claim that a burgeoning interest in semiotics in the seventies represented a depoliticising retreat from the arena of politics into discourse following the defeats of 1968, she argued instead that the aftermath of 1968 'led to the interrogation of discourse, of modes of identification and of structures of role formation', which could be understood 'not as a flight from politics but as an expansion of the political'.[29]

Former Red Therapy members Sheila Ernst and Marie Maguire, who went on to work at the Women's Therapy Centre in North London, reflected in 1987 on how experiences of political organising had led to their interest in the unconscious: 'Psychic distress might be formed and determined by external factors, but it existed in its own right and had to be responded to in its own terms.'[30] Rose confronts the complexity of this relation between politics and the individual in her 1989 essay 'Where Does the Misery Come From?', returning to a disagreement between Wilhelm Reich and Sigmund Freud, which she takes to exemplify the limitations of many left-wing accounts of psychic life: communist psychoanalyst Reich accused Freud of mistakenly locating the origins of misery inside the subject, while Reich situated them in external social conditions. The problem with carving out such a stark dichotomy, Rose points out, is that it robs both the psychological and the social of their complexity while downplaying their entanglement:

> For a theory that pits inside and outside against each other in such deadly combat wipes out any difference or contradiction on either side: the subject suffers, the social oppresses, and what is produced, by implication, is utter stasis in each.[31]

Misery and violence, Rose suggests, cannot be located in either the psyche or society but instead appear 'as the effect of the dichotomy itself'.[32] After all, the 'outside' is a social world populated by other people, each with their own inner lives, each shaped by their past experiences in that social world, which they also participate in shaping. Though this argument may lack the seductive neatness of Reich's proposition and has far murkier implications for how individuals committed to political change conceptualise psychic experience, it helps to make sense of the frustrations to which Red Therapy responded, and it articulates this book's animating tension between individuals and the social conditions in which they live and against which they struggle. Urgent demands can be difficult to enact, and subjective transformation requires patience – it's hard to change.

Anti-adaptive healing

Examining historical attempts to address the psychological toll of political struggle necessitates contending with contradictory relationships between the transformative and the restorative, between revolution and healing, between rupture and repair. What I call 'anti-adaptive healing' refers not only to the contradictory endeavour of striving to heal psychic wounds in a wounded and wounding social reality (without affirming its structures in the process), but also acknowledges the psychic damage that can be incurred by fighting to transform social reality (so as to make it less psychically wounding). If political revolt can be interpreted as a deviation from a norm, then how to understand and treat the psychic suffering of rebels and revolutionaries without diagnosing political rebellion itself as a form of mental illness?

The final chapter of Frantz Fanon's *The Wretched of the Earth* (1961), 'Colonial War and Mental Disorders', consists of a series of case histories based on clinical work he conducted with colonisers and colonised people during the Algerian War of Independence (1954–62), demonstrating the damaging psychological effects of living under colonial rule and of the fight to end it. Fred Moten identifies the paradoxical task faced by the 'militant psychopathologist' through a discussion of a contradiction between internal healing and external political transformation that twists through these case histories.[33] For Fanon, colonial society produces pathologies in two senses: by incurring psychic distress and by applying scientific models that uphold the 'sanity' of existing social norms. Colonial psychiatrists with a racially essentialist understanding of colonised people labelled as pathological behaviour that which could instead be understood as conscious forms of resistance to colonial oppression.

If pathologies are both created by and understood in relation to oppressive social structures, how can psychic damage be treated without simply assimilating people back into the oppressive and damaging world that wounded them in the first place? 'How can the struggle for liberation of the pathological be aligned with the eradication of the pathological?' At stake in Moten's reckoning with Fanon's ambivalent relationship to the pathological and the normative is a tension between woundedness and healing, which is in turn entangled with a relationship between the social and the individual (wounded by what? healing into what?): 'What', Moten asks, 'does or should the liberation struggle have to do, in the broadest sense, with the "rehabilitation of man"?'[34]

Fanon crashed into these issues while working at the Blida-Joinville psychiatric hospital in Algeria between 1953 and 1956. Following the example of his mentor François Tosquelles, with whom he had worked at the experimental psychiatric hospital Saint-Alban in France, upon arrival at Blida, Fanon and his team of interns sought to establish social activities among patients and staff in the hospital. They eliminated staff uniforms and constraining clothing for patients and introduced activities such as a film club, ward meetings, festive celebrations, theatrical evenings and a newspaper, alongside group therapy sessions. A 1954 paper co-written with Jacques Azoulay describes their attempt to introduce methods of *socialthérapie* they had learned in France to patients in Algeria. They discovered that while their techniques were successful with a group of European women patients, they 'lamentably failed' with three groups of Muslim men. They eventually realised that the kinds of activities they had introduced were unsuited to the specificities of the culture and society in which they were now working: 'A revolutionary attitude was essential, because it was necessary to go from a position in which the supremacy of Western culture was evident, to one of cultural relativism.'[35] They had rejected a therapeutic approach based on restraint in favour of one based on sociality, but had failed to notice that the social activities they introduced were culturally specific and hence relied on a colonial logic of assimilation. *Socialthérapie,* they concluded, required therapeutic techniques attentive to the specificities of different social environments, as Lucie K. Mercier discusses, 'by interrogating the universality of Tosquelles' revolutionary therapeutics, they ended up exploring the boundaries of the very category of the "social."'[36]

The social world within the hospital was not, however, isolated from the social realities of war. Fanon eventually resigned from his post at the hospital in 1956 as the conflict was escalating and in the wake of the repression of a series of strikes. He declared that although he had hoped to 'attenuate the viciousness of a system' and strive for the 'emergence of a better world' through his psychiatric work with Algerian people, he had come to view this as an impossible endeavour:

> If psychiatry is the medical technique that aims to enable man no longer to be a stranger to his environment, I owe it to myself to affirm that the Arab, permanently an alien in his own country, lives in a state of absolute depersonalization ... The social structure existing in Algeria was hostile to any attempt to put the individual back where he belonged.

Healing was not possible in a situation in which 'belonging' perversely meant oppression rather than a feeling of congruity. Fanon came to see that persevering in such circumstances would entail 'the illogical maintenance of a subjective attitude in organized contradiction with reality'.[37] He did not quit psychiatric work altogether, however, but after his expulsion from Algeria in early 1957 took up a post in Tunisia, which had gained its independence in 1956. There he became more involved with the *Front de Libération Nationale* (FLN) and participated in a convoy of doctors sent to the border to treat Algerian refugees. His therapeutic work in this context formed the basis for some of the cases contained in 'Colonial War and Mental Disorders'.[38]

In his famous preface to *The Wretched of the Earth*, Jean-Paul Sartre declared that Fanon's work shows that anti-colonial violence 'can heal the wounds it has inflicted': 'The native cures himself of colonial neurosis by thrusting out the settler through force of arms.'[39] For Fanon, 'total liberation' is subjective as well as social; a new social order would ultimately be inhabited by new people. The fight against colonialism is not only a fight against external social structures, but is also a fight against the internalised logics of colonialism and the 'hatred of self', 'implanted' through years of living in a racist society:

> The fight carried on by a people for its liberation leads it, according to circumstances, either to refuse or else to explode the so-called truths which have been established in its consciousness by the colonial civil administration, by the military occupation, and by economic exploitation. Armed conflict alone can really drive out these falsehoods created in man which force into inferiority the most lively minds among us and which, literally, mutilate us.[40]

But although Fanon perceived the necessity for armed struggle against colonial rule and envisioned a liberated future, his case histories make clear that for combatants engaged in that struggle it could not function as an immediate cure with the speed or ease Sartre's proclamations imply. Mutilated minds take time to heal and the fight against mutilation can be wounding in its own right.

His clinical examples in *The Wretched of the Earth* not only discuss the psychological damage inflicted by colonial violence – they also attest to the psychic toll of the militant struggle to end colonial violence: 'The future of such patients is mortgaged.' The first case Fanon discusses in 'Colonial War and Mental Disorders' is of a man in his thirties who was active in the resistance in 'one of those African countries which have been independent for several years' and had sought out help to deal with insomnia, suicidal thoughts and anxiety that he had experienced since planting a bomb that killed ten people. In a footnote, Fanon notes that since independence the man had become friendly with people from the former colonial power who were enthusiastic about independence and celebratory of the combatants who fought for it. The patient, who had never regretted his actions and had performed them in the knowledge that he would 'pay the price of national independence', began to worry that he might have been responsible for killing similarly sympathetic people, rather than the 'notorious racists' known to frequent the target of his attack. This reflection provokes in the former militant an 'attack of vertigo'. Fanon writes that

> we are forever pursued by our actions. Their ordering, their circumstances, and their motivation may perfectly well come to be profoundly modified *a posteriori*. This is merely one of the snares that history and its various influences sets for us. But can we escape becoming dizzy? And who can affirm that vertigo does not haunt the whole of existence?[41]

This short case history does not contradict the political arguments concerning violence made elsewhere in *The Wretched of the Earth*, but the patient's vertigo results from the necessarily unsynchronised relationship between psychic and social transformation with which Fanon's clinical work brought him into close contact. People's relation to the past is also unstable, liable to change. In this example, the man's cause was ultimately victorious and Fanon passes no judgment on his actions, but the process of trying to create a future social world in which healing might be possible was individually wounding nonetheless; a price was paid.[42] The militant clinician is situated between the transforming and the transformed world.[43] The feelings of psychological dizziness and vertigo that Fanon describes, the difficulties of escaping from past experiences, and the paradoxes that characterise the role of the anti-adaptive revolutionary psychotherapist that his work grapples with are all pertinent to this book.

Personal politics

Traced backwards, this book could probably be understood as an oblique response to some of my own experiences. Rather than emerging from any single event, however, its origins are tangled and overdetermined. Stuart Hall claimed that the New Left in Britain contained people from two distinct political generations, whose differences were 'not of age but of formation'.[44] Although my personal biography is uneventful and insignificant compared to the lives of the New Left figures discussed by Hall, my perspective on the psychological toll of political struggle has nonetheless been shaped by my political formation in specific historical conditions. 'Geriatric millennial' is the moniker given to my micro-generation in the mainstream media. Politically I belong to a cohort sandwiched between anti-globalisation movement Gen Xers and younger millennials who had no experience of adulthood before the financial crisis in 2008. I am old enough to remember when the World Trade Organisation protests took place in Seattle in 1999 but too young to have participated in 'summit hopping', just about young enough to have participated in the 2010–11 UK student movement but old enough to have left university in England with much less student debt than people of a similar class position a decade younger than me.[45]

Born in Middlesbrough in 1983, although I cannot recall anything about the 1984–85 Miners' Strike or the closure of the last shipyard in Teesside in 1987, I do remember growing up in an anti-Thatcher household playing with a box of colourful badges emblazoned with slogans like 'Coal Not Dole' and 'Free Nelson Mandela'. I watched people on the news queuing for food in what, until very recently, had been called the USSR. When I was fourteen, I wrote 'New Labour, New Britain' in my diary the day after Tony Blair won the 1997 general election. The constituency I lived in at the time (Shrewsbury and Atcham) elected its first and to date only Labour MP that year, but he defected to the Liberal Democrats in

2001 due to his opposition to Labour's support of military action in Afghanistan. I owned a copy of Naomi Klein's *No Logo* and fretted about buying a pair of Nike trainers. By the time I started university in London in 2002, the anti-war movement was underway. In the months leading up to and following the invasion of Iraq, I joined demonstrations, rallies and meetings that I recall being characterised by a feeling of outraged futility. In a sense, my first experience of a political movement felt defeated from the beginning, but if futility can demotivate and provoke cynicism, anger at such flagrant injustice endures.

Though I spent a lot of time in anarchist friends' squats – friends who, unlike me, joined protests against the G8 summit at Gleneagles in 2005 and protested outside the Mexican embassy in London in 2006 after a filmmaker from the US was murdered during a teachers' strike in Oaxaca – in the New Labour years I spent more time reading dense, jargon-laden Marxist theory than I spent engaged in any kind of political praxis. I was much more interested in partying than in party politics, workplace organising or activism, but after the 2008 financial crisis the themes of the theoretical talks by ageing French '68ers I had been attending for years suddenly seemed more urgent and their audiences grew. Some of my neighbours, who lived in a squat on my street in Hackney, were students involved in the occupation at Middlesex University to resist the closure of its philosophy department in spring 2010.

In late 2011, by which time I was already in my late twenties, I had the strange experience of entering a political movement that was on the cusp of defeat and disillusionment. In winter 2010 a student movement began in parts of the UK in response to the recently elected Conservative–Liberal Democrat coalition government's announcement that it would scrap the Education Maintenance Allowance for college students and increase the cap on tuition fees for undergraduates to £9,000 in England and Wales. I was not a student in autumn 2010. Working in an administrative role for a small theatre company, as that especially freezing winter melted into spring, I watched global political events unfold on my office computer screen: in Sidi Bouzid, in Cairo, in Tripoli, in Athens. I was at work when protestors stormed the Conservative Headquarters at Millbank. I did not get kettled by police on Westminster Bridge. I attended the national Trade Union demonstration in March 2011 on my own and was away on holiday when rioters tore through London that summer. I went to demonstrations when I could, but I was not involved in the meetings, the actions, the marches, the enthusiastic auto-didacticism, the antagonisms with the police, the banner making, the arguments about strategy, the mass arrests, the collective writing processes, the shared meals, the occupations.

In autumn 2011, I quit my office job and started a PhD in London. I would sometimes drop by the Occupy encampments at St Paul's and Finsbury Square on my cycle home. A building down the street from my department was occupied that autumn, but the space – briefly known as the Bloomsbury Social Centre – was raided by police that December. The movement was waning. For the next few years my time was filled with life-altering collective discussions, endless meetings and reading groups that were far more enriching than anything I ever encountered at university, but I also found myself joining a fraying political milieu, as many activists awaited or stood trial, friendships unravelled, and people were breaking up and breaking down. We read poetry on university picket lines, organised in solidarity with outsourced cleaning and security staff, painted huge anti-police banners, attended anti-fascist demonstrations, joined packed talks on struggles in Montreal, Istanbul, Madrid, Rojava and Santiago, and engaged in seemingly interminable debates about social reproduction, the value form and capitalist crisis in the cramped living rooms of shared rented houses.[46] But it was also a time punctuated by the panic attacks of friends who had experienced police violence and by hastily improvised and always insufficient-seeming forms of care.

I spent the summers of 2012 and 2013 in Moscow, where I met people who described the brutal police tactics during the anti-Putin 'Occupy Abai' (named after the Kazakh poet Abai Kunanbayev, whose statue stood at the centre of the encampment in May 2012), and in spring 2013 I visited Oakland, another city that had been caught up in the fleeting global ripple of social 'movements in the squares' in the wake of the Arab Spring in 2011. Defeats were still fresh, but the energy of the movements felt within reach. We followed the scenes in Gezi Park unfolding from afar. Everyone seemed to be going through similar things and we compared notes feverishly. In summer 2014 I spent five months on a library fellowship in Washington, DC, where I attended protests outside the White House against Israel's attack on Gaza. Crowds at rallies called for justice after black teenager Michael Brown was shot and killed by the cop Darren Wilson in Ferguson, Missouri, on 9 August 2014. A visiting comrade from the Bay Area gave me a zine filled with translated articles, poems and interviews reflecting on experiences of Maidan in Kyiv and the uprisings across Ukraine, covering the period between November 2013 and February 2014 (prior to the annexation of Crimea). Earlier that year I had met Ukrainian leftists in Lithuania who had just returned from Maidan Square.

Back in London, many people I knew who had been politicised in 2010 threw themselves critically but decisively into parliamentary politics after Jeremy Corbyn's election as Labour leader in 2015, while others continued to organise against the continuing impact of austerity and the UK's violent border regime. I left the UK for a job in Berlin a couple of months after the Brexit referendum in June 2016. My calendar in the months before I moved was stuffed with political engagements: regular shifts volunteering at a centre providing legal advice to migrants; feminist political meetings and skill shares; trips accompanying people to housing offices and social services in an attempt to resist councils' gatekeeping practices; demonstrations at Yarl's Wood detention centre and at Holloway Prison; a trip to the island of Chios in Greece to volunteer preparing food for mostly Syrian refugees who had recently arrived on boats from Turkey; a short trip to Paris during which friends talked about protests much larger, more consistent and more militant than anything I had ever experienced in Britain.[47] It was during that period that I encountered the kind of burnout that forms the focus of this book's second section: the exhaustion that can come from prolonged engagement in organising.

I started writing this book at the start of the first Covid-19 lockdown in March 2020, following Jeremy Corbyn's 2019 election defeat and the defeat of Bernie Sanders in the Democratic primaries. The uprisings that erupted across the US and around the world in response to George Floyd's murder in summer 2020 briefly shattered the prevailing despondence but now seem to mark the end of a cycle of struggle.[48] It is hard to know how to characterise the current conjuncture; the list of crises is so long – climate catastrophe, far-right ethnonationalist resurgences, war in Ukraine, economic stagnation, high inflation, low wages, ever-more precarious working and housing conditions, rampant transphobia, attacks on reproductive rights, and so on – that the term 'polycrisis' does seem apt. Of course, resistance is already happening, but the scale and varied nature of the crises can seem overwhelming. At the time of writing, in autumn 2023, Israel's genocidal attack on Gaza has only just begun and the struggle for Palestinian liberation continues with renewed urgency.

In early 2020, in the wake of the Corbyn defeat and just before people retreated into the isolation of lockdown, Gargi Bhattacharyya wrote that being heartbroken was a painful but necessary condition for a revolutionary: 'Only we, the heartbroken, . . . can truly battle and long for a world where no-one ever feels like this again.'[49] But how to unbreak our hearts in the context of a still broken social reality?

'Hurt People' by Bobby London, an article published in *The New Inquiry* in 2018, begins by identifying

> an untold story of what happens away from the streets, the rallies, the skillshares, and the gatherings. When our attempt to hold onto the connection has failed, and dirty dishes become as destructive to movements as state co-optation. The wave of insurrectionary hope has reached a lull, and another world no longer feels possible.[50]

Reflecting on the author's own experiences of political despair without identifying any events in particular, the piece calls for people in political movements to reflect on loneliness and isolation while their movements are still ongoing, not only in their fractured and defeated aftermaths. The article captures the magnetic rush of street movements and the 'inner change' they provoke, but it concludes sombrely, reflecting on the reproduction of racist hierarchies in supposedly horizontal anti-racist groups and affirming solitude over collectivity. *Burnout* is an attempt to tell such untold stories by placing these despairing sentiments in historical perspective, in the hope that doing so might point to ways – both practical and theoretical – beyond despair.

Note on method

The more I read about different historical movements, the more emotional questions and psychological problems seemed ever-present. Even revolutionaries who were dismissive of psychological questions in theory often described, in practice, being surrounded by people breaking down, falling out, sinking into depression or seeking psychotherapeutic help in response to their political engagements. Despite all the historical examples I encountered of revolutionaries or activists describing their experiences in terms that resonated with those to which I had been proximate, I could not find any texts that brought together spatially and temporally disparate examples to thematise political burnout. This book is an attempt – however partial and tentative – to do that.

Today it is commonplace for people in political movements to acknowledge burnout, advocate self-care and promote developing forms of mutual support. Discussions of the need for spaces of respite and times of recovery are accorded a prominent place in activist milieus.[51] Organising WhatsApp groups buzz with mutual concern for the 'capacity' of others, an ambiguous term that seems to encompass the quantitative register of time and the qualitative register of emotions. In the wake of deinstitutionalisation and with the rise of a bio-medical paradigm for understanding mental illness, there has also been something of a rapprochement between the mainstream psy-disciplines and the left, as well as a renewed interest in psychoanalysis and psychotherapy among many activists, arguably symptomatic of the current political and historical moment.[52] I have not therefore felt the need to address my arguments to people who might be inclined to dismiss a concern with psychological questions as 'bourgeois individualism'. But if burnout and the sometimes corrosive effects of political organising are now frequently acknowledged in social movements, self-published materials that circulate within them, detailing practical techniques for dealing with personal and interpersonal issues, can sometimes be uncritical of mainstream psychiatric or neurological concepts and self-help techniques. I hope that historicising, and hence denaturalising, experiences of political burnout can suggest alternative ways of approaching emotional difficulties that arise through struggle in the present.

Tracing histories of political burnout involves retreating from the streets to the enclosed spaces of the home, prison or hospital, from large public arenas to scattered smaller-scale interactions. I have attempted to describe phenomena sometimes located in the afterwords, margins and epilogues of historical accounts, experiences often alluded to but usually glimpsed only peripherally. Although my examples are historical, I make no claim to have produced a work of 'history from below'. I did not burrow into dusty archives, speak to people sidelined by existing historical accounts, uncover forgotten materials. Instead, I drew on an array of published sources available in English – secondary histories, memoirs, novels, films, as well as works by psychiatrists, psychologists and psychoanalysts – that enabled me to think conceptually about how people trying to make history were unmade or remade in the process.

As the examples already discussed indicate, the approach I have taken is intensive rather than extensive, microscopic rather than synoptic, fragmentary rather than synthetic: case studies are selected to illustrate distinctive angles on key concepts. This is neither a definitive nor an exhaustive account. Indeed, I hope that readers might extend, expand, supplement and interrogate the concepts, artworks, key texts and historical moments I have selected, by bringing them into dialogue with others. Having said that, the choices I made were by no means arbitrary – I strove to find case studies that would help to elucidate particular conceptual questions – but in making choices I was guided by my own subjective interests and limitations. While I consider the medical alongside the spiritual, my own background as a historian of the psy-disciplines, for example, led me to focus on understandings of mental life developed in 'expert' scientific contexts, even while pointing to their limitations. Similarly, while the case studies cover a period from 1871 to the present, they reflect my interest in movements of the long 1970s, and while I discuss histories that unfolded in different parts of the world, I include far more examples from Western Europe and the US than I can comfortably defend.

Burnout is addressed to ongoing movements on the left; hence my examples are also from left movements, broadly defined. I discuss anti-imperialist, anti-racist, anti-war, feminist, environmentalist and queer movements alongside workers' movements that emphasised class struggle, but I am well aware that many of the motley array of anarchists, social democrats, socialist feminists, Maoists, Communist Party apparatchiks, black nationalists, ultraleft militants and libertarians that populate these pages would have vehemently disagreed with one another on many issues. I also consider extreme experiences (murder, torture, incarceration) alongside far more mundane ones (interpersonal strife, tiredness, disillusionment) without implying equivalencies between them. I consciously sought to engage with an expansive and internally contradictory set of examples to provide different angles on my object of analysis.

Revolutionaries and activists have sometimes sought out psychological treatment and framed their experiences in terms consistent with mainstream medical discourse. It is also possible to find examples of movements and individuals who rejected or reworked existing psychiatric paradigms or those who advocated militancy as a therapeutic endeavour in its own right. The themes I discuss thus necessitate engaging with a fraught interplay between expert and lay practices, between professional and amateur forms of psychological care, and between formal and colloquial diagnostic categories. The book's time span and geographical scope also necessarily engage with historical shifts and cultural differences in both mainstream and marginal understandings of psychic life – from psychiatry to antipsychiatry, psychoanalysis to neuroscience, and psychotherapy to spiritual healing.

Although examining historical encounters between political struggle and theories of psychic life involves grappling with the question of how, whether or which understandings of mental health could be consistent with left-wing political agendas, I approach this through a discussion of sources that respond immanently to particular political struggles, rather than applying existing theories of psychic life to those struggles (if you want to read, say, an application of the theories of psychoanalyst Wilfred Bion to group dynamics among cadres in the Cuban Revolution, you'll need to find another kind of book). Here I describe diagnoses rather than propose them. Structured around emotional responses to social movements and revolutionary uprisings, this book does not provide an overview of the historical encounters between Marxism and the psy-disciplines, whether framed as an intellectual or clinical history; it provides neither a history of the diverse approaches to treating and understanding mental illness developed in the former 'Second World', nor a history of radical psychiatry, though the episodes it recounts were traversed by these histories in various ways. Some of the sources I discuss were written by psychoanalysts, psychologists or theorists who drew on particular medical traditions or models to make sense of particular political movements or moments, but I also analyse depictions of political experience in novels, films and memoirs.

By bringing disparate events into dialogue with one another and by focusing on the meaning of distinct concepts in the context of different political movements, I hope to preserve particularity while demonstrating echoes, harmonies and rhymes between nows and thens, heres and theres. The ways political defeat and exhaustion have been understood, described and worked through historically are as variable as the events that provoked them. While this book seeks experiential resonances across time and space, it also underlines the specificity of different movements' psychological impacts and the varied theories used to make sense of them: exiled Paris Communards diagnosed themselves with 'nostalgia' (a pathological homesickness), Bolsheviks in the aftermath of the October Revolution said they suffered from 'nervous exhaustion' (a physiological depletion of vital energy), while today activists are more likely to engage with diagnostic categories found in the works of Freud or in the *DSM-V*, the latest edition of the *Diagnostic and Statistical Manual of Mental Disorders*.

Burnout's eight chapters, each focused on a particular concept, are divided into three sections, which circle around the book's core themes: the complicated relationships between individuals and their social conditions (and between the past and the present), the necessity for patience even in urgent political struggles, and anti-adaptive understandings of healing. The first section, 'Historical Symptoms: Past Attachments', probes how the left relates to past attachments and experiences, asking how it might be possible to make sense of the leaps of scale involved in considering individual memories in relation to collective histories. The second section, 'Survival Pending Revolution', borrows a slogan from the Black Panther Party and addresses the emotional difficulties of sustaining political action over long periods. The chapters in this section reckon with the asynchronicity of individual and social transformation – the fact that people's behaviours and desires often fail to transform at the pace demanded by their political ideals – an experience that I propose demands 'patient urgency'. The question of how to heal without affirming or adjusting to social structures that inflicted and continue to inflict harm is central to *Burnout*, and its final section, 'Concepts Transformed: Anti-Adaptive Healing', examines historical moments in which existing psychiatric or psychoanalytic concepts were transformed to account for the politically repressive contexts in which suffering people were attempting to feel better.

For many on the left today, it remains axiomatic that individual suffering originates in sick societies and that true psychological well-being requires social change, but simply stating that all mental suffering is caused by capitalism leaves the problem of fighting to transform social conditions in the meantime unsolved. As Rose perceived in her analysis of the conflict between Freud and Reich, which Fanon confronted in his discussions of vertigo among militants, such an argument risks downplaying the social implications of the formative impact of external conditions on subjectivity by existing social structures and skips over the annoying and painful intermediary stages. After all, the only people who can enact social change in the present are the people who live in it already. Making sense of emotional experiences of political defeat involves confronting the ravelled and mutually shaping relationships between psyches and society, the personal and the political, individuals and history. The people this book both discusses and addresses are not newborn babies in an already transformed world; they are fucked up people trying to transform their fucked up realities and often getting even more fucked up in the process.

Although negative emotions are the subject of this book, my intention in excavating despairing experiences is not to prompt feelings of doom in the reader, but to open up questions about how to confront, overcome or ameliorate such feelings. It is a book addressed to burnt-out comrades – past, present, future – and to all the fires that are yet to be lit.

PART I

Historical Symptoms: Past Attachments

1

Melancholia

Catastrophe – to have missed the opportunity.[1]

– Walter Benjamin

In the wake of Labour's crushing defeat in the UK's 2019 general election, I walked home weeping from a friend's flat at 6 a.m., with already peeling 'Vote Labour' stickers covering my coat. A sodden, rose-festooned flyer floated in the gutter. When I finally woke up after that dismal night, I found myself reaching, bleary-eyed, for texts written in the wake of earlier election defeats. Jeremy Corbyn first became an MP in 1983, the year I was born, in an election in which Margaret Thatcher, who had swept to power in 1979, increased her parliamentary majority to 144 against the left-wing Labour leader Michael Foot.

When I read the closing words of the dedication to Stuart Hall's *The Hard Road to Renewal: Thatcherism and the Crisis of the Left*, a collection of essays written between 1978 and 1988 that take stock of Thatcher's appeal and the left's failures to offer an alternative, I started to cry again. The book is dedicated to Hall's children, 'who spent their adolescence under the shadow of "Iron Times" – in the hope of better things to come'.[2] As part of a younger generation who had grown up under Thatcher and Major and protested against the war in Iraq under New Labour and then against Tory austerity, it seemed as if the Iron Times had never really ended. After a surreal interlude of strained hopefulness, in which many people I had first encountered as masked-up anarchists at student movement protests in 2010 had abruptly swerved into parliamentary politics, it once again seemed that things would never get better.

Hall provided insights into the left's incapacity to make sense of, let alone respond to, the phenomenon of Thatcherism. Hidebound by outmoded analyses that applied sclerotic ideological formulations to the world, rather than developing theories that grasped the changing realities of class relations in contemporary Britain, the left, Hall contended, was more attached to tradition and to a nostalgic image of the past than the right. Thatcher's social conservatism was combined with an economic vision that sought to tear the foundations of British society up by the roots, while the left clung helplessly to a tattered status quo. But an essay near the end of Hall's collection (co-written with Martin Jacques), which castigated the left for failing to embrace Bob Geldof's Live Aid and Sport Aid projects, gave the book a bathetic arc. Despite Hall's diagnosis of the anachronistic qualities of the left's theoretical models elsewhere, the arguments he made in this essay felt suddenly anachronistic. The sharp blades of Hall's criticisms of both the Conservative and Labour parties appear blunted as soon as he cited a concrete alternative. Were things really so bad that Live Aid could be hailed as the most significant event for the British left in years?[3] I had started flipping desperately through Hall's essays to find an antidote to feelings of disappointment, yet I finished the book feeling deflated and disoriented. The left's problems in 2019 didn't quite seem to match those outlined by Hall in the 1980s. What did resonate was a fear that in defeat – tired, battered, divided, self-recriminatory and without a single new project to unite around – the temptation would be to look back nostalgically to a moment of near-victory in 2017 or to unite in anger at the sneering centrists who blocked any further success. What happens when hope curdles? Reading Hall's essays, I felt a vertiginous fear about the length and depth of the doldrums that lay ahead.

Written in the aftermath of Thatcher's third election victory in 1987, Jacqueline Rose's 'Margaret Thatcher and Ruth Ellis' responds to Hall's reflections on Thatcher's continued successes. Rose praises Hall for acknowledging that Thatcher's victories could not be explained solely in material terms – they also appealed to the imagination. According to Hall, the left neglects at its peril the political power of images, symbols and fantasy. In recognising these factors in the right's appeal to people whose material interests right-wing policies do not serve, Rose observes that Hall returned to a problem concerning the entanglement of the psychological and the political that was also central to theorisations of the rise of fascism in early twentieth-century Europe. For Hall, there were rational explanations for the kinds of identifications that led working-class people to vote Tory, but for Rose a 'rationalist concept of fantasy' was insufficient for making sense of the ambivalence at work in how people related to the image of Thatcher. Vehement hatred might, paradoxically but precisely, have been part of Thatcher's appeal: 'The attempt of the social order to secure its own rationality, and its constant failure to do so, may be one of the things that Thatcher brings most graphically into focus.⁴ Sometimes historical circumstances demand that Marx be read alongside Freud.

The psychoanalytically informed theories of the unconscious appeal of right-wing politics that Rose invokes – from Wilhelm Reich's *Mass Psychology of Fascism* (1933) to Theodor Adorno et al.'s *Authoritarian Personality* (1950) – gained new audiences in the wake of the UK's Brexit referendum and the election of Donald Trump in 2016. The psyche returned as a key political site in mostly unconvincing attempts to make sense of the appeal of the right and far-right to a vaguely imagined 'white working class', or sometimes in efforts at lay diagnoses of Trump himself. But what about the psychic life of the defeated left? In the UK and US, the resurgence of the right coincided with the brief resuscitation of the left in electoral politics. Weeks after Corbyn's defeat, I went on a research trip to the US where my friends were travelling to distant states to go knocking on doors for Bernie Sanders. It felt like a nightmarish form of déjà vu. Alone in hotel rooms, transfixed by endless TV coverage of the Democratic primaries while scrolling through friends' social media posts that had a familiar tone of jangling, frantic optimism, I felt ashamed of my cynicism and sense of doom.

This is not a book about social democracy being defeated at the ballot box, but it struck me in the aftermath of those two defeats – in which many of my friends and peers had been fervently, if critically, involved – that while people on the left had quickly amassed and circulated theoretical materials from the past to help make sense of the role of psychic life in the right's ascendency, there seemed to be no equivalent resources for enabling people on the left to work through our own psychological experiences. Yet the need seemed more urgent. It is one thing to speculate at a distance about other people's mental motivations, but quite another to address psychological pain and suffering in our own movements. And it's not as if there isn't a whole repertoire of defeats and disappointments to draw from, many far more deadly and devastating than those I've just mentioned. Could anything be gleaned from those historical experiences that might help to make sense of the psychological toll of political defeat? One existing frame for approaching this question and for highlighting the perils of over-identifying with histories of defeat might be provided by theorists of 'left melancholy'. Constructing a partial anatomy of that concept helped me to elucidate how the object I try to describe in this book – burnout – is actually something slightly different.

Anatomy of left melancholy

In summer 2017, I went to see Wendy Brown deliver a talk in Berlin on 'Apocalyptic Populism' in which she asked, like Hall and Rose before her, why people were drawn to vote for right-wing authoritarians. The first of the three 'strains or energies' she identified behind white support for Trump was psychic: 'fears and anxieties'.[5] But I was more interested to discover that these two feelings also appear as key terms in her 1999 essay 'Resisting Left Melancholy' and in that earlier essay they are associated with the left rather than the right. She begins her 1999 essay by returning to Hall's writings on Thatcherism and the crisis of the left, asking if it might be possible not only to identify left-wing 'fears and anxieties', as Hall does, but to understand their 'content and dynamic'.[6] To do this she explores the phenomenon of 'left melancholy'.

The term 'left melancholy' should not be confused with understandings of melancholia in medicine and psychiatry, which have a complicated history stretching back to ancient Greece; its origins are more recent and can be traced to a strange book review by Walter Benjamin. 'Left-Wing Melancholy' (1931) is a scathing review of a book by poet Erich Kästner, and it is addressed to a specific phenomenon that Benjamin identifies in the supposedly radical literature of Weimar Germany. Despite proclaiming themselves sympathetic to the working class, poets like Kästner address themselves to a 'middle stratum' of readers, producing a body of work Benjamin derides as 'the decayed bourgeoisie's mimicry of the proletariat'. Distant from political action, with 'little to do with the labour movement', writers like Kästner transform political struggles into pleasant objects for the titillation, consumption and amusement of a bourgeois public, resulting in a nihilistic poetry of 'tortured stupidity'. Rather than depicting the masses in anticipation of revolutionary moments, Kästner's poems, in Benjamin's analysis, present flabby stereotypes, ignoring the realities of mass unemployment. The left-wing melancholic is a reactionary figure, politically complacent and nihilistic, who would 'trample anything and anyone in their path'.[7] Benjamin likens left melancholy to constipation. In Brown's gloss, which transforms Benjamin's circumscribed definition of the concept into something more general: 'Left melancholy ... is ... a mournful, conservative, backward-looking attachment to a feeling, analysis, or relationship that has been rendered thing-like and frozen in the heart of the putative leftist.'

Left melancholy is not just an incapacity to move on from loss; it involves converting something that had belonged to someone else in the first place into a hollow, deadened thing. Proletarian action is replaced by bourgeois routine. Here Benjamin's proximity to Hall is apparent: in his view, the (pseudo) left has become too attached to its outdated and hollow ideological apparatus to apprehend the surging realities of the actual world and its living inhabitants. Brown expresses her fears about the comforts and seductions offered by left melancholy:

> It is a Left that has become more attached to its impossibility than to its potential fruitfulness, a Left that is most at home dwelling not in hopefulness but in its own marginality and failure, a Left that is thus caught in a structure of melancholic attachment to a certain strain of its own dead past, whose spirit is ghostly, whose structure of desire is backward looking and punishing.[8]

Paradoxically, loss itself becomes the lost object. A dusty case is all that remains when its once sparkling contents have disappeared: 'Now hollow forms are absent-mindedly caressed.' As Benjamin observes, left melancholics are myopic and only position themselves to the left of 'what is in general possible'.[9] There is something strange about the temporality of left melancholy. Marx and Engels' spectre haunting Europe counterintuitively came from the future, whereas the left-wing melancholic grieves for the loss of something that was never fully realised. And that ossified grief becomes a permanent political disposition.

In Brown's account, published ten years after the fall of the Berlin Wall, the losses are many – of theories, of movements, of faith, of certainties. Yet her analysis is zoomed out and intellectual, devoid of references to localised struggles or particular instances of defeat. Another twelve years later, Jodi Dean pointed out key differences between Benjamin's definition of left melancholy and Brown's: his targets were hacks who peddled revolutionary ideas to a bourgeois audience at the expense of proletarian action (implying the existence of a non-melancholic left still committed to class struggle), whereas Brown, elaborating on Hall, describes a left clinging to outdated orthodoxies in the absence of ongoing revolutionary movements. Dean's own diagnosis is different again. She describes a left that has abandoned the totalising goal of revolution for smaller, more dispersed activities, 'sublimat[ing its] goals and responsibilities into the branching, fragmented practices of micro-politics, self-care, and issue awareness'. She proposes that left 'melancholia derives from the real existing compromises and betrayals inextricable from its history', from capitulations and accommodations with capitalist reality as much as from defeats that have external origins.[10] However, in a paper that was first delivered in New York in autumn 2011 and ends with a discussion of Occupy Wall Street, she suggests that times had changed – insufficiently and tentatively but decisively – since Brown's essay and that a process of collective working through had begun.

Enzo Traverso's 2017 book on the concept is more explicit in identifying left-wing melancholia as an epochal condition, but he does not share Dean's sense that the economic crisis of 2008, the Arab Spring and the Occupy movement shifted anything. Although he acknowledges that 'the history of revolutions is a history of defeats', he distinguishes the defeats that punctuated the nineteenth and twentieth centuries from the more definitive capitulation marked by the fall of the Berlin Wall.[11] Traverso treats communism as a finished project and speaks of the paralysis of the utopian imagination and the hollowing out of the emancipatory promises of liberation movements of the sixties and seventies. In his account, history has been displaced by memory, meaningful struggle by vapid contemplation. Unlike the revolutionary defeats of the past, which nourished future radical movements, generated pride and provided an inspirational repertoire from which current revolutionaries could draw, 1989, in Traverso's view, was not just the end of history, but the end of the capacity for people to make their own.

Melancholia in these varied theoretical accounts is framed as a shared disposition or mood, but it does not really convey anything about defeat as something people actually experience. Historical events feature in these texts, but the impasse of the left is narrated at a grand, epochal level, rather than as a plethora of messy, often painful events lived through personally and interpersonally. The desires seem abstract, the losses distant. These accounts all lack any sense of genuine emotional distress. Having read these theories of left melancholy, I thought again about that walk home in the rain in December 2019. I thought about waking up in tears on a cold mattress and reading about the 1980s, not wanting to get up, sending and receiving endless broken-hearted messages. I thought about the meandering, hungover walk I took with a friend in the park later that day. I thought of the helpless anger we incoherently exchanged. I thought about another friend who had joined us for the last rounds of desperate door knocking before leaving to go to another friend's funeral. I thought of our dead friend who wrote poems about hating cops and watching swans, about blackbirds and comrades, who wrote: 'Next time they shoot us, we'll refuse to die.'[12] So many people I knew were sad, angry, disoriented and so, *so* tired. In the hollow months that followed the election, it became increasingly clear that the losses were not only located in an unrealised future (that was already more of a compromise than a utopia), but in actual experiences of collectivity, however fleeting, rain-soaked and fractious. Whatever those experiences were, they didn't seem to have much in common with the phenomenon theorists of left melancholy I had read were trying to describe. Who had theorised that kind of experience? What name would it have?

After the morning after

Between the elections of 1983 and 1987, the 1984–85 UK miners' strike, which the Labour Party under Neil Kinnock had shamefully not supported, was defeated – an event just beyond the edges of my memory. My mother, whose father had been a miner in Teesside, worked as a social worker in County Durham mining villages during the strike and gave my pram to a striking miners' family. Hall's intellectual analysis of the strike reiterated arguments about the left's hopelessly outmoded rhetoric and class analysis, but he contrasted this poignantly with the solidarity the strike generated among black, feminist and gay groups 'far removed from any pit-head'. This aspect of the strike, as well as the leading role women played in it, he characterised as belonging 'instinctually with the politics of the new'.[13] Retrospective accounts of the strike by women in mining communities, who organised soup kitchens, pickets and fundraising, described how the strikes fundamentally changed them: throwing them into public-facing roles beyond the home, bringing them into contact with people and places they would not otherwise have encountered (from East German miners to Greenham Common feminist peace activists), enabling them to forge relationships with one another, and making them aware of the unjust structures of the British state with its violent cops, lying media and punitive welfare system. A joke was repeated by striking miners who would say they wanted their wives back after the strike was over, adding, 'Not this one, the one I had before.'[14] But the women they had been before no longer existed.

On 4 March 1985, the *Guardian* reported that the end of the strike had been announced the previous evening in 'a mood of bitterness and tears'.[15] In the immediate aftermath of defeat, Vicky Seddon's *The Cutting-Edge: Women and the Pit Strike* (1986) gathered together accounts from women involved in the strike. She spoke to miners' wives, women from mining villages, feminists in cities who offered solidarity (including Communist Party and peace movement activists and those involved in support groups like Lesbians and Gays Support the Miners), and striking workers employed in mines in cleaning, catering and clerical roles. In its pages I found accounts that came closer to conveying what I had been hoping to find in writings on 'left melancholy': the expression of a rawer and more ambivalent range of emotions. The feelings that accompanied defeat were never narrated entirely in isolation from the profound and positive personal shifts the strike had brought about. Barbara Drabble, who participated in the strike as a member of the National Union of Miners (NUM), joined the picket lines outside the National Coal Board's building throughout the year and was active in Sheffield Women Against Pit Closures, conveyed the sense of shock and sadness that followed the announcement that the strike was over:

> On Sunday night when the announcement was made by the NUM that we were to return to work on Tuesday I just couldn't believe it. It *couldn't* be over; we *hadn't* won, we *couldn't* give up. For my part, I could have stayed out for as long as it took to win and so could all the activists I spoke to. We were stunned. For a year now we built another way of life which was, by turn, hard, depressing, exciting, exhilarating, new. We never knew what each day would bring . . . That Sunday night I wept and wept and despaired.

Tears and despair surface again and again in accounts of that night and the days that followed. Margo Thorburn, who had been active in Fife Women Stand Firm in Scotland, recalled: 'We were all feeling down, I shed buckets that night and for days, weeks after it.'[16] Although many people cried alone, the phenomenon of simultaneous widespread weeping could also be understood as a collective experience. People were falling apart together.

Eventually, however, people began to drift apart. Though many women reflected on the permanent subjective changes they had undergone, recalled times of joy and elation, expressed no regret for having participated in the strike, and declared how much they hoped to continue with political activism in some form, this did not mean they therefore found it easy to carry on fighting straight away. These contradictory feelings are captured in reflections by Dorothy Phillips, who set up a soup kitchen for miners at the Celynen Collieries' Miners' Institute in Newbridge, Wales.

She separated the immediate emotions associated with Sunday, 3 March – 'I haven't spoken to one woman who didn't tell me she cried on that day' – from transformative solidarity during the strike – 'that sense of togetherness . . . is an experience I cannot forget'.[17] The defeat disrupted a whole infrastructure and a set of routines that had sprung up to support the striking workers. The political roles and forms of support that were described as precipitating changes in subjectivity were material. Solidarity was a practice. Just as the strike had transformed the rhythms, routines and relationships of people's daily lives, so the emotions associated with defeat were not just a response to a loss located in the future but also to the loss of an existing context of struggle.

Although Phillips' reflections were overwhelmingly positive – 'we gained such a lot, we learned such a lot' – she nonetheless described feeling unable to continue immediately with her women's group or other political activities: 'I want to stand back and take a breathing space. When it was all finished I felt physically and mentally drained . . . It just went "whump".' Cath Cunningham from Fife Women Stand Firm struck a similar note:

> Everything isn't rosy in the women's groups now. In the strike we were all saying how the women's groups are going to go on and on forever, we were never going to stop. It isn't like that. The women are tired, a lot of them are shattered.[18]

To rid itself of melancholic attachments to the past, according to Hall, the left needed to engage with the material realities of the present and dispense with outmoded assumptions. History does nothing inevitable, defeats guarantee no final victory. Benjamin perceived this: 'The experience of our generation: that capitalism will not die a natural death.'[19] But what about emotional experiences of political defeat, exhaustion or disillusionment that *are* realities in the present tense? The accounts of the aftermath of the miners' strike gathered by Seddon make clear that the losses and shatterings were not abstract but material, not intellectual but experiential. The question of how to prevent such forms of despair from hanging around indefinitely is a different one when framed on the level of psychological experience. Of course, the capacity to engage in political struggle should not be reduced to a question of feelings, dispositions and moods but cordoning off psychological questions from political struggle altogether risks prolonging the impasses.

Treating political defeats as bombastic cinematic events that unfold in history with a capital 'H' makes it harder to understand them as particular experiences, which sometimes dramatically rupture and sometimes fold awkwardly into the rhythms of people's everyday lives. People make history, after all. I'm not sure I would claim that one person lying in a bed in Glasgow crying on a cold December morning in 2019 was a political event, though it was an experience with definite political causes. And despite being physically isolated in that moment, the experience, like the weeping and despairing on Sunday, 3 March 1985, was connected to scenes unfolding simultaneously in many rooms, which, taken together and traced forwards through time, had real effects, however diffuse, differentiated and difficult to trace.

In the concluding paragraph to 'Resisting Left Melancholy', Brown half-jokingly asserts that she is not proposing therapy as a solution to the issues she identifies but is instead insisting on the importance of examining the negative feelings that often sustain attachments to left-wing theories and movements. Dean, meanwhile, is scathing about the left's increasing emphasis on self-care. Both thinkers offer valuable interpretations of Sigmund Freud's 'Mourning and Melancholia' (1917), but they approach psychoanalysis theoretically rather than as a clinical practice. I would not blithely propose some one-size-fits-all therapy or self-care as a solution to experiences of political disillusionment, exhaustion and despair either, but I am less inclined to brush therapeutic questions or the issue of care aside altogether. Indeed, therapeutic questions form part of these historical experiences, whether integrated into political struggles or pursued in response to them. Treating psychic distress and attempts to ameliorate it as extraneous to political struggle neglects the gravity of the mental strains that arise from living in the world and striving to change it. It is worth analysing why many people have turned to therapies of various kinds, withdrawn from collective projects, or struggled to continue living their everyday lives in the aftermath of political defeats or prolonged periods of political engagement. It is also worth asking whether they developed methods, concepts or techniques for working through those experiences that helped them keep going or enabled them to reengage in future struggles.

What are the psychic effects of defeat? How have people historically made sense of and attempted to work through these effects? What did defeated people do with their days and nights? How did they feel when they woke up in the morning? Did they seek solace with their comrades, throw themselves into new fights, disappear into solitude or renounce their former political commitments altogether? What concepts did they use to describe what they were feeling? What methods did they try to make themselves feel better? Are histories of exile and incarceration, funerals and fugitivity also histories of renewed hope? By excavating specific accounts of the emotional impact of defeat or disillusionment, and by approaching them as lived events and psychological phenomena, I have attempted to think about epochal histories of the left in relation to smaller, more mundane experiences, however big they might have felt to those who lived through them.

Seeking a foil to the stuffy left melancholia epitomised by Kästner, Benjamin reached for the committed poetry of Bertolt Brecht, with whom he had recently become friends when he wrote the essay and who, he declared, fulfils the 'task of all political lyricism'.[20] In 'Experience and Poverty', published five months after non-Nazi parties were formally outlawed in Germany in July 1933, Benjamin mentions Brecht among a list of artists who demonstrated a 'total absence of illusion about the age and at the same time an unlimited commitment to it'.[21]

Brecht, who outlived Benjamin by sixteen years, came to the end of his days in the 1950s, splitting his time between East Berlin and a light-filled lakeside house in the countryside of the German Democratic Republic (GDR). His final collection, *Buckow Elegies* (1953), reflects bitterly on the violent suppression of a construction workers' strike that began in East Berlin in June 1953 before rippling across the nascent socialist state. Although laced with sadness, guilt and regret, Brecht's late poems do not forsake his earlier convictions, nor do they dwell solely on the failures and losses of the past. Benjamin accused Kästner of suffering from a 'heaviness of heart' that 'derives from routine',[22] whereas Brecht's heart seems broken by what he names in 'Dialectical Ode', 'the pain of experience'.[23] Kästner suffers from the tedium of the status quo, Brecht from a lifetime of struggle against it. Brecht nonetheless retains a faith that hearts 'torn to pieces in the struggle' will be reassembled in the future. In Benjamin's description the feelings of the left melancholic once lay in 'dusty heart-shaped velvet trays' that are now empty, while Brecht describes revolutionary hearts that have been broken but remain full of feeling. The sliver of difference between the empty heart and the broken one may seem negligible, but it is the difference between resignation and commitment or between left melancholy and mournful militancy (the concept with which this book concludes). The chapters that follow dance in the sliver of light between these two heart-shaped images.

2

Nostalgia

> *What happens to a dream deferred?*
>
> *Does it dry up*
> *like a raisin in the sun? . . .*
> *Or will its blood*
> *make you drunk*
> *fermented*
> *like syrup?*
>
> *Maybe it just sags*
> *like a heavy load?*
>
> *Or does it explode?*
>
> – Alaa Abd El-Fattah and Ahmad Douma
> (adapted from Langston Hughes)[1]

In a paper on poetry and revolution, Keston Sutherland argues that the climaxes of all revolutionary moments – whether realised or defeated – share an emotional dimension, which he designates 'revolutionary subjective universality':

> People never in their lives feel so fully and really alive as they do in revolutions. There is not a single revolution since 1789 whose annals and fictions are not overflowing with repetitions of that single testimony. It is the constant song, infinitely reprised, from St. Petersburg to Cairo, from the Paris of 1968 even to the London protests of 2003 and 2011.[2]

Sutherland's linkage of distinct political uprisings across time participates in a tradition of leftist hagiography. Revolutionary moments are lifted out of the ebb and flow of time and inserted into a still pool of emancipatory feeling. Alain Badiou similarly draws connections between disparate historical events, which he claims are all characterised by the 'communist invariant'.[3] Sutherland imagines these moments as transcendent, almost mystical. Revolutionary commemoration seeks to reignite that emotional flare in the present, linking past moments of victory – however brief – to the praxis of aspiring revolutionaries in the present. Karl Marx discussed the 'radiant ... enthusiasm' unleashed by the Paris Commune of 1871, stating that emancipation would only be achieved through an arduous struggle that would transform both circumstances and people, a social revolution that would precipitate a psychological revolution.[4] But if historical circumstances change the people who make them, what becomes of the feelings and subjective transformations wrought by revolutionary defeats?

Between 18 March 1871 and the Commune's brutal defeat just seventy-two days later on 28 May, Paris became a laboratory for a revolutionary experiment in self-governance. The dates of the Commune's foundation and defeat both subsequently became significant anniversaries in left-wing calendars, the former as celebration, the latter as lament. The Paris Commune became a powerful yet malleable symbol for future revolutionaries. This chapter explores a tension between the Commune's afterlives in the collective imaginary of the left and the actual lives of surviving Communards, between the Commune as eternal image and as fleeting experience. My discussion is animated by a tension between two concepts: moribund nostalgia (backward-looking, stultifying) and political nostalgia (forward-facing, energising).

Following the Commune's defeat, over 4,000 surviving Communards were tried and sent into exile in New Caledonia, a colonial archipelago in the southwest Pacific. The 241 deported Communards who died in exile were said to have been suffering from 'nostalgia', understood as a form of pathological homesickness, a diagnosis the French penal authorities contested. By contrasting the nineteenth-century medical definition of nostalgia, which some surviving Communards used to describe their own experiences, with the nostalgia still evident in left-wing attachments to the image of the Commune, I ask how examining subjective experiences of defeat might add nuance to how the left relates to its past and how that might in turn inform its relation to the future. Following Svetlana Boym's injunction to treat nostalgia as an 'historical emotion' symptomatic of an era, I also ask whether it has a radical political inflection in this context or if it remains stubbornly backward-looking and conservative.[5] Susan Stewart claims that nostalgia is 'always ideological'. Nostalgia's longed for object, imagined as 'an impossibly pure context of lived experience at a place of origin', is inauthentic by definition; an ideal image of past authenticity that blots out the immediate present.[6]

By invoking historical moments when hegemonic structures were shattered, however briefly, revolutionary commemorations could be said to reverse the temporality Stewart presumes is inherent in nostalgia: the authenticity of a past moment of glimpsed liberation breaks through the complacent ideological sheen of the present state of things.[7] But does a nostalgic relation to the revolutionary past risk reifying historic struggles? Does nostalgia close off the more psychologically difficult aspects of historical experience from scrutiny? Does it sever connections to immediate circumstances by elevating past events to the status of myth and converting their participants into heroes and martyrs?

This dilemma applies not only to events located in the distant past. Recent events can transform with remarkable speed. In a piece written to mark the first anniversary of the 2020 George Floyd rebellions, Jason E. Smith already cautions: 'We must . . . be sure not to slip into the bad habit of commemoration, the rituals of monumentalization, whose effect is to consign them to the bygone past, to stitch them into a solemn tapestry of poignant defeat.'[8] Although Smith identifies this danger inherent in the memorialisation of historic uprisings, he does not see maudlin monumentalisation as their only or inevitable outcome. Indeed, he identifies restoring the vibrancy and ruptural energy of the original events as an urgent task. Smith articulates the two poles of nostalgia that this chapter wrestles with: the enlivening and the deadening. Following on from my discussion of left melancholy, this chapter asks if an attachment to the past that stifles future action (moribund nostalgia) can be distinguished from a mode of engagement with revolutionary history that harnesses the energies of past experiences for the present (political nostalgia).

In shifting attention from the euphoria felt at the height of a political uprising to the despair and disillusionment following it, as well as in considering how the mythological legacy of an event might be complicated by returning to the event's more immediate emotional ramifications, I do not follow Sutherland in assuming that revolutionary subjectivity is universal. Emotions are historically contingent, feelings varied and contradictory. The actual emotions felt by long dead people cannot be accessed in a direct, unmediated fashion. I'm conscious that the 'experience' I'm attempting to counterpose to a mythological image is just another image, but by trying to perceive the sombre strokes sketched beneath the inherited portrait, perhaps a different picture can emerge that smudges the lines of both triumphant and tragic historiography. This chapter will explore the psychic lives, deaths and afterlives of the Commune in reverse, beginning with a discussion of its function as an emotive symbol before analysing its more immediate psychic aftermath.

Forever enshrined

The Paris Commune has a particular status in the collective memory of the left.[9] Though it is not the earliest historical event that has been posited as a mythical communist or anarchist origin point – its own participants located themselves in a revolutionary tradition stretching back to 1793, 1830 and 1848 – the short duration and delimited space of the Commune, its working-class character and the brutality of its defeat all contributed to its being treated as a tragic yet inspiring emblem. Georges Haupt argues that the various legacies and mythologies of the Commune have a history of their own: 'Through the prism of the Paris insurrection was born a new historical consciousness.'[10] Reflecting on the historiography of the Commune since the 1980s, Karine Varley similarly notes that 'more attention has been devoted to the memories and representations of the Commune than to the events and actions of March to May 1871'.[11] The image of the Commune – its function in subsequent political movements, its role in shaping class consciousness, and the rituals associated with its commemoration – has a reality that exceeds the existence of the Commune itself. Commemorations of the Commune also have a psychological aspect, stirring pride and fostering bonds of solidarity in their participants.

In her discussion of the significance of the Paris Commune for socialists in Britain, Laura C. Forster notes that by the 1880s, British commemorations, which took place on 18 March, were less sombre than their French and Belgian counterparts, where 27 May was the more significant date. In Britain, the events had a festival atmosphere 'with a great deal of emphasis on singing and dancing and drinking'.[12] Commemorations in Britain that took place in the immediate aftermath of the Commune's defeat had a different tenor, as exiled Communards themselves played an important role in them, but over time the event became detached from individuals' experiences. It began to form part of the collective memory of the left in a more abstract sense, transforming into a more generalised uplifting and inspirational symbol in the process.

In the France of the Third Republic, the Commune's public memory was officially suppressed: references to the events were strictly censored and an alternative 'conservative, counter-revolutionary and reactionary' myth of French history was constructed in its place.[13] Of the Communards who survived, most were either in prison or in exile during the 1870s. Though there were smaller commemorative banquets and ceremonies in earlier years, mourning rituals and commemorations focused on honouring dead martyrs began following the partial amnesty that was granted to former Communards in 1880. In April of that year, around 2,000 socialist mourners met to lay a wreath on the grave of Communard Gustave Florens. This was followed by a mass demonstration in the Père Lachaise cemetery in May to commemorate the defeat of the Commune, which became an increasingly significant annual fixture.[14]

In 1918, seventy-three days after the October Revolution, V. I. Lenin (who was born just a year before the Commune's birth and death) famously danced in the snow to celebrate the fact that the Bolshevik experiment had outlived the Paris Commune. In her last known piece of writing, penned just before she was killed by right-wing paramilitary officers and thrown into the Landwehr Canal following the defeat of the January Uprising in Berlin, in 1919 Rosa Luxemburg defiantly proclaimed:

> What does the entire history of socialism and of all modern revolutions show us? The first spark of class struggle in Europe, the revolt of the silk weavers in Lyon in 1831, ended with a heavy defeat; the Chartist movement in Britain ended in defeat; the uprising of the Parisian proletariat in the June days of 1848 ended with a crushing defeat; and the Paris commune ended with a terrible defeat. The whole road of socialism – so far as revolutionary struggles are concerned – is paved with nothing but thunderous defeats. Yet, at the same time, history marches inexorably, step by step, toward final victory! Where would we be today without those 'defeats', from which we draw historical experience, understanding, power and idealism? Today, as we advance into the final battle of the proletarian class war, we stand on the foundation of those very defeats; and we can do without any of them, because each one contributes to our strength and understanding.[15]

In the kind of litany later echoed by the likes of Badiou and Sutherland, Luxemburg framed political defeat as noble and heroic – a necessary sacrifice on the difficult but inevitable journey to triumph. Luxemburg believed that historical defeat could still act as a source of knowledge and inspiration. On the occasion of the seventy-fifth anniversary of the Commune in 1946, C. L. R. James echoed this sentiment, pronouncing that 'the Commune, *despite its failure*, was a symbol of inestimable value' (my emphasis).[16]

Like Lenin before him, Leon Trotsky placed the October Revolution on a continuum with the Paris Commune. Framed as a lesson to improve upon rather than a model to replicate, the Commune became a flawed yet inspiring example of class struggle that would soon, it was assumed, spread across the world.[17] Young activists experimenting with new domestic arrangements and modes of living in the aftermath of the October Revolution turned to the Paris Commune as 'a model of direct democracy, mutual cooperation, and collective reorganisation': the Baku Commune of 1918 was framed as a 'reincarnation' of the Paris Commune, while a commune group based at the Stalingrad Tractor Factory a decade later proclaimed their intention of emulating the Communards.[18] Though such Soviet initiatives may have relied on a romanticised image of the past, the example of the Paris Commune nonetheless inspired concrete practices in the present. The Paris Commune in these cases did not ossify into a relic for sober museal contemplation but inspired vibrant new forms of social relation; the political triumphed over the moribund. Soviet babies were even named *Parizhkommuna*: newly born yet linked to a revolutionary inheritance.[19]

In the aftermath of the October Revolution, the annual anniversary marches to the Mur des Fédérés (Communard's Wall) in the Père Lachaise cemetery in Paris were reinvigorated, indicating that revolutionary inspiration flowed in both directions.[20] When Lenin died in 1924, a local section of the French Communist Party sent the red flag of the 67th Battalion of the Paris Commune to Moscow.[21] But as with Lenin's mausoleum, in which the flag was displayed, the symbolism was ambiguous. Was the red flag a symbol of proletarian struggle or revolutionary mourning? The slogans 'Vive la Commune!' and 'Lenin lives!' make jarring accompaniments to an embalmed corpse. When the remains of Communard Théophile Ferré were exhumed from the Levallois-Perret cemetery in July 1881, eulogies were read over them. Attendees could see that his skull had been shattered by his executioners, and after the exhumation, Ferré's sister offered hanks of his hair to mourners as souvenirs.[22]

The Commune's significance waned in the Soviet Union under Stalin, but it remained a touchstone for revolutionaries elsewhere. In Western Europe, anniversary commemorations continued to be observed, and they functioned as significant rituals for the Popular Front in the 1930s, in which surviving Communards were sometimes involved. In the Spanish Civil War, International Brigade battalions were named after both the Commune and the Communard Louise Michel. Like the Guangzhou Commune five decades earlier, the Shanghai People's Commune of 1967 proclaimed itself to have been built on the model of the Paris Commune. In May 1968 thousands of people in Beijing marched to express their solidarity with students and workers in Paris, chanting the slogan: 'Long live the revolutionary heritage of the great Paris Commune!' As well as being a historical inspiration for those on the barricades in Paris in May 1968, on the Commune's centenary in 1971, high school students in the city went on strike. Another forty years later, Cairo's Tahrir square was likened to the Paris Commune, an Occupy Oakland activist gave their name as 'Louise Michel' to a *New York Times* journalist, and in New York, a version of Bertolt Brecht's 1949 play *The Days of the Commune* was performed in locations across the city in solidarity with Occupy Wall Street.[23] In contrast to macabre rituals fixated on deadly remains, these examples evince a vital relation to the revolutionary past aiming to transmit something of the euphoria of the original event into new contexts of struggle. The revolutionary past here functions more like a sonic vibration than a catalogued object under glass.

Kristin Ross argues that the afterlives of the Commune should be read as the ensuing chapters of the actual event, rather than an epilogue or afterword: 'The thought of a movement is generated only with and after it: unleashed by the creative energies and excess of the movement itself.'[24] For all that the Commune inspired and galvanised, how does collective memory contend with the scale of violence and suffering that accompanied its defeat? Haupt concludes his discussion of the legacy of the Commune on an uneasy note, reflecting that the image of the Commune has come to displace 'the complex reality of history'.[25] Without wanting to crush the hopeful example of the Commune, it is important to ask what can be gleaned from returning to the history of its aftermath, not as a transcendent image or symbol, but as something that people lived through and survived (or, in many cases, didn't).

Dead birds, stranded jellyfish, ridiculous hopes

The entanglement of image with reality is also at stake in accounts of the *semaine sanglante* or 'Bloody Week' of 21 to 28 May, which put a brutal end to the Commune. Adolphe Thiers' army, which gradually came to outnumber the amateur army defending Paris, closed in on the city and invaded on 21 May, with orders to shoot any armed insurgents on sight. Firing squads were set up across the city. Communard retaliation was notably muted, though the killings that did occur, particularly the execution by Blanquists of the Archbishop of Paris, were used to justify a brutal purge.[26] By 24 March anarchist Communard Élie Reclus, who acted as director of the Bibliothèque Nationale during the Commune, could reflect that Communards were left 'floating like the unfortunate jellyfish left aground by the ravages of a storm, our willpower is useless, our efforts in vain, our hope has become ridiculous . . . our little lives are engulfed by these incredible events'.[27] Many thousands of Communards were executed or killed in battle.[28] Buildings burned. Barricades hastily constructed with paving stones were soon covered by the corpses of people who had built them. The air smelled of rotting flesh. Around 35,000 Communards were arrested and incarcerated in horrendous conditions. Paris remained under martial law. Military trials spanned several years: 12,500 were tried, 10,000 convicted.[29]

In the aftermath of the Commune's defeat, photographs of ruined buildings circulated as souvenirs. Tourists visited the rubble.[30] As Karl Marx remarked: 'The Commune knew that its opponents cared nothing for the lives of the Paris people, but cared much for their own Paris buildings.'[31] Photographs were also taken of detainees and of dead Communards in the morgue; images of dirty, swollen, bloodied, decaying corpses provided a stark contrast to the defiant barricade figures that had circulated in the press weeks previously.[32] In anti-Communard accounts, overblown mythological and animalistic metaphors abound. Wild furies, Amazons, viragoes, hyenas, witches: Communards were depicted as unnatural, as dangerously transgressive of social norms, as gender nonconforming and over(t)ly sexual. During the last days of the Commune, women who came to be known as '*les pétroleuses*' were rumoured to have lit fires across Paris. Though the phenomenon seems to have been largely imaginary, caricatures of wild-eyed, saggy-breasted women circulated in the conservative press, an aberrant allegorical counterpart to Liberty, Justice, Marianne and various other female figures used to symbolise the French nation.[33] The Commune was also often associated with madness, characterised as a pathological outbreak performed by sick, perverse or deranged people.[34]

Written in exile in London and first published in French in Brussels in 1876, prior to the amnesty granted to surviving Communards in 1880, Prosper Olivier Lissagaray's *History of the Commune of 1871*, which was translated into English by Eleanor Marx, became a foundational left-wing account of events. Lissagaray had fought for the Commune and was said to have been the last man remaining on the barricades at the moment of defeat.[35] Lissagaray perceived that recounting what he called the 'balance-sheet of bourgeois vengeance' would be insufficient to convey the qualitative suffering a violent state repression of this scale incurred. His account of the final days of the Commune is full of morbid details – swarms of flies hovering over rotting bodies, streets full of dead birds, corpses bloated by rainwater staring with open eyes at passers-by – as if conveying the putrid materiality of the aftermath might render its horrors tangible to the reader. He also describes the emotional toll of the defeat and the mental suffering deliberately inflicted on the vanquished: 'The Versaillese want more than the body; they must attaint the rebellious mind, surround it with an atmosphere of stench and vice, in order to make it fail and founder.'

Lissagaray claimed that the conditions of imprisonment that accompanied the torment of defeat among arrestees had dramatic psychological effects: 'Some, going mad, dashed their heads against the walls; others howled, tearing their beards and hair.' 'Many went mad', awaiting trial; 'All passed through their hours of madness.'[36] As Communard Louise Michel recalled of the period of incarceration prior to her exile: 'The cries of the insane, uncertainty about relatives and friends whose fate was unknown, mothers left alone – all that I feel even now.'[37] Though he insisted that efforts to break the will of Communards failed and that revolutionary faith remained undimmed, the closing pages of Lissagaray's book nonetheless recount numerous deaths and suicides, as well as citing letters from survivors describing utter hopelessness:

> I have suffered much ... How many times have I been discouraged! What despair, what doubts have seized me! I believed in mankind, and all my illusions have been lost one by one; a great change has come over me, and I have almost failed to resist so many disillusions.

Far from invoking rousing dreams of the future, Lissagaray concludes by imploring readers to dwell on the fate of the survivors: 'Remember the vanquished not for a day, but at all hours . . . let the agony of the prisoners haunt you like an everlasting nightmare.'[38]

No news from home

Among those convicted, over 4,000 were sent into exile in New Caledonia, on long and arduous voyages that took between four and six months. Only twenty of the exiles were women. Communards fighting on the barricades during Bloody Week were reported to have shouted 'Better death than Cayenne!'[39] Political exiles had been sent to the penal colony in Cayenne in French Guiana following the 1848 revolution, but the islands of New Caledonia, situated in the South Pacific to the east of Australia, which had been formally declared a French colony in 1853 and opened as a penal colony a decade later, were selected as the site for the Communards. They became the first large group of prisoners to arrive on the islands.

Though similar metaphors were applied to the Versaillese by sympathisers of the Commune, including Marx, in right-wing publications Communards were frequently likened to savages, barbarians and cannibals.[40] Yet when the metaphorically savage Communards were sent to New Caledonia as exiles, they were intended to become a civilizing influence on indigenous Kanak people, who were perceived by the French government as literal savages. As Alice Bullard discusses, Communards were viewed as 'subjects of moralization and agents of civilization'.[41] Life in the penal colony was envisaged as a process of mental and moral reorientation, an 'engineered redemption', in which the corrupt Communards, through agricultural labour on a supposedly 'virgin earth', would be transformed. Having reformed themselves, the colonial logic went that their labour would transform their surroundings and New Caledonia's indigenous inhabitants in turn.[42]

Provided with meagre food rations, the exiles built simple huts in which to live. The colonial administration attempted to devise incentives to colonise, promising family reunification, but in practice very few family members joined their spouses or parents on the islands. In 1874, following a successful escape by a small group of Communard prisoners, harsher rules were imposed by the penal authorities, making daily life on the islands even more difficult for the deportees. Constant rumours of an amnesty led to restlessness among the prisoners, which discouraged them from investing in their immediate surroundings. Lacking purpose, family, friends or an active political or intellectual milieu, they complained of loneliness, boredom, hunger, sadness, destitution and ultimately despair.[43]

Lissagaray notes of those exiled to New Caledonia that the 'condemned hoped to make themselves a home in this far-off land'. But he goes on to describe the emotional collapse that many suffered on arrival: 'In the beginning endless reveries, then discouragement and sombre despair; cases of madness occurred, then death.' He gives the following account of Albert Grandier, who died at the age of thirty in November 1873:

> His heart had remained in France, with a sister he adored. Every day he went to the sea-shore to wait for her; so he became mad. The Administration refused to admit him to an asylum. He escaped from the friends who guarded him, and one morning was found dead in the swamps, not far from the road that heads to the sea.[44]

After disembarking from the long voyage to New Caledonia on the Ducos Peninsula, Louise Michel sought out her comrade Augustin Verdure, to find he had already 'died of grief at receiving no news from home'. Like Lissagaray, Michel described causes of death among the exiles, including homesickness, distance from loved ones (particularly young children) and a misplaced belief that they would soon be permitted to return to France: 'Premature hopes which disillusionment later crushed... they preferred to dream those fallacious dreams that killed them rather than to listen to the voice of reason.'[45]

The failure to make a new home, a preoccupation with absent people and a continued attachment to France were all characteristic features of pathological nostalgia. The deaths of 241 political prisoners between 1873 and 1876 were all attributed to nostalgia by the Communards, whose newspapers also published advice for those suffering from the illness. The penal administration did not accept the diagnosis. Constant waiting for news from loved ones in letters that were sometimes withheld by the authorities exacerbated the psychological sufferings of the deportees, as did the belief that amnesty was imminent. They sometimes distracted themselves with heavy drinking and also exhibited physical symptoms: sleeplessness, a lack of appetite, strange itching. In contrast to the vividness of the remembered past of their distant homeland, their immediate surroundings in the present struck them as empty, void-like.[46]

Nostalgia has medical origins. The term was introduced by Swiss doctor Johannes Hofer in 1688 to describe a form of pathological homesickness with a range of symptoms, including difficulty sleeping, weakness, heart palpitations, sighing, hunger, thirst and a 'continued sadness' that could lead to organ failure and death.[47] The nostalgic withdraws from their immediate environment due to a preoccupation with their longed-for homeland, which they meticulously reconstruct in their imagination. In eighteenth- and nineteenth-century France, the illness took on shifting meanings connected to social upheavals. The young male soldier was the archetypal case. During the French Revolutionary Wars (1792–1802), an epidemic of often fatal nostalgia broke out among soldiers, particularly among conscripts from rural areas. Unable to return all soldiers back to their homes, doctors proposed a cure that was both medical and political, in that it relied on a redefinition of patriotic attachment so that 'home' could mean something abstract rather than concrete, an ideal nation rather than a physical land mass.[48]

Nostalgia involved a pathological attachment to the past and was defined in relation to progress. Understood as a symptom of modernity, it was assumed that nostalgia would diminish as civilization progressed, people learned to adapt to new environments and methods of communication across long distances advanced.[49] Lisa O'Sullivan discusses ambiguities inherent in the definition of nostalgia that meant it could accommodate different definitions of 'home' – physical, cultural or emotional – with varied political valences and a concomitant range of implications for understandings of patriotism and the nation. By the mid-nineteenth century, the prevalence of nostalgia as a diagnosis had declined. It also began to acquire a broader set of meanings beyond the clinical sphere. In the work of Balzac, for example, according to O'Sullivan, 'nostalgia was not linked specifically to the past, but referenced the fantastical, a thwarted passion that could be directed toward any number of, often impossible, dreams'.[50] Yet the disease resurfaced briefly during the 1870–71 siege of Paris, prompting a flurry of interest in nostalgia as a medical phenomenon during the Commune. Its definition shifted to absorb some of the associations it had acquired in literary accounts along the way; fantasies of imaginary situations were given precedence over reconstructed memories of actual experiences. The nostalgic was no longer said to reconstruct a lost world, but instead to create a new one in their imagination. By the time Communards were sent into exile in New Caledonia in the 1870s, nostalgia was already anachronistic and marginal as a medical diagnosis. Indeed, their exile coincided with the disappearance of nostalgia from the medical sphere.

As an illness provoked by displacement, nostalgia was a pathology of both space and time. The nostalgic longed for a distant place and a lost moment. In the more expansive definition that had emerged by 1870, however, the ambiguities O'Sullivan identifies with nostalgia as a concept were compounded. Did nostalgic Communards long for a concrete time and place from their own pasts, or did they suffer from the lack of an abstract ideal located in a future that had never come to pass? The definition of nostalgia as it evolved in France was entangled with understandings of patriotism, nationalism, citizenship and inheritance. Backward-looking and resistant to change, nostalgia seems conservative by definition. It is difficult to reconcile nostalgia as a fatal longing for a homeland with the radical political vision of the Communards, particularly given their role in the colonial environment, but could the form of nostalgia with which they diagnosed themselves instead be understood as a temporally paradoxical yearning for the future society that had not come to pass? Louise Michel, who did not share her comrades' sense of despair in exile, wrote in her poem 'Song of the Captives':

> In our hearts hope survives,
> And if we see France again,
> It will be to fight anew![51]

Framed as a commitment to a just future that was glimpsed in the Paris Commune, nostalgia among the Communards could be understood not as resulting from a continued attachment to the France of the Third Republic, family or even the Commune as a historical entity, but rather from the loss of the emancipated society they had hoped to create.

In the aftermath of the July Revolution of 1830, political exile Pierre Urbain Briet proposed a definition of 'political nostalgia', in which symptoms arise not from a yearning for a lost home, but from a longing for freedom. 'Political nostalgia' looks to the future rather than the past. It does not result from a displacement from a preexisting home, but instead evinces a desire to feel at home in a just world.[52] By this period, the archetypal nostalgic was passive, introverted, lethargic and often bed-bound, but Briet instead envisioned a nostalgic who looked outwards and desired social transformation. The concept of political nostalgia addresses the paradox – central to this book – of healing while living in a wounding social world, and it does so by suggesting the possibility of psychological healing in a socially just future.

A similarly double meaning arising from experiences of exile is articulated in the first volume of Peter Weiss's epic novel *The Aesthetics of Resistance*, set between the late 1930s and the outbreak of the Second World War, by a character who, before the novel's start, engaged in antifascist organising in Switzerland, Norway and France and fled Nazi Germany; now he is fighting with the International Brigades in the Spanish Civil War. The distinction between moribund and political nostalgia is here expressed as a distinction between the émigré and the political exile:

> The émigré feels he has been forced into an alien world, a vacuum, that he painfully lacks familiar things, the things of his homeland, that he often cannot or will not grasp what has happened to him, and that he tussles either with his personal sufferings or with the difficulties of reorienting himself and trying to adjust to the new country. On the other hand, the political exile never accepts his expulsion, he always keeps his eye on the reasons why he was driven out and he struggles for the change that will someday enable him to return. That is why, he said, we have to fight against the fatigue manifested in exile, against the first signs of psychosis caused by functionlessness, we must always view ourselves as activists who are merely assigned to different venues under the demands of historical events.[53]

Were Communards in New Caledonia still struggling for change as political exiles or were they falling prey to the 'psychosis caused by functionlessness' associated with émigrés? Were nostalgic Communards suffering from political nostalgia or the fatigue of moribund nostalgia? Was their rejection of their immediate surroundings partly a refusal to become 'civilizing' settler colonists in the mode envisioned by the French authorities?

In Alice Bullard's detailed discussion of fatal nostalgia among the Communards deported to New Caledonia, the answers to these questions are ambiguous, but they resist being read as political in Briet's sense. Communard testimonies have more in common with the émigré described by Weiss than with the political exile still struggling for change. Indeed, Bullard describes exiled Communards motivated by a 'deep love of France': 'Time in the penal colony passed in ceaseless dreaming of the beneficent republic and pining for the day of reconciliation with *patrie* and family.'⁵⁴ They remained attached to their national identity, even if it differed from the one promulgated by the authorities who imprisoned them. Their encounters with anti-imperialist rebels from Algeria and New Caledonia further tested their loyalties and identifications, and they raise broader questions about the limits of solidarity, the collective memory of the left and the historiography of political defeat.

Anti-imperial insurgencies

After the 1848 revolution, political exiles were sent not only to Cayenne, but also to Algeria. Kristin Ross stresses the internationalism of the Commune and also situates the virulence of the reprisals against it in a global context. French troops sent to crush the Commune were then sent to Algeria to put down another uprising. After the Commune's defeat, Communards were exiled to New Caledonia rather than Algeria partly because it was farther away than North Africa, but also due to the political upheavals taking place in Algeria at that moment, where settlers had declared their own Commune, independent of the metropole, in autumn 1870, and where in the east of the country, just two days after the declaration of the Commune in Paris, between 100,000 and 200,000 Kabyle insurgents, led by Muhammad al-Mokrani, rose up against their colonial rulers.⁵⁵ Like the defeat of the Paris Commune at the hands of the French state, the uprising was brutally crushed and, like defeated Communards, Kabyle rebels were sent into exile to New Caledonia, joining Communard prisoners on the Isle of Pines. Massimiliano Tomba notes that 'the vast literature on the Paris Commune has often disregarded the link between the events in Paris and those in Algeria', but he also observes that those links were fraught, revealing continued colonial and racist attitudes among Communards, alongside moments of solidarity.⁵⁶

Michel admired the 'strong sense of justice' among those exiled from Algeria.⁵⁷ Communard Jean Allemane, who was among those deported to New Caledonia, wrote in his memoirs of an encounter between Communards and Algerian political prisoners. The two groups sat together in their shared defeat, 'thinking of those they loved, of the unravelling of their existence and the destruction of their dream of liberty'.⁵⁸ Ross extols the cosmopolitan, anti-colonial character of the Commune and cites this anecdote from Allemane's memoirs as evidence of transnational solidarity, but a less celebratory narrative is presented by

Niklas Plaetzer, who argues that 'the communards' language of universalism foreclosed rather than enabled a dialogue between European and non-European experiences of struggle.'[59] Dislocated from its origins, the Communard understanding of the universal proved to be particular and racialised. For the French deportees, the values they fought for on the barricades in Paris did not automatically extend to the colonised islands of the Pacific. And Communards' nostalgic identification with France also blocked identification with the political concerns of the people they lived alongside.

In 1878, a large-scale Kanak uprising further tested the limits of Communard solidarity, while underscoring their ambivalent identification with the French state. Set off in response to delimitation commissions through which the French confiscated land from tribes for European settlers, conflicts over cattle and complex interclan alliances and rifts, the insurrection was swiftly and violently quashed by the French. A thousand Kanaks were killed, villages and crops burned, stolen land was given to settlers, and many arrestees were deported to other islands.[60] Michel identified commonalities between the political struggles of the Communards and Kanaks, who she saw as being propelled by the 'same hope' and united by a desire for the 'same liberty'.[61] Michel drew on her existing experiences of political engagement to help the Kanak cause by cutting telegraph wires, disrupting the communications network relied on by the French authorities.[62] She also tore the red scarf she had worn during the Commune in half to give to two Kanak insurgents. In contrast to the red banner displayed in Lenin's mausoleum, this is an example of an artefact from the Commune connecting to the vibrancy of a new movement, rather than functioning as a deathly relic.

But Michel was unusual among the deportees in her support of the insurrection. Her fellow exiles held dismissive and patronising attitudes toward Kanak culture and were also largely unsympathetic to the uprising, failing to discern the political grievances that lay behind it. One Communard declared himself 'part of a European society lost some six thousand five hundred leagues from our France, subjected to all of the brutalities of a people a bit too primitive', while another proclaimed 'it was our duty not to sleep a cowardly sleep, but to defend the French government'.[63]

Nostalgia is an illness fixated on an imagined past, but in colonial New Caledonia, French civilization was imagined as historically ahead of the existing societies in the 'primitive' colonies, which were not understood as strictly historical at all but situated in timeless nature. Colonial nostalgia is not simply moribund; it further scrambles linear temporality by romanticising past experiences located on the progressive frontiers of advanced history, while consigning the present context to prehistory or ahistorical nature. Though there were fleeting expressions of solidarity and recognitions of shared repression between Kanaks and Communard exiles, in the Communard press, racialised interpretations of the insurrection that relied on assumptions about the biological and cultural 'backwardness' of Kanak people came to dominate.[64] Communards located class struggle in a historical time in which oppressed people could actively intervene to propel time forwards, but they imagined Kanak people occupied an evolutionary time that progressed in natural stages. This precluded the possibility of recognising the actions of colonised Kanak people rising up to reclaim their stolen land as properly political or historical.[65] Locating New Caledonia in a different time, unsynced with and even external to the civilizational march of progress (or the teleological march of history towards communism), also implied that Kanak people did not share a psychological disposition with French Communards. The Kanak uprising, like the Paris Commune, was brutally defeated by the French state, but what were the psychic consequences of its defeat? What would it take to include such a rebellion in the rarified canons of the vanquished? Would it be better to dispense with such hagiographies altogether or could they be reconfigured? Accessing the subjective experiences of any historical actor is necessarily mediated and incomplete, but some such histories are more difficult to access than others.

In the absence of first-hand accounts, writers of anti-imperialist histories and histories 'from below' have traditionally read official documents produced by those in power in the hope of glimpsing ripples of dissent, points where the agency of resisting subjects pokes through the formal prose of those seeking to contain them. Adrian Muckle traffics in these familiar tropes in an article on colonial fears of Kanak rebellion in New Caledonia, declaring that he had tried to 'read against the grain for signs of Kanak agency', but his focus still remains trained on the feelings and fears of the coloniser rather than those of the colonised.[66] In passing, he suggestively cites Ranajit Guha's *Elementary Aspects of Peasant Insurgency in Colonial India*, a work that discerns 'the presence of a rebel consciousness' in documents produced by colonial administrators. Guha insists that 'it is not possible to make sense of the experience of insurgency merely as a history of events without a subject' insisting that peasants were political rather than 'prepolitical' actors.[67] In Guha's Marxist account, a subject is understood as a person with a will, capable of intervening deliberately in the course of history. Would it also be possible to talk about something like a rebel unconscious, or would that be pointlessly anachronistic when analysing the 1870s? What were the Kanak concepts for making sense of human agency and psychological distress in this historical moment? It may not be possible to reconstruct the emotional experience of Kanak defeat as easily as that of Communard nostalgia, about which there are numerous published accounts, but that difficulty, that inaccessibility, that imbalance is important to acknowledge. If revolutionary remembrance can enliven ongoing movements without petrifying into moribund nostalgia, then the failures and limits of past revolutionaries should not be glossed over. History can be prised open so the subjectivities and struggles of people not traditionally included in left-wing canons can rush in and stir up the dust.

Mute bones and cosmic agency

Surviving Communards may not have identified similarities between their mental lives and those of Kanak people, but in death both groups were subject to scientific scrutiny and classified as physically and psychologically 'backward' by medical experts whose narratives bolstered those of the ruling class. In the aftermath of the Kanak defeat, the decapitated head of the leader Ataï, who had been killed in battle, was sent back to Paris by a colonial governor for study by the physical anthropologist Paul Broca, who placed Kanaks between apes and white men on a racist evolutionary ladder. The head was only returned to New Caledonia in 2014.[68] Similarly relying on a science that analysed external features to make assumptions about biological hierarchies and innate characteristics that linked criminality with 'primitivism', criminologist Cesare Lombroso analysed photographs of Communards to draw conclusions about their atavism and supposedly natural propensities for crime based on the shapes of their skulls.[69] Their suffering, he claimed, was exacerbated by their excessively passionate commitment, which he compared to that of religious martyrs.[70] The power of diagnosis that led to the posthumous pathologisation of both groups lay with the vanquishers. Mute bones were unable to resist the authority of scientific classification.

Among Blanquists, rituals of revolutionary commemoration began as political demonstrations that often involved clashes with the police, but as belief in the possibility of imminent revolution receded they ossified into formalised cult-like rituals. Louis Auguste Blanqui's funeral was held on 5 January 1881, which was subsequently observed as an anniversary in increasingly packed revolutionary calendars of remembrance. Blanqui's followers spent years raising money for an elaborate statue to honour his memory. These efforts to 'apotheosize' Blanqui in death, as Patrick Hutton points out, ran contrary to the revolutionary's own 'spirit of simplicity' and pursuit of anonymity.[71] Further deaths of significant Communard figures followed. Funerals were attended by thousands, who set aside their political differences regarding society's present ills to unite in grief over the past. Nostalgia began as a mode of reinvigorating political energies and sustaining solidarities but transformed from a means into a (dead) end. Mute bones were unable to stipulate what they would signify to the living.

Blanqui is a major figure in Walter Benjamin's posthumously assembled collection of notes for a work on nineteenth-century Paris, *The Arcades Project*. Benjamin reads Blanqui's strange late work *Eternity by the Stars*, which he wrote while incarcerated in a fortress on the coast of Brittany as the Commune was unfolding in Paris, as a document of political defeat: 'Resignation without hope is the last word of the great revolutionary.' Blanqui depicts a vast cosmos in which infinite parallel worlds are endlessly unfolding. Any new star is a copy of an old one, every person just one version of a self whose life is also unfolding in every possible iteration on multiple simultaneous planets. Benjamin sees this universe, in which everything repeats but nothing progresses, as 'the complement of that society which Blanqui, near the end of his life, was forced to admit had defeated him'.[72] Blanqui's depiction of the cosmos represents for Benjamin an 'unconditional surrender'.[73] The cosmos Blanqui describes is, Benjamin declares, a 'vision of hell',[74] which is to say a vision of the world as it already is, a reflection rather than a rebuttal of the dominant society in which Blanqui was imprisoned and in which he died: 'Blanqui yields to bourgeois society'.[75]

Blanqui's cosmic tract, as Peter Hallward discusses, might strike a reader as baffling when compared to his political writings and actions, which, since his student days in the 1820s, consistently rejected fatalism: 'How could this ultra-voluntarist revolutionary come to embrace a vision of the cosmos based on endless repetition and the eternal recycling of monotonous variation?' Hallward admits that a vision of an infinite universe in which all 'past barbarisms' repeat and in which the humanity on one planet cannot intervene in the lives of their twins on another, does indeed seem like a melancholic political vision.[76] But if Blanqui pictures dead stars gathering in the cemetery of the sky, he also talks of their resurrection. The apparent tranquillity of the corpse-filled universe disguises the possibility of transformation. And stars are not its only inhabitants. Hallward rebuts Benjamin's comparison of Blanqui to Nietzsche, insisting that Blanqui's presentation of nature as an indifferent and immutable context in which lives infinitely unfold does not imply that those lives therefore unfold in preordained ways. Blanqui's endless universe may seem impervious to change, but it is still one in which human fates remain unsealed. Nothing is preordained.

> The turbulences of man [sic] never affect the natural workings of physical phenomena in any serious manner, but they do turn their own kind upside down. We must therefore factor in this subversive influence that changes the course of individual destinies, destroys and modifies the animal species, tears nations apart, and collapses empires.[77]

Blanqui was concerned with the living not the dead; with the present, not the past; not even, Benjamin perceived, with the future:

> The activity of a professional revolutionary such as Blanqui does not presuppose any faith in progress; it presupposes only the determination to do away with present injustice. Indeed, it is just as worthy of humane ends to rise up out of indignation at prevailing injustice as to seek through revolution to better the existence of future generations.[78]

Rising up out of indignation and making history are always possibilities, but Blanqui's voluntarist vision relies on a conception of a willed subject capable of rising up.

Sometimes it is not possible for people to act in accordance with their commitments. Sometimes prevailing injustice is too great. A nostalgic attitude to the past that retains a connection to life in the present is preferable to a deathly attachment. Sometimes, however, the past shapes the present in ways that make conscious action feel impossible. That sense of impossibility is the theme of the next chapter.

3

Depression

During depression the world disappears.[1]

– Kate Millett

In summer 2016 I moved from London to Berlin for work. During the next few years I sunk into what I would retroactively call depression. At the time it just felt like an unpleasant new texture accompanied my days, something like static on an old TV but duller, grittier and less electric. Every metaphor I can think of to describe the feeling falls apart in this way because everything I can think to compare it to sounds too vivid, too much like a tangible something, while comparing it to nothing sounds too dramatic and abyssal. Invoking the void would be way too interesting.

I didn't feel sad. I felt bad but – I'm aware how nonsensical this sounds – I felt neutral about feeling bad. I just felt bad and that was my reality. I often wondered who would notice if I disappeared. Doing even the most routine things required great effort that I had no interest in expending. Days would pass and I would pass through them. Even that sounds too dynamic. It might be more accurate to say that the days passed over me, like the clouds that passed above the room in which I spent so many of them. Sometimes in the late afternoon I would think that maybe the next day was going to be different. This recurrent thought implies that I knew something was wrong and that I wanted it to change, but it never occurred to me that there was anything that could be done to bring a change about. I didn't seek medical advice. I didn't have a therapist. I didn't even talk to my friends about how I was feeling because I couldn't really think of anything to say.

During this time, though I found it hard to make myself think about anything, I was ostensibly working on a project about histories of radical psychiatry and beginning to think about what would eventually become this book. Unable to read more than a few pages at a time, I instead tried and mostly failed to write about theories of mental illness that insisted on the social origins of psychological symptoms. Meanwhile, I slowly gathered sources about the aftermaths of political uprisings and revolutions, trying to compile examples of people describing psychological responses to experiences of political defeat. In the period immediately before I left London, political organising had taken up much of my time, more than at any other point in my life. When I arrived in Berlin, in the months between the Brexit referendum in the UK and the election of Donald Trump in the US, I didn't get involved in any organising. I decided I needed a break. Yet to claim that my former experience of intense political engagement had any causal relationship to the depression that followed it seems facile. Almost as meaningless as the claim – made by a doctor in London just before I left – that various physical symptoms I was experiencing were likely caused by stress about Brexit (in fact I had a large ovarian cyst exacerbated by endometriosis that went undiagnosed for the next two years). Nor did it ever occur to me to relate my subjective stagnation to leaving the city I had lived in for my entire adult life, to my ongoing physical symptoms, to my disappointments in love, frustrations at work or to the disorientating historical circumstances through which I was living.

The enveloping texture of depression seemed to arrive from nowhere. Being in it felt atemporal; it muffled any sense of past and present. The future existed only as tomorrow, which functioned as an alibi for giving up on today. This all also coincided with a dramatic *improvement* in my personal material circumstances, which made me feel something other than nothing: guilt leading to flamboyant self-recrimination. I had longed for a situation like the one I was now in, felt acutely aware that I was in a much more comfortable situation than most people and felt disgusted at my incapacity to make anything of my days. When it eventually began to cross my mind that I might be depressed I would convince myself it was just a sham, incomparable to the real sufferings of others. After all, everything I was reading persuasively argued that mental distress was exacerbated by economic hardship, not caused by its absence. I felt haptically hyper-aware of the physical objects in my immediate environment, but that awareness did not seem to have anything in common with what the Marxist authors I was reading had in mind when they invoked materialism. Indeed, the objects seemed to stand between me and a world of social relations and structural historical forces beyond them.

The depression I experienced seemed to have nothing in common with arguments I read and wrote about in my academic work concerning the social, historical and political origins of mental illness and psychic distress. It did not even occur to me to think of it in those terms. Effects (or symptoms) that seem to have no causes (or aetiologies) are not even experienced as effects but as states. Feeling inert and finding everything pointless for no discernible reason – not that I was trying to discern a reason – was antithetical to everything I could have imagined arguing about the relationship between psychic life and social forces, experiences of political exhaustion or living through history. This book is about the psychological toll of political struggle; it explores mental states prompted by experiences of defeat, disillusionment and despair. But what about bad feelings that feel causeless? This chapter is about the relationship between politics and depression, but it takes as its starting point my subjective experience of the non-relationship between my depression and my withdrawal from political activism.

My original starting point had been sources by three women – Kate Millett, Shulamith Firestone and Luisa Passerini – who were all politically active in and around 1968 and in the women's liberation movement, and who all later experienced and wrote about depression and other forms of psychological distress. I took for granted that depression should be understood in the context of a depressed person's particular social conditions – and did not assume that medical or therapeutic treatments were therefore unnecessary or unhelpful – but I intended to explore something with more narrowly defined political causes: experiences of depression that accompanied experiences of political disillusionment, despair or defeat. The former contextual definition understands 'the political' spatially, as the historically contingent environment in which a subject lives, while the latter causal definition distinguishes temporally between a politicised before and a depressed after (both of which could be understood as spatial environments in the former sense).

I had assumed that these texts recounting individual experiences of the aftermath of political movements could also be read in relation to a broader historical shift from politicisation and collectivity to apathy and increasing individualism, a meta-narrative that links histories of the aftermath of 1968 with histories of the medicalisation of depression, which began to take hold in the 1970s.[2] As with my own subjective experience of depression, however, I found that my attempts to impose narratives that pinned personal experiences to particular political events or that drew arrows pointing from individuals to epochs failed. The relationships between past and present, cause and effect, symptom and aetiology, individual and history, depression and politics described in these sources were far more tangled and overdetermined than such an argument implies. Although Shulamith Firestone's semi-autobiographical *Airless Spaces* (1997) may be of interest to many readers due to their familiarity with her earlier polemic *The Dialectic of Sex: The Case for Feminist Revolution* (1970) and her key role in radical feminist groups in New York City, her short second book resists being read as having any neat causal relation to her engagement with and disappearance from the women's liberation movement. Its characters are instead submerged in a strip-lit present cut off from past and future, cause and effect. As Sianne Ngai notes, the temporality evoked by Firestone's second book is distinctly depressive: 'The most deeply depressed persons are unable to say that they are depressed about any particular thing, political situation X or life event Y; rather, they view themselves as just depressed.'[3]

This chapter attempts to bring a spatial understanding of depression into dialogue with a temporal one by emphasising that the experiential non-relationship between politics and depression could also be thought of as a problem of scale in which an individual loses all sense of their connection to larger structural forces (which should not be confused with actually being disconnected from them). Before turning to a discussion of those post-'68 texts, I will first discuss two more recent theories of depression's relation to the political, theories to which this chapter attempts to provide an alternative.

Depression, politics and depoliticisation

Ann Cvetkovich's *Depression: A Public Feeling* (2012) begins with an autobiographical section, 'The Depression Journals (A Memoir)', before switching into a more conventionally academic register. Her memoir describes a white, middle-class woman in her thirties who, in the early stages of an academic career, fell into a state of inertia and hopelessness. She evocatively describes the difficulty she had getting out of bed, buying groceries or finding meaning in her intellectual work, and she recalls activities, like swimming or seeing friends, that helped 'hold the despair at bay'.[4] Structural systems and historical forces remain a distant backdrop before which thwarted routines, strained quotidian habits and quiet feelings of despair play out. Conscious of avoiding the redemptive structure that has tended to characterise the depression memoir as a genre, and sceptical of reductive medical approaches to depression, she instead seeks 'to track what it's like to move through the day' while at an impasse.[5]

Cvetkovich introduces her book as emerging from a collective intellectual project called 'Public Feelings' through which the concept of 'political depression' was developed. 'Political depression' was coined in the early 2000s to articulate a sense that traditional forms of political engagement were no longer effective; the concept aimed to 'depathologize negative feelings so that they can be seen as a resource for political action rather than its antithesis'. Although Cvetkovich succeeds in her declared goal of finding a way to write about depression that 'captures how it feels', her memoir does not deliver her related intention of providing 'an analysis of why and how its feelings are produced by social forces'.[6] Cvetkovich's emphasis on the lived textures of depressed life with its unwashed bedsheets, uncooked meals and unbought groceries, while vivid and sometimes moving, seems at odds with her goal to locate depression in the wider social world. Depression is declared to be a public feeling, but, beyond the fact of appearing in a published book, it is narrated as a private one.

It is not that the 'small' everyday things she focuses on are intrinsically cordoned off from 'large' systemic issues. She is well-versed in feminist theories that refuse to situate domestic concerns outside of history proper. In her third chapter, she justifies her decision to focus on the 'intimate', 'material' and 'humble' sites in which depression is lived, describing the home as 'the soft underbelly of capitalism,' but describing an experience of depression under capitalism does not necessarily constitute a political analysis, just as her autobiographical reflection on the feeling of inhabiting a domestic space is not a treatise on socially reproductive labour. Of course, her housing and work situations, her family history, her subject position, her queer friendship groups, her access to health care could all be understood as being in some sense 'political', but they are not discussed in such terms in the memoir, which could instead be read as the basis for a theory of the *depoliticising tendency of depression in spite of its always politicised context* ('apolitical depression' would be a catchier term but it fails to capture the contradiction I am attempting to articulate). Though she occasionally references her relative comfort and discusses the centrality of the figure of the white middle class woman to the medical history of depression, I was struck by a moment in which she likens her apartment to a prison, indicating her detachment not only from the social forces that shape her own experience but from a broader social world full of people whose subjective experiences are shaped by material circumstances very different from her own – a social world that includes non-metaphorical prisons full of actually incarcerated people.[7]

The memoir opens in the mid-1980s with an anecdote about a university protest camp for divestment from apartheid South Africa being brutally cleared by cops. Anxious about pending job applications, Cvetkovich had missed much of the recent protest activity leading up to this event and also went home early on that day rather than joining friends at the police station where they were providing support to arrestees. On her way back, mulling over police violence alongside job applications, she sprained her ankle on the street. The anecdote is accorded significance because she ignored the pain, only noticing her injury hours later, while her decision to focus on her own individual job security over collective solidarity seems almost incidental. She expresses mild regret at leaving the protest but does not accord the decision any broader significance – what it implies about the political *effects* of depression, for example – nor does she reflect on the apartheid regime in South Africa against which her friends were protesting.

Later in the memoir, she begins to take Prozac and briefly emerges from depression and enters a manic phase during which she attends ACT UP meetings and a Pride march. This experience of political engagement contrasts with her subsequent inability – due to the recurrence of her depression – to provide support to a friend and his partner who is dying of AIDS-related illnesses. She narrates her inability to do anything more than turn up at their house and confesses to feeling envious that their 'crisis had a tangible shape that seemed to give them a power and agency that I lacked'. 'The Depression Journals' consistently demonstrates the contradiction that characterises political depression as a concept: the inability of the depressed person to act politically is in turn related to an inability to perceive the experience of depression as political. But Cvetkovich neglects to identify the contradiction because she suggests that simply existing in a room under capitalism is already 'political'. If the gap between the realms of the individual and the social, between 'the micro-level of everyday life and the macro-level of organized collectivities and politics', remains unbridgeable, then is 'politics' reduced to a nebulous force that surrounds individuals but which they have no capacity to analyse let alone influence?[8]

In one of her book's non-autobiographical chapters, Cvetkovich discusses Gregg Bordowitz's video *Habit* (2001), which intersperses footage of his domestic daily routines while living with HIV with footage of South African AIDS activism. Unlike in the memoir, in these pages she does confront what she calls the 'problems of incommensurability' that characterise political depression, which she glosses as 'the difference in scale between our political goals and what we're actually feeling'. The video, she argues, enacts 'depression as the failure to be able to mediate between widely disparate worlds'.[9] This statement perfectly articulates the contradiction that I have identified at the heart of the concept of political depression, offering an alternative to her memoir's insistence that the daily routines that can make depressed life more liveable are modest political practices in their own right.

Mark Fisher's arguments offer an alternative way of framing the relationship between depression's origins in material conditions, the need for political action that would change those conditions, and the individual depressed person. He approaches the problem of incommensurable scales from the opposite direction. Like the concept of 'political depression', Fisher's concept of 'capitalist realism' was born in the Bush-Blair years to describe the impasse of the seemingly endless 'end of history', the experience of living in a world in which all possibility of radical political change seemed to have disappeared and, despite exploitation and immiseration under capitalism, a sense of resignation to current conditions prevailed; in those years, it was easier to imagine the end of the world than to imagine the end of the impasse of political depression.

Rather than staying with the granularity of individual experience, in his 2014 essay 'Good for Nothing', Fisher leaps from individual depression to the diagnosis of a pervasive social malaise: 'Collective depression is the result of the ruling class project of resubordination.' Cvetkovich dwells on the 'small' while Fisher jumps to the 'large'. In a manner analogous to Karl Marx's discussion of the mystical character of commodities in *Capital*, in which value (socially necessary labour time) is hidden behind exchange value, for Fisher, the experiential remoteness of depression from politics can be understood ideologically, as a product of living under capitalism, in whose interests it is to individualise suffering, obscure its systemic origins and encourage people to blame themselves for feeling terrible; the political is impersonal. Curing socially induced unhappiness would therefore involve 'converting privatised disaffection into politicised anger' through the revival of political institutions and class consciousness.[10] Here an individual and temporal experience of depression is elided into a social and spatial understanding of depression. Depression becomes a metaphor for contemporary capitalist society, which causes non-metaphorical depression in some working-class and oppressed people who live in it (implying that members of the ruling class are immune).

Although they reach the problem from opposite directions, Cvetkovich and Fisher both get stuck in a hamster wheel. As Johanna Hedva asks in 'Sick Woman Theory': 'How do you throw a brick through the window of a bank if you can't get out of bed?'[11] It's all very well to proclaim the political origins of depression or to describe what it feels like to be depressed under capitalism, but doing so does not change subjective experiences of self-recrimination, stasis and disengagement that can both obscure any sense of cause being related to effect and obstruct the capacity for political action. Stating that depression has social causes does not enable someone to throw a brick through them.

Building political institutions and class consciousness requires people capable of going to meetings, picket lines and demonstrations or at the very least people capable of taking an interest in their social surroundings, while Cvetkovich's emphasis on small shifts in daily routines that can gradually help make life more bearable seems to imagine a depressed person insulated from the kinds of economic hardship that can make such action difficult or impossible. Just as anti-depressants or therapy can only help people who have access to them, the suggestion that swimming, yoga or crafting can help ameliorate feelings of depression is ultimately an apolitical prescription if it is isolated from a demand to create a society in which such activities, and the time and space in which to pursue them, are available to all. This is where Cvetkovich's arguments differ from those made by disability justice activists and scholars who conceptualise the bed as a site of struggle.[12] Think simply of all the kinds of beds that a person might not be able to get out of (if they have a bed at all): a comfortable bed in a property they own, an uncomfortable bed that belongs to a landlord in a rented room they could be evicted from at any time, a hospital bed, a prison bed and so on.

Cvetkovich's descriptions of the depoliticising qualities of depression acknowledge that sometimes it is impossible to act, but beyond going swimming or taking up knitting – as beneficial and necessary as such activities may indeed be – her analysis does not suggest how to move beyond diagnosis. By claiming the immediate daily experience of depression as political, she side-steps the question of how to move *between* the disparate scales she identifies in her discussion of Bordowitz. Depression obstructs political action, but if depression is *already* political then there is no problem to be solved. Surely the everyday individual experiences of depression are only political insofar as they are shaped by and enmeshed with larger systems and structures in the first place? The isolation of the micro from the macro might *feel* like a fact from the depressive's perspective and, yes, sometimes depressed people really cannot get out of bed, but making these observations is a diagnosis, not a cure. Can an analysis of the depression that follows periods of intense political engagement help to unlock the concept of political depression from this impasse?

Dialectic of airlessness

The year 1970 saw the publication of two landmark feminist texts written by authors active in the women's liberation movement in the US, both of which became canonical works of the second wave: *Sexual Politics* by Kate Millett and *The Dialectic of Sex* by Shulamith Firestone. These fiery polemics have shadowy counterparts in later autobiographical works: Millett's *Flying* (1974) and *The Loony Bin Trip* (1990) and Firestone's *Airless Spaces* (1997). *Flying* charts the movement's unravelling, while the other two titles discuss experiences of mental breakdown, political withdrawal and institutionalisation.

Firestone was found dead in her East Village apartment in summer 2012. At the memorial service at St Mark's Church in-the-Bowery, Millett, nine years Firestone's senior, addressed the assembled mourners. She read a passage from a section of *Airless Spaces* entitled 'Emotional Paralysis', in which a character – who is incapable of reading, writing or feeling the emotions she once had – surveys her ruined life. After finishing the passage Millett said: 'I think we should remember Shulie, because we are in the same place now.' In an argument that recalls Fisher's slippage from individual to collective depression, Millett treated an individual experience as a metaphor for a far-reaching depressive cultural mood. As Susan Faludi remarked: 'It was hard to say which moment the mourners were there to mark: the passing of Firestone or that of a whole generation of feminists who had been unable to thrive in the world they had done so much to create.'[13]

Kathi Weeks resists reading the relationship between Firestone's two books as 'a cautionary tale' or 'tragic narrative' about the fate of Firestone herself and, by extension, of the women's liberation movement more broadly, many of whose participants refused the norms of patriarchal society only to find it impossible to live. Instead she reads the contrast between the two books allegorically, as instances in the history of feminist theory: not only symptomatic of 'feminist theory's retreat from structural analysis, tendency toward methodological individualisms, and abandonment of visions of radical change ... but also of the narrowed and largely backward-looking temporalities and affects that have been cultivated in tandem with them'.[14] Weeks observes how interpretations of Firestone's legacy echo the increasingly individualising trajectory of the movement she had participated in creating:[15] 'Brutally cast out of the revolutionary history she tried to live and imagine, she was left to live on the margins as a lone individual responsible for her own – once again merely private – "failures."'[16]

According to Weeks, Firestone is often cast as a casualty of her own utopia, serving as a reminder of the impossibilities of revolutionary transformation in the present. Weeks yearns to resuscitate the spirit if not the content of Firestone's early utopianism, while remaining alert to the numerous omissions and flaws in *The Dialectic of Sex*: her 'inability to think adequately about race', her essentialism, her neglect of questions of sexuality.[17] Weeks's argument proposes reading Firestone's two works in relation to a broader historical trajectory that saw the macro abandoned for the micro, the political displaced by the personal, structural analysis relinquished in favour of an emphasis on emotions. This account of feminist intellectual history could itself be mapped onto accounts of the emergence of a particular brand of post-'68 individualism.

This argument is exemplified by *The New Spirit of Capitalism*, first published in French in 1999, in which Luc Boltanski and Eve Chiapello famously argue that the 'waning of critique' that occurred in the 1980s and 1990s was not merely a consequence of the crushing of the movements of 1968 but also involved the recuperation of their demands.[18] The rejection of hierarchy and embrace of individual autonomy, liberation, authenticity, informality, 'conviviality, openness to others and novelty, availability, creativity, visionary intuition' all became central to the new spirit of capitalism. Such uncertain, unstable and short-termist conditions, they claim, have emotional effects, evidenced by rising suicide rates and increasing diagnoses of depression.[19] As historian of depression Jonathan Sadowsky also argues, medicalised depression, and a concomitant increase in dependence on anti-depressants such as Prozac, flourished during a historical moment in which psychological well-being was framed as the responsibility of the suffering individual.[20] Self-actualisation took the place of collective struggle.

Proclamations about the dissolution of master narratives that characterised definitions of postmodernism post-'68, which have themselves been read on the left as 'theoretical forms that validated defeat', constitute a master narrative in their own right.[21] Meaning evaporates. Telos falls. Everybody hurts, but nobody really knows why or what to do about it anymore. This taken-for-granted-ness of capitalist reality is precisely what Fisher designated 'capitalist realism'. A particularly fatalistic version of the well-worn narrative appears in many of Adam Curtis's television series, glossed by Alberto Toscano as follows:

> The failed revolutions of the 1960s accelerated the collapse of mass democracy into an individualism that left traditional political parties and elites without a people, sending them into the arms of financial operators and behavioural psychologists to manage and monetize these social atoms.

For Curtis the age of individualism, like the age of depression outlined by Sadowsky, is an age of fragmentation and disorientation. Curtis may not relish this outcome, but he nonetheless presents it as being as uncontrollable as the weather. His goal is to evoke the textures of the clouds, not to explain where they came from or suggest how they could be dissipated. Yet Toscano argues that in the most recent series, *Can't Get You Out of My Head* (2021), Curtis's archival materials and the emotional histories they document threaten to burst through the seams of the tightly woven master narrative, allowing for the 'glimpse of a politics, and of a political emotion, that refuses to be shoehorned into a story about depoliticizing individualism'. Toscano cites a scene in which an undercover agent who conspired against the Black Panther Party is confronted by the former Panther Afeni Shakur and admits that he had found the group's militancy 'powerful, inspiring and beautiful'.[22] Such moments, Toscano claims, brush against the grain of Curtis's account, suggesting messier emotional realities latent in the histories he is excavating, as well as gesturing towards other possible outcomes.

Weeks, meanwhile, proposes taking a 'selective' approach to the feminist past, using it 'as a standpoint from which to see the present from a different angle of vision'.[23] Her characterisation of the contrast between Firestone's two books seems to follow the contours of the post-'68 master narrative I have just sketched, but her essay proposes a valuable methodology for approaching radical thought from the past in a manner that challenges neat, sequential understandings (though I will contest her reading of *Airless Spaces* as concerned with 'therapeutic adjustment', precisely because the book is so unremittingly depressing). Depression can seem inconvenient, anti-utopian, an obstruction to those hoping to stir and organise exultant political movements aimed at transforming the totality. But lamenting the displacement of a more politicised mode neglects the realities of psychic, and hence of social, life and neglects to probe how the two conditions are linked. Depression might feel apolitical and might encourage depoliticisation, but accepting this diagnosis neglects to ask whence depression arises and how it can be shifted. After all, in both the politicised before and the depressive after, individuals live in history; the problem of incommensurable scales is present in both periods, regardless of the narratives applied to them. What political emotions can be glimpsed in accounts of depression? Is it possible to think political transformation and emotional paralysis as enmeshed rather than antithetical? Could the airless space paradoxically ventilate utopia?

Cell windows

In Shulamith Firestone's second and final book, the sparse and slim *Airless Spaces*, nothing and nobody seems to move or be moved. Where *The Dialectic of Sex* was bombastic, acerbic and far-reaching, *Airless Spaces* is abbreviated, morose and constricted. At first glance, it makes perfect sense to characterise the former as political and the latter as depressed. The pathologised subjects who populate *Airless Spaces* are often sedated and inert. Firestone writes of a mental 'paralysis [that] was stubborn and lingered for years'. Suicides. Wakes. Coffins. Hospital wards. Valium. Disconnected telephones. In the fragment 'Swooning', a character called Lucy takes a forty-two-milligram dose of Trilafon and feels herself fainting: 'If only she could faint all the way, blackout, and never wake up again.' Elsewhere a character called Rachel is involuntarily institutionalised in a mental hospital and says she feels 'submerged, as if someone were holding her under water for months'. For Holly, sleeping all day and all night is a way to escape imprisonment until it became its own trap – 'she was in a permanent state of drowse' – while Bettina tries to overcome sleeplessness by lying 'still as a corpse'. In the passage Millett read from at her memorial service, Firestone writes of a character that: 'She could not read. She could not write . . . Nor could she hang out . . . she couldn't care about anything and love was forgotten . . . Her life was ruined and she had no salvage plan.'[24]

When characters in *Airless Spaces* return from hospital, they wrestle with everyday objects: cauliflowers that can't be cut, deodorants that can't be bought, clothes that no longer fit. Though the novel is written primarily in the third person, some of the characters seem to be versions of Firestone herself. The book begins in a hopeless register by recounting a dream of a sinking ship, a luxury cruise liner like the Titanic. Everyone on the ship will die but the dreamer stows herself away in a fridge 'hoping to live on even after the boat was fully submerged until it should be found'. Upon waking, she finds this hope for survival crushed when she reads of a real disaster in the Bermuda Triangle where no attempt will be made to recover the ship.[25] Living on isn't possible.

One of the book's shortest chapters describes a woman who receives a Reichian treatment for cancer which is effective, though she then realises that 'there was nothing, no one in her life for her to reach out towards'. The book closes with a fragment reflecting in the first person on the narrator's brother Danny, her almost-twin (they were only one year apart in age), who committed suicide in his early thirties by shooting himself in the head. She writes that she 'spent some years trying to find Danny in the spiritual realm, but . . . was told by more than one medium that his violent death had shattered his ethereal body so he couldn't be reached'.[26] There is nothing to be salvaged here, not even a fridge to hide in. The minimal hope offered by the dream cannot be sustained when confronted with reality. A cure for cancer cannot cure a lonely life. And not even a ghost can survive in a mutilated corpse. All that lies ahead are the characters' psychological shatterings. 'If only she could faint all the way, blackout, and never wake up again.'

The Loony Bin Trip, which is more explicitly autobiographical than *Airless Spaces*, describes Millett's experience of withdrawing from lithium. Soon after doing so she ends up being committed to an asylum in Ireland, which leads her to recall her previous experiences in a psychiatric institution in the US in 1973. Millett describes the repetitive and stultifying routines of institutional time in the psychiatric hospital:

> The blur of days in this place. I no longer know how many. Hours marked only by the tease of tablets, the cheat of the watered tea, the fat rubberoid slices of white bread . . . Years have passed already in preview. Always the same room, these chairs. The same women or replicas.

Even when she acts compliantly, she is never resigned to her situation but continues to dream of insurrection, 'of witches by the fire, uprisings, the whole gang of us building the fire high and higher and defying the doctors and nurses . . . the wretched of the earth in an incendiary fever'. Though much of *The Loony Bin Trip* is concerned with betrayal – at the hands of the various relatives, lovers and friends who contacted psychiatric institutions or professionals about Millett without her consent – it does not exclusively dwell there but also yields vivid descriptions of Millett's attempts to forge connections with others. Indeed, she even views the injustice of betrayal in collective rather than individual terms, seeing it as connected to 'every other quivering soul who ever saw these bastards coming'; in her experiences of psychiatric institutions the personal is explicitly framed as being political.[27] Her experience of being in hospital is not narrated as a time outside of history or the social; indeed, the experience itself is politicising, prompting her to challenge how people diagnosed with mental illnesses are treated under capitalism.

Millett describes her efforts to forge solidarity among the patients at the asylum, envisioning a collective resistance to the institution, which sought to keep them apart: 'United, we will refuse to cooperate at all. There will not be enough of them to control us even with their drugs.'[28] Similarly, although *Flying* recounts numerous arguments and antagonisms between Millett and other women in the women's liberation movement, she also describes how the surfacing of ambivalence among them, and the limits of liberation they crashed into, created a new kind of bond, which she describes as the 'solidarity of disappointment'.[29] For Millett, both the disintegration of the movement and her later psychiatric breakdown are accompanied by ongoing connections, discussions and contested political commitments, rather than by total isolation or withdrawal.

Millett ends *The Loony Bin Trip* back on lithium and back in New York, where her mania gives way to a depression which she finds harder to bear, even though society finds it easier to accommodate. A form of publicly unacceptable mania is replaced by a private 'craziness that reeks worse than old socks, more than a ten-day-old corpse'. Slow, sedated, lonely, 'submerged' but 'passably normal', Millett's constricted and defeated experience coincides with a breakup with her partner Sophie, the possible disappearance of her experiment in collective living at her farm (which she can no longer afford), and the loss of the dream of feminist collaboration that it represented: 'The vision failed.' She is left contemplating death with time stretching before her in a dirty apartment full of broken things and imagines herself passing years as a 'decrepit woman living alone on toast or canned soup or cocoa or whatever requires the least effort'.[30]

'During depression', she observes, 'the world disappears.'[31] In contrast to Cvetkovich's memoir, Millett captures something of the contradiction of a depression with political origins: her experience of the disappearance of the world is at least partly connected to the perceived failure of a particular political project and an experiment in collective living, but her symptoms include the vanishing of any meaningful connection between cause and effect, external events and internal feelings. Depression may have origins in her political disappointments, but Millett makes clear that a depressed person can be incapable of really feeling or acting on that awareness, even if they can articulate the intellectual claim that they are braided together. Breaking through the walls dividing the internal from the external, reaching out from the individual to the social, feels impossible.

In these pages Millett's descriptions of her mental state as a vacuum echo the hopeless fragments that comprise *Airless Spaces*, but ultimately she and Sophie find a way to stay together and she emerges from her depression. The book ends with her beginning to write the book. The act of writing, as in Cvetkovich's memoir, is presented as part of a gradual healing process, but for Millett it is not only an individual therapeutic exercise. She also reiterates her desire to connect with 'the multitude who like me have known the cruelty and irrationality of the system', calling for an end to forced hospitalisation and a more empathetic understanding of the experiential realities of 'madness'.[32] The healing she advocates here is an anti-adaptive healing that refuses adjustment to the existing state of things. The process is therefore not 'therapeutic' in the adaptive sense implied by Weeks, which would imply a disinterest in the structural causes of mental illness or in the political dimensions of mental health care diagnosis and provision. Indeed, Millett discusses her engagements with the mental patients' liberation movement that saw ex-patients organise against their oppression by the psychiatric establishment.[33] Her experiences of breakdown and depression form part of a renewed engagement in political activism and enable her to form new bonds of solidarity. Can any similar traces of hope or continued collective engagement be discerned in *Airless Spaces*?

Empty shelves

The final chapter of Firestone's *The Dialectic of Sex* is entitled 'Ultimate Revolution' and concludes bombastically, as if teetering on the edge of a precipice: 'We now have the knowledge to create a paradise on earth anew. The alternative is our own suicide through that knowledge, the creation of a hell on earth, followed by oblivion.' Firestone proposes that technological advancements could free women not only from socially reproductive labour but also from reproductive sex, gestation and the 'tyranny' of childbirth altogether. For Firestone, the distinction between the sexes may be natural, but nature, she contends, is not immutable: 'To grant that the sexual imbalance of power is biologically based is not to lose our case.'[34] Firestone places all her cyber eggs in the artificial uterus basket of future technological transformation, but, as Stella Sandford argues, her 'insistence on the overwhelmingly monolithic nature of natural sex oppression suggests that nothing had significantly changed from prehistory to the second half of the twentieth century'.[35] Despite the title of Firestone's book and her professed admiration for the dialectical method which allowed Marx and Engels to avoid a '"stagnant" metaphysical view',[36] for Firestone, the 'female *is* stagnant, mired in sex, and sex does not change or develop, at least until the revolutionary period'.[37] Women's liberation, in Firestone's view, remains contingent on technological revolution – nature could change and *become* historical, precipitating social transformation in turn, but history in that sense paradoxically lies only in the future. The stakes are perilously high and the only alternative Firestone imagines is catastrophic: suicide, hell on earth, oblivion.

Is *Airless Spaces* a document of the impossibility of living out the insights of *The Dialectic of Sex* in a still intolerable world? Can reading the two books together generate any illumination of the depressive by the political, or of the political by the depressive? Firestone's airless spaces are mostly rooms (both domestic and institutional); only occasionally are they streets, rarely cities, never worlds. Yet for all this there are specificities – textures, colours, feelings – that are absent from the pages of *The Dialectic of Sex*. And there are people too – individuals with proper names, particular t-shirts, fluctuating body temperatures. Weeks claims that genre distinguishes Firestone's two books from one another, arguing that the manifesto (*The Dialectic of Sex*) is oriented to the political, the collective and the militant, while the diary (*Airless Spaces*) is concerned with the personal, the therapeutic and the individual. The contrast might also be expressed as one between the abstract and the concrete, the future and the present, the ideal and the actual, or even in terms of incommensurable scales. *Airless Spaces* is certainly not militant and does not retain the explicit orientation to collective political action expressed in *The Loony Bin Trip*, but neither is it strictly therapeutic either. It is way too depressed for that.

The Dialectic of Sex is dedicated to Simone de Beauvoir, a feminist forebear, whereas *Airless Spaces* is dedicated to 'Lourdes Cintron – as promised in the hospital', expressing a bond of friendship, rather than an impersonal intellectual debt.[38] Firestone's characters remain isolated in their separate chapters, each cut off from the others, like patients enclosed within the curtains of their hospital beds, but some of the vignettes describe friendships developing on the wards and moments of solidarity between patients who save cigarettes or candy for one another and provide advice about navigating the hospital's systems. Instances of 'unaccustomed tenderness' occur between patients and their visitors, while a whole section is dedicated to 'Losers'. These 'losers' are old, poor, ill, marginalised, isolated and forlorn people adrift in a cruel world. They are mostly not productive on capitalism's terms and some have failed in their creative aspirations as writers or musicians, but Firestone's descriptions obliquely suggest that these lives need not be so difficult, and that they should not be treated as expendable. Marlene, friendless, widowed and poor, fractures her foot in a supermarket and wonders, 'What if it doesn't heal?'[39]

That no healing is possible in a damaged and damaging world is an implicit conclusion that *The Dialectic of Sex* and *Airless Spaces* share. In this respect, each is as uncompromising as the other. Many of the characters in the latter struggle with the bureaucracies and institutions of the present, and it is here that moments of resistance and refusal emerge: against the oppressive social world of cops, doctors, social workers, lawyers, immigration officials, health insurance policies, bosses, landlords. A punk patient rejects the hospital's pyjamas. The temporalities of depression, mania, insomnia and psychosis clash with the strict routines of the hospital ward and the demands of the society in which it is situated. The sense of dull antagonism between the external world and the individuals struggling to live in it also distinguishes *Airless Spaces* from Cvetkovich's memoir, where she is more insulated from broader economic forces than some of Firestone's characters (in that Cvetkovich seemed able to spend time depressed in bed without being evicted, fired or sent to hospital against her will). Though stifled, muffled, overcome with inertia, incapable of action, restrained by external forces, there is never an acceptance of the existing situation in *Airless Spaces,* nor a desire to function smoothly within it. It seems strange to describe as 'therapeutic' a book in which no one seems to get any better. Ultimately, for all its hopelessness, the book cannot be characterised as apolitical.

In the fragment 'Emotional Paralysis', Firestone writes of a character recently discharged from hospital who cannot shop: 'Her shelves were lined with missing objects she needed and had almost bought.'[40] These physical gaps are matched by unfilled hours in her time, which were once spent reading and writing. The mental health professionals with their 'self-esteem' classes think in terms of progress and describe a 'road to recovery' which links future health with reintegration into the normative rhythms and structures of society. Health would mean having full shelves and busy days. But the empty spaces on her shelves do not seem identical to the airless spaces elsewhere in the book. The missing objects evince the impossibility of action and stand as weird anti-monuments – void-like, invisible – to a 'healthy' existence that cannot be fulfilled, at least not within the frameworks of society as it is currently organised. There is air in the spaces if nothing else. Could they be filled with something else? Could the objects around the spaces be moved, removed, rearranged? Should the shelves be destroyed?

The Dialectic of Sex is euphoric, angry and visionary but so uncompromising it can seem stifling. By its standards, anything less than everything would be considered a failure leading to oblivion, whereas the friction generated by reading Firestone's two texts together opens a space of ambivalence and strained solidarity among the disappointed, similar to that expressed by Millett in *Flying*. Between the future-oriented politicised past and the intractability of the depressed present – between the social and the individual, between the totalising and the granular – something begins to stir. The seemingly incommensurable scales of the political and the depressive strain towards one another.

Emergency and inertia

1968: A Student Generation in Revolt, based on interviews with former activists in the US and Western Europe, surveys the student rebellions of that year from a distance of twenty years. The book's postscript on the 1970s sketches the aftermath: student movements collapse, new movements and political parties emerge, then wane. Trade unions are assaulted, militants incarcerated, radical groups infiltrated by cops. Some former student activists get involved in community organising or experiment with communal living, some throw themselves into emerging liberation movements, some attempt to get respectable professional jobs in the kinds of institutions they had previously attacked, while others turn to terror and violence. Amid this litany of consequences is a fleeting reflection on the emotional fallout from the crushing and crumbling of groups and movements post-'68: 'There were many instances of personal disillusionment, despair, breakdowns and even suicides among former student radicals.'[41] These subjective effects are reported in a cursory, matter-of-fact manner without pausing to convey their emotional weight.

Among the book's contributors was Luisa Passerini, whose *Autobiography of a Generation: Italy, 1968* refuses to skate over such phenomena so swiftly. Instead, her book grapples with the difficulties she experienced while conducting interviews for the oral history collection that would become *1968: A Student Generation in Revolt*, exploring how the process of talking to her peers about their relationship to their militant youths opened up a relationship to her own personal history. *Autobiography of a Generation* intersperses excerpts from oral history interviews conducted as part of the collaborative book project with autobiographical reflections on Passerini's own experiences of the sixties and seventies, alongside diary excerpts written during her psychoanalysis, which she undertook between 1984 and 1990.

Once she sits down at her desk to review the material she has gathered, Passerini deems her interview transcripts 'unusable' and she is convinced that the project is a failure. She is disappointed with the interviews and so too are her interviewees, who react with 'disappointment, irritation, rejection' upon reading them. The transcripts seem incapable of conveying the emotion of the original historical experience or of its oral retelling. She finds her interviewees' narratives simultaneously 'too full and too empty', and upon being interviewed by a researcher about her life similarly pronounces the story she produces to be 'too much and too little'. When visiting archives in Turin to research the university occupations, she encounters images of her interviewees as young, impassioned people, but she reflects on how remote and 'securely ensconced' the documents seem, lying quietly in their folders.[42] *Autobiography of a Generation* confronts these difficulties by departing from the conventions of social history to create a hybrid form appropriate to the intertwining of the personal and the political that characterised both the events of 1968 and the author's subjective relationship to them. By constantly switching scales from individual anguish to collective joy, from personal to historical, Passerini's collective autobiography preserves the distinct intensities associated with different experiences without suggesting they are therefore disconnected. The past shaped the present and revisiting history and memory can be transformative in its own right, like opening a window in an airless room.

The formal ambiguity of the book, which switches between genres and registers, responds to the frustrations Passerini encountered while attempting to write about the fraught entanglements and stark disjunctions between history, politics and subjectivity. Explorations of memories that surface in her analysis help to unlock her relation to her past and eventually enable her to write about the history of her generation, with whom she identifies without being identical. The title of the chapter 'Mirrors' metaphorically captures this sense of simultaneous affiliation and difference, of an experience both shared and divergent, as well as referring to the mirroring of the analytic encounter.[43] This is a narrative of individuals mourning the splintering of collectives and their failure to achieve their political goals, but it also reflects on rifts within those collectives and describes people, particularly women, who never felt they fully belonged to them in the first place.[44] Politicisation was both enlivening and disappointing.

Passerini resists any attempt to pull disparate threads into a neat account of 1968, nor does she reduce the collective to the individual or attempt to place history on the couch. The book shuttles between past and present, and it simultaneously shifts between scales, moving between personal memory and collective history. It is this latter aspect that interests me most. The individual does not remain unable to locate herself in relation to the social world (as in Cvetkovich's memoir), nor does the individual become a metaphor for society (as in Fisher's polemics). Instead, the book's montage-like form enables Passerini to explore the contradictory and conflicted ways she and her peers variously registered, reflected upon and repressed the shared loss of their past convictions in the present.[45] This is a history of subjectivity and intersubjectivity that constantly foregrounds the troubled relation between history and the subjects who were made – or were unmade – by it. She does not deny the incommensurability of different scales but foregrounds the problem of accessing the individual from the perspective of the historical and vice versa. By constantly shifting perspective and refusing to either dwell in the impasse or romanticise euphoria, the politicised and the depressive begin to seep into one another.

The contrast between the moods of the elated, politicised past and the depressed, isolated present is stark, paralleling the distinction Weeks identified between Firestone's two books and the two eras in which they were written. Gradually, however, the moods and the eras in Passerini's book begin to interpenetrate. Initially, the difficulty of gathering adequate testimonials is entangled with Passerini's feelings of depletion and isolation. She reflects on the 'dissipation – of resources and energy'. After conducting the first interviews, she is confronted with her own memories, which render her immobile and lead her to question her current romantic relationships and career: 'I lie defeated, under the weight of my own contradictions.' She describes her 'sense of loneliness, of having erred, lost, failed'.⁴⁶ She partly attributes these feelings to being single without having chosen it and expresses regret for having spent so much of her time prioritising political activities over others, but she does not identify a single definite cause of her current malaise. By remembering, repeating and working through in analysis and by assembling the collage of memories gathered from her peers, Passerini probes the relation of now to then. The boundary between the politicised and the depressive becomes porous.

The flatness and inertia evoked in her early diary entries stands in contrast to the dilation of time associated with the movements that erupted in 1968, during which 'the temporal dimension was expanded'. Her interviewees recount a temporal shift and a sense of euphoria that rushed through them when they were swept up in the movement: 'There was no room for the depressed in '68.'⁴⁷ The individual self melted into the collective: 'It was an all-encompassing universe in which the private and public got mixed up.'⁴⁸ Politics soaked into the fibres of the quotidian: 'The cause lay in the very form of the new politics, tied to the everyday, to subjectivity, less separated from life.' She describes people passing from 'tormented and depressed isolation to feeling themselves part of a whole, to communication and appropriation of new times and spaces'. She also describes their recollections of past exhilaration mingling with the torment that followed: 'Alternating with these lively tones are the sombre tones of mistakes made, the evocation of feelings of defeat long shunted aside by collective pride, the emptiness after comrades have scattered.'⁴⁹ The transformation of the individual psyche was central to the movement in which they were immersed, but the statement of there having been no room for the depressed is ambiguous, suggesting that depression was disavowed rather than absent. This hints that the images of pure elation, of pure politicisation, summoned up in retrospect, were always shadowed by more ambivalent feelings.

She likens her own experience of joining migrant workers' struggles at Fiat in the early 1970s to stepping into a 'swirling river', in which she shivered not from cold but from 'the emotion of seeing rules and social barriers, which seemed insurmountable, overcome'. The atmosphere of being submerged in struggle with others is described as exhilarating, exhausting, all-encompassing. She and her comrades lived urgently, in a 'permanent state of alarm'. The stultification she describes experiencing in the present is a slow, stuffy, curdled time devoid of certainties and lacking a clear purpose or shared goal, whereas the insurrectionary moment hurtled towards a cliff edge – cataclysmic, thrilling, breathless, apocalyptic:

I experienced a sense of the end of the world, a mental state of emergency, like an inner perception of an imminent end, with the urgency to act before it was too late. The rhythm of daily life accelerated in order to live up to the circumstances, absorbed in the approach of the eschaton, which might be a triumphant outcome or a catastrophic result. Time curled like a wave repelled by a dike, life was marked by continual deadlines; but what was supposed to fall due? The final hour, the encounter between our time and the time of the definitive uprising of the downtrodden masses.

The memory of mental emergency clashes up against the present time of defeat when no definitive uprising seems imminent. But as with the oblivion Firestone invokes in *The Dialectic of Sex*, the sense of emergency Passerini recalls was perilous.

Moving back and forth between the past of lively collectivity and the present of lonely defeat prises open a space for reflection that lightens the heavy weight of loss: 'One also glimpses, next to the tones of mourning, of bewilderment, of uncertainty, those of the reunification between living and narrating with the necessary detachment that allows for self-representation without shirking the painful and unresolved points.' Like Millett in *Flying*, though Passerini describes social rifts and broken friendships emerging from political movements, 'leaving remnants of bitterness and things unsaid', she also reflects on the many significant friendships that long outlived the movements in which they were forged.[50] The solidarity of disappointment may not be a straight-forwardly joyful bond but it provides an alternative to atomisation. Working through personal difficulties with others can provide mutual support in the present and form the ground for future action.

The confrontation Passerini describes between two moments in time – and between their associated experiences of temporality – injects some of the urgency of the past into the inertia of the present, while intervening experiences serve to slacken the perilous sense of emergency to stave off apocalypticism. The political shakes up the depressive without fully negating it. The process of going back through history, of going back through Passerini's own memories and those of her peers, eventually precipitates a shift in consciousness. Oscillating between times and, more significantly, between scales, precludes this collective autobiography from being either an account of individual depression in the present or a lament for a collective history. Rather the spark generated through the encounter unseals the future: 'It is this very alternation that I now think can be considered as a contribution to the history of subjectivity and indeed the history of intersubjectivity.'[51]

Throughout her diary entries, Passerini recounts dreams. Initially these are dominated by bleak images characterised by obstruction. She dreams of 'a gray, turbulent sea'.[52] She dreams of murky waters. She dreams of cockroaches. She dreams of being stuck on a rock and unable to climb away. Sometimes she finds it difficult to sleep at all. But towards the end of the diary the tone of the dreams shift. She dreams of reaching the end of a path at night where she sees fog lift before her. She dreams of mailboxes made of crystal. She dreams of an old man showing her the map of an island. She dreams of huge heaps of snow melting. These more hopeful dreams follow the slow and painful process of working through the past both in psychoanalysis and through writing the history of her generation, which she describes as a generative depression: 'Loss, depression, collapse . . . I begin to understand that depression is necessary in order to get to the bottom and fish something out, something at times too heavy. And it's very different from torment.' Towards the end of her diary she talks with a friend and reflects on the psychological transformation she has undergone. She does not claim that this shift is political in its own right, but hopes it could help make political change in the future possible because it has made her feel capable of action again: 'Even the journey from the external to the internal, if you break the scheme dividing and hierarchizing them, can find roads for changing the world and reducing injustice.'[53]

Suffering from delay

As the deaths of Fisher and Firestone attest, not everyone emerges from depression in the manner of Cvetkovich, Millett or Passerini. During the process of conducting her oral history interviews, Passerini describes gathering life histories in Naples that seemed haunted by 'the presence of those more defeated than we, who can't talk about '68 because they're strung out on drugs, emarginated [sic], lost'.[54] Kristin Ross's *May '68 and its Afterlives* concludes by dwelling on similarly ghostly and anonymous figures, figures who haunt the official narratives of May '68, which are dominated by those who were more easily accommodated by – or who actively participated in creating – the 'new spirit of capitalism' that emerged the wake of '68.

Ross cites a scene from a novel by Jean-François Vilar: in a photograph of students outside the occupied Sorbonne in May '68 stand two figures who recently married – a man called Marc and a woman called Jeanne. While Marc is easily identifiable in the middle, Jeanne stands to the side, 'hard to make out' and unnamed in the photo's caption, her face partly obscured by her hand which is holding a cigarette.[55] Marc went on to become a 'professional revolutionary' in the 1970s and later the editor of a major newspaper (the character and his trajectory from militant *gauchiste* to powerful and respectable professional, Ross explains, are based on real-life *Libération* editor Serge July). Marc's post-'68 experience not only conforms to the 'collectivity to individualism / revolution to reform' meta-narrative sketched in this chapter – he was also instrumental in creating it. Ross is more interested in the figure of Jeanne, once in the midst of the movement, but now forgotten and excluded from its official history. Ross cites Vilar's description of Jeanne's post-'68 experience:

> As a result of the crises, the suicide attempts, the running away, the encroaching gesticulations, the fastidious depressions, a habituée of all the psychiatric couches and all the cures, she was committed [to a psychiatric institution] . . . Jeanne was doing badly, like everyone. She used to say, laughing, 'I suffer from communism's delay.'[56]

The novel's narrator calls Marc to inquire about Jeanne and is told that she committed suicide. For Ross,

> She represents the anonymous militants of May and those lost in May's aftermath: the suicides, depressions, and despairs of those who became derailed, horrorstricken or dumbfounded by the reversals and recuperations that transpired after May – those who didn't embrace the forward march of modernity, those who were inexorably caught between trying to make something continue that had lost its momentum and trying to reintegrate back into a society they had so forcibly rejected and tried to bring down.[57]

Figures like Marc may have come to exemplify the movement, but they do so at the expense of figures like Jeanne, whose histories have been steamrollered into oblivion by the master narrative. Ross insists that Jeanne's suicide and the breakdowns and depressions of many others were not due to 'psychological fragility', but to an unwillingness or incapacity to synchronise with the victors. Not everyone embraced or was embraced by capitalism's new spirit. The chapters in the next section of this book take suffering from the delay of a transformed world, the problem of trying to survive in the present while trying to transform it, as their subject.

PART II

Survival Pending Revolution: Patient Urgency

4

Burnout

> *The very existence of the clinic is political.*[1]
> – Volunteer, People's Free Medical Clinic

'Burnout' has become ubiquitous as a term to describe the exhaustion that comes from working too hard in a cutthroat capitalist world. I hesitated to give this book the title *Burnout* for that reason, but I had first encountered the word in activist contexts and continue to think that the colloquial way it is often used by activists captures something specific about an experience that results from prolonged engagement in political groups or movements. Though widely recognised and pervasive, the phenomenon is rarely placed centre stage. When people say they are 'burnt out' from excessive organising, do they mean that they are physically exhausted or does the term also convey something emotional? Does burnout in these contexts have any connection to the content or trajectory of political projects, so that it could be understood as a symptom of a broader political malaise? Or is political burnout a form of depletion identical to those arising from other kinds of tiring activity?

I also hesitated to use the word 'burnout' as a title because my intention was to emphasise the historical specificity of particular concepts for describing psychic life, rather than implying some transhistorical understanding of subjectivity. Examining the historical emergence of the concept of burnout helps to shed light on the simultaneously physiological and psychological valances of the term. Excavating the particular meaning given to burnout when it was first identified by the psychologist and psychoanalyst Herbert J. Freudenberger and tracing how that meaning morphed over time will in turn help to illuminate the distinction between forms of mental suffering that arise from living in the given structures and systems of the world and those that arise from fighting against those structures and systems, a distinction that is key to all the chapters in this section.

Neoliberal burnout

Imogen Daal's *Burnout Survival Kit* – to pick one example at random from the many recent self-help books on the topic – proclaims on its cover that it 'provides instant relief from modern work'.[2] The author describes switching from a career in advertising to one in screenwriting and recalls developing symptoms such as chest pain as her work began to overwhelm her. Sprinkled with jaunty drawings and inspirational quotations from authors including Gandhi, Maya Angelou and Ursula K. Le Guin, the book offers practical solutions to dealing with the toll of taking on too much as a busy and ambitious white-collar worker: breathe deeply, get more sleep, drink water, go outside, smell something nice, wash, cry, watch TV, say no, do yoga, stop looking at your phone, lower your expectations, write a list, make a cup of tea, eat some chocolate, get an accountant. The closing image depicts a cartoon woman relaxing in a bubble bath. The symptoms of burnout are presented as arising from particular kinds of time-consuming but potentially lucrative non-manual work. Self-care is the cure.

In *Can't Even: How Millennials Became the Burnout Generation*, a book that builds on a viral *Buzzfeed* article published in 2019, Anne Helen Petersen describes how her exhaustion from overwork as a journalist manifested in 'errand paralysis', an incapacity to do small daily chores like going to the post office. She argues that burnout is pervasive among millennials (people born between 1981 and 1996), which she attributes to increasingly precarious working conditions in the aftermath of the 2008 financial crisis. Burnout, she claims, is 'our contemporary condition'.[3] Her emphasis is on workplace exhaustion, which she sees operating across class divides. People juggling retail work with gig economy work experience burnout, as do startup workers, academic adjuncts and freelance graphic designers. According to the World Health Organisation (WHO), burnout is a syndrome resulting from workplace stress; they specify that it does not apply to other kinds of exhaustion.[4]

Accounts of burnout by contemporary philosophers do not offer wildly different perspectives on the condition. For Pascale Chabot, burnout 'is a disease of civilization' produced by the 'unsustainable values' of capitalism, while for Byung-Chul Han a 'burnout society', the successor to the disciplinary society identified by Michel Foucault, is one in which discipline has been replaced by achievement.⁵ In a burnout society everyone is compelled to take an entrepreneurial approach to their own lives. In Petersen's model, neoliberalism produces burnout among bosses and workers alike, whereas in the burnt-out world of 'office towers, banks, airports, shopping malls, and genetic laboratories' described by Han, capitalism persists but class divisions seem to have been internalised; the 'achievement subject' is compelled by an internal rather than external force.⁶ Exploitation is replaced by self-exploitation.

Petersen explains that the term 'burnout' was first introduced by Herbert J. Freudenberger in 1974 to describe 'cases of physical or mental collapse as the result of overwork'.⁷ Sarah Jaffe, in a review of Petersen's book, notes that the concept 'emerged around the same time as neoliberalism', positioning it as a diagnosis symptomatic of shifts in wage labour.⁸ But the origins of the concept are more in tune with the themes of this book than these accounts imply.

Freudenberger escaped Nazi Germany at the age of twelve and settled in New York, completing a doctorate at NYU. He trained at the National Psychological Association for Psychoanalysis (NPAP) and in 1962 completed his training analysis with Theodor Reik who had trained with Freud in Vienna. He worked as a training analyst at the NPAP from 1970 until his death in 1999. In an essay from 1989, Freudenberger looks back on years spent analysing manifestations of burnout among different workers, primarily though not exclusively in the 'helping professions' – social workers, teachers, nurses, librarians, vets, pharmacists, air traffic controllers, psychotherapists. He also discusses working with corporate clients to advise them on how their workplaces might better address 'stress management' and praises businesses for embracing 'philosophies of wellness'. He defines the burnt-out person as an 'impaired professional', but cautions: 'We need to be careful that we do not place so many concepts under burnout that [the term] becomes meaningless.'⁹

Freudenberger's initial publications on burnout in the 1970s did not focus on waged workers, however, let alone on those working in corporate boardrooms. They drew instead on his experience as a volunteer in the free clinic movement. Burnout originated as a term to describe people exhausted from helping others 'in free clinics, therapeutic communities, hot lines, crisis intervention centers, women's clinics, gay centers, runaway houses'.¹⁰ It was explicitly addressed to the phenomenon of fatigue and encroaching cynicism among people who devoted their spare time to projects that sought to transform society. Freudenberger worked in private practice with wealthy clients in uptown Manhattan by day, then would travel downtown to work as a volunteer at a free clinic in the East Village in the evening, until eventually he was forced to take a six-month break, 'burnt out' from devoting his time to providing care to marginalised people.

Burnout, a term he borrowed from hippie drug-users he encountered through his voluntary work, was not seen to result from overwork in general, but from feelings of guilt and disappointment specific to working as part of a project with broader social justice aims. Burnout in Freudenberger's articles from this period is not just defined in terms of physical tiredness as a result of doing too many things; rather, it emerges from emotional investment in a cause and from the disappointments that arise when flaws in a political project become apparent. Freudenberger's concept not only describes physical exhaustion but also acknowledges the need to deal with anger caused by grief brought about by the 'loss of an ideal'.[11] Burnout in the context of social justice projects thus often involves a process of mourning, according to Freudenberger. Returning to his earliest writings on burnout makes clear that when understood as a malaise arising from politically committed activities, burnout cannot be equated with tiredness or stress.

Militant compassion

The free clinic movement was a grassroots initiative that began in San Francisco in 1967, in an attempt to provide free, non-judgmental health care to people in the local community. By the 1970s there were over 300 free clinics across the US.[12] Freudenberger had spent a summer volunteering at the original free clinic in Haight-Ashbury, which was set up in 1967 to help people experiencing bad LSD trips. David E. Smith, who founded the clinic after witnessing drug addicts and hippies being denied medical care in conventional institutions, situated its emergence in the context of the social movements of the 1960s and the California counterculture. Looking back on the development of the free clinic movement in 1976, Smith summarised:

> The free clinic has evolved as a symbol for nonjudgmental, humanistic health care delivery to alienated populations in the United States including hippies, commune dwellers, drug abusers, third world minorities, and other 'outsiders' who have been rejected by the more dominant culture.[13]

Often set up in former shop fronts, free clinics opened across the US in the late sixties. They aimed to serve local communities or specific minority groups and tended to be democratically and non-hierarchically run. Their emphasis on offering services to drug users meant that they were often targets of police raids, especially in the early years of the movement. Vietnam veterans with medical training were prominent among volunteers, and some clinics became sites where conscientious objectors could volunteer to avoid the draft. Historian of the movement Gregory L. Weiss describes the free clinics as 'militantly compassionate', a phrase that sounds like an oxymoron but captures the paradoxical qualities of anti-adaptive healing.[14] Though part of a politically heterogeneous movement, the clinics combined a commitment to radical social change with a valorisation of care, placing issues of sickness and health at the heart of the era's liberation struggles, while fundamentally problematising how those terms should be defined and where their origins should be located. The free clinics provided health care that offered an alternative to mainstream, profit-driven and exclusionary medical institutions. They were also prefigurative, offering glimpses of a radically different future society organised in a way that placed people before profit.

After returning to the East Coast, Freudenberger became director of psychological services at the St Mark's free clinic in the East Village, which opened in early 1970 and offered treatment to drug users, as well as STI treatments and mental health services in the evenings.[15] Volunteers dressed no differently from patients to reflect their non-hierarchical approach and suspicion of medical expertise. Freudenberger described the waiting room as a relaxed space in which music played, community notices were hung, and people could gather: 'We try to create an all-important atmosphere of ease and acceptance.'[16] In a 1973 essay discussing the role of a psychologist in a free clinic, Freudenberger stresses the importance of connecting health care to broader social issues in the community, such as housing shortages, declaring: 'We need to see the free clinic as a possible center for social activism.'[17] Freudenberger clearly defines the free clinic in opposition to mainstream medical practices and institutions, describing it as 'an alternative model for bringing health care, as well as political change within a community'.[18]

The needs of people who came to the clinic for treatment demanded that volunteer psychologists deviate from conventional diagnoses and therapeutic methods: 'Categories will become useless and meaningless.'[19] The clinic's purpose was to heal, but healing was defined as an anti-adaptive process that could proceed without conventional definitions of health or sanity, without, that is, demanding that people seeking treatment conform to prevailing social or cultural norms. For example, Freudenberger describes the case of a Cuban man who came to the clinic seeking help with hallucinations that had a religious content. Ignorant of Cuban culture and unable to interpret the symptoms' meaning through conventional one-on-one therapy, Freudenberger suggested that the man join a rap group of Spanish speakers at the clinic, who were better placed to discuss and make sense of the man's experiences. The man eventually made friends through the group, including someone who accompanied him home to help him sleep. In this case, non-expert collective support was of more therapeutic value than contact with a professionally trained clinician. Free clinics not only theorised an anti-adaptive model of health care and elaborated a socially grounded understanding of the origins of mental distress, but they also sought to put that understanding into practice.

While in 1974 Freudenberger claimed that those most at risk of burning out were 'the dedicated and the committed', by 1989 he linked burnout to 'the externally imposed societal values of achievement, acquisitions of goods, power, monetary compensation and competition'.[20] Burnout shifted its meaning: from a symptom experienced by people struggling to change society to one experienced by people trying too hard to succeed within it. Historian Matthew J. Hoffarth traces this trajectory. He also discusses the role of Christina Maslach in popularising the term 'burnout' and expanding its definition. Maslach conducted research with mental health workers and other 'helping' professionals in the 1970s, partly in response to the cruel behaviour she witnessed during her experience working on the Stanford Prison Experiment in 1971. Her emphasis, according to Hoffarth, was on encouraging individual workers in 'helping' roles to guard against their emotionally demanding clients, ultimately reinforcing the 'notion that self-interestedness was not only suitable, but perhaps an even more effective way of helping others than engaging in more demanding forms of social change'.[21]

Freudenberger, who Hoffarth points out similarly complained of clients who '"continually take, suck, demand"', also began to argue that 'self-awareness' and 'self-protection' were needed to ameliorate burnout.[22] The non-hierarchical understanding of care discussed in Freudenberger's earlier idealistic works on free clinics was displaced by a more suspicious relationship between givers and receivers of care that reasserted the importance of expertise and accepted the relationship's asymmetry. This shift in the understanding of both the causes and cures of burnout follows Freudenberger's professional trajectory from politically engaged free clinic volunteer to corporate consultant, which also fits neatly into a familiar historical narrative of recuperation (a meta-narrative glossed in the previous chapter), that saw radical initiatives set up in the late sixties gradually become part of the establishment they had originally sought to challenge. As Hoffarth argues, the biography of burnout as a concept conforms with Christopher Lasch's analysis in *The Culture of Narcissism* (1979). Indeed, despite his involvement in the free clinics, in the same period Freudenberger was already making arguments that questioned youthful revolt's political content, interpreting student militancy as a reaction to a lack of paternal authority rather than as a response to broader material conditions.

Absent fathers

In addition to his publications on burnout, in the late 1960s and early 1970s Freudenberger also published articles advancing general arguments about young people in the US at a historical moment characterised by youth revolt. He identified a form of '*dis*relation' within families in the US, claiming that despite living in close proximity to their teenage children, parents were unable to understand or emotionally support them. Young people, he argued, felt lost and sought to 'fill up the empty spaces within themselves'.[23] To address the hollowness at the heart of their lives, they let themselves be drawn into close relationships with their peers and turned to drugs, sex and political militancy. In his own therapeutic encounters with young people, he said, he abandoned the psychoanalyst's clinical neutrality in favour of more informal forms of support, as well as offering his patients a model of 'rational authority' that he believed their families had failed to provide. He gave reproachful advice on drug-taking and sex, for instance – he did not look favourably on LSD or 'promiscuity' – and discussed political issues such as the American war in Vietnam and the student rebellions at Columbia University. The radical arguments evident in his writings on free clinics from this period that eschew hierarchy and question his role as a psychiatric 'expert' sit uneasily alongside the more conservative assumptions underpinning his contemporaneous texts about the psychic lives of adolescents.

His 1970 essay 'The Case of Missing Male Authority' bemoans the absence of fathers as authority figures, claiming that, unlike in the past, fathers now worked in places removed from the home and were thus not around to instil a sense of reality in their children. These passages echo concerns about distant, absent or 'invisible' fathers articulated by various psychoanalytic and sociological thinkers (including Erik Erikson, Erich Fromm, Kenneth Keniston, Herbert Marcuse, Alexander Mitscherlich and David Riesman) in the fifties and sixties.[24] Mothers, according to Freudenberger, had taken the place of fathers in the family and hence felt resentful about taking on disciplinary responsibilities, leading them to become more intolerant of their children. Nestled within the paper's hand-wringing about the absence of paternal authority, however, is a vignette of a group therapy session in which Freudenberger's patients challenged him about his positions and refused to trace the political commitments of radical young people back to their family relationships.

In the fraught therapy session described by Freudenberger, a patient turned up 'upset and angry'; he was on bail after having been arrested during a university protest earlier in the day. The man attacked others in the group for failing to attend the protests, leading to heated arguments that threatened to erupt into physical violence. Freudenberger intervened to point out to the man that his violent outbursts could have negative consequences for his life. The man's furore, Freudenberger suggests, arose from his attitude to authority, of which his recent arrest was another example. Freudenberger's interpretation of the situation was met with protest by the group: 'I was accused of being a dictator, of not permitting the patient freedom of expression, of feeling threatened by his strength of conviction, and of being, among other things, "an archconservative representative of the middle class."'[25] The contestation indicates that some of the people present recognised a personal need to pursue therapy but nonetheless refused to accept that political commitments and actions could be addressed solely in a therapeutic context. Freudenberger responded to this mini-coup by doubling down. He claimed that the patient's insistence on 'the rightness of his behavior and position' was a form of self-destructive denial. He then describes how he took on the role of an authoritative father figure within the room; a role, he tells the reader, that the patient's actual father could not perform. Freudenberger thus reduced the patient's concern for unjust social conditions to an unresolved internal conflict grounded in his relationship to his father.

The article concludes by speculating that 'juvenile delinquency, street gangs, drop-outs, and the hippie phenomenon' might all be explained in similar terms: 'As a young man's venting his anger on society because the reality-and-value giving man had not been available to him in childhood.'[26] Although he describes the patient as ultimately amenable to his interpretation, the uproar in the group demonstrates how contentious Freudenberger's interpretation was. It is instructive to compare Freudenberger's views to those of psychoanalyst Robert Liebert in his contemporaneous analysis of youthful militancy in New York City, *Radical and Militant Youth: A Psychoanalytic Inquiry*, a study more in tune with the rebels in Freudenberger's therapy group than with Freudenberger himself. Assessing a series of interviews with student radicals in the immediate aftermath of the occupations at Columbia University in 1968, Liebert explicitly rejects the arguments about paternal figures advanced by Freudenberger and other psychoanalysts, asserting instead the rationality of the students' convictions. The book concludes by appealing to psychoanalysts to embrace demands for social transformation so they can help 'conflicted people of all generations' achieve their political goals.[27]

Freudenberger's early writings on the free clinics, by focusing on the effects rather than the causes of political engagement, did not interpret volunteers' commitments in terms of their family issues; he suggested rather that their commitments could have psychologically damaging *consequences*. Would it be possible to retain this aspect of Freudenberger's early writings and combine it with an understanding of political motivations that acknowledged their grounding in material conditions? Indeed, although the free clinics may have caused burnout, their history also – ironically, given some of Freudenberger's own arguments and his subsequent career trajectory – provides one possible answer to this question.

Small flames in the darkness

In her review of Helen Petersen's book on workplace burnout, Sarah Jaffe acknowledges that 'movement burnout is real', but she suggests that collective action can be an antidote to the grinding burnout of living under capitalism. She also invokes the 'structures of community care' – what M. E. O'Brien has called 'insurgent social reproduction' – that were built up by activists in Ferguson in 2014 and the spontaneous forms of mutual aid enacted by protestors on the streets during the Black Lives Matter uprisings in 2020.[28] Freudenberger's original definition of burnout, by contrast, implied that these very activities – aid, care – could be the sources of burnout rather than its antidote. Despite Freudenberger's emphasis on challenging hierarchies and medical expertise, he nonetheless conceptualised the free clinic as relying on a sharp distinction between givers and receivers of care, which segued neatly into something closer to a charitable or welfare model of service provision. Jaffe highlights a reciprocal model of care, a model which, against some of Freudenberger's own arguments, can be identified as having operated in the free clinics movement.

In an essay situating the origins of burnout in the specific urban environment of the East Village, Bench Ansfield cites a metaphor from the opening pages of Freudenberger's *Burn-Out: How to Beat the High Cost of Success*:

> If you have ever seen a building that has been burned out . . . you know it's a sight. What had once been a throbbing, vital structure is now deserted. Where there had once been activity, there are now only crumbling reminders of energy and life.

This analogy, Ansfield points out, had relevance to the neighbourhood where Freudenberger volunteered, a neighbourhood where arson was commonplace and was generally committed – at the behest of landlords – in the hours Freudenberger would have been leaving the clinic for his home uptown. Freudenberger's analogy, in Ansfield's reading, is telling because just as burnt-out buildings in the East Village 'generated value by being destroyed', 'Freudenberger's burnout likewise telegraphed how depletion, even to the point of destruction, could be profitable.' The gentrification of the city was mirrored, according to Ansfield, in the 'displacement of tenants from the ranks of those eligible for the diagnosis' as Freudenberger shifted from free clinic volunteer to corporate consultant.[29]

In their discussion of the emergence of free clinics in LA, Mike Davis and Jon Wiener make an argument that suggests an alternative, less despairing possibility for narrating the history and possible futures of burnout. Funded by the Monterey Pop Festival, the second free clinic in the US opened in LA in 1967. Like the original clinic in San Francisco, it focused on drug treatments and sexual health services, mostly serving a young white clientele of dropout drop-ins. Subsequent initiatives broadened the kinds of services offered and more clinics were established, including the Brown Berets' El Barrio Free Clinic (originally called the East LA Clinic), the Long Beach Free Clinic and the Alprentice 'Bunchy' Carter Free Clinic down the street from the Black Panther Party's headquarters. Eventually there was a council of free clinics across

Southern California. The Saban Community Clinic, which continues to provide community health care today, seeing up to 100,000 patients a year, traces its origins back to the free clinic movement, which Davis and Wiener frame as a concrete, positive legacy of the movements of the sixties.[30]

The Black Panther Party's survival programmes and free health clinics were set up in the context of the broader radical health movement at a moment when the US health-care system was in crisis.[31] The party's clinics, as Alondra Nelson has shown, operated as a significant part of a heterogeneous 'decentralized aggregate of groups, collectives, and organizations with distinct missions that sought to transform medicine, institutionally and interpersonally'. Inspired by the role health workers played in struggles in what was then referred to as the 'Third World' and by the medical writings of Che Guevara and Frantz Fanon, the Panthers' clinics held to a totalising, holistic understanding of 'health' that connected individuals' well-being to their social environments. The forms of care, services, advice and education offered by the clinics were also prefigurative: 'Activists enacted the better world they imagined.'[32]

Freudenberger left the free clinic at St Marks behind to embrace a more adaptive understanding of healing, and many of the communities the clinic served have since been displaced from the neighbourhood, but the St Marks Clinic continued. A lesbian group called the Women's Health Collective took over the St Marks Clinic in the late 1970s. In 1983, in response to the AIDS crisis, the St Marks Clinic merged with the Gay Men's Health Project Clinic, which had been set up in 1972 to offer therapeutic support to gay men and lesbians, to form the Community Health Project, which was later renamed the Callen-Lorde Community Health Center.[33] As Katie Batza traces in her history of gay community clinics in Boston, Chicago and LA, gay health activists were inspired to set up clinics in the late 1960s and early 1970s by the Black Panther Party and the women's movement. They coined the term 'oppression sickness' to articulate the social origins of their illnesses. Gay community clinics were then the 'first responders' to the AIDS crisis, offering care and advice in a non-judgmental environment that mainstream medical institutions were failing to provide.[34] Artist Gregg Bordowitz recalled going to the Community Health Project for an examination and advice in 1986, where he felt he could talk freely and ask questions about HIV that were impossible to pose elsewhere: 'That was a very profound experience for me and it changed a lot of things.'[35]

The history of the St Marks Clinic acts as a reminder that the politically committed targets of Freudenberger's theory are not just historical relics of a more politicised time which burnt out. However marginal and small-scale, they have continued to exist even if the causes to which they were dedicated have shifted. Spaces set up to provide health care outside of mainstream medical facilities do not just address gaps in existing provisions; they can also challenge the damaging ideological underpinnings of mainstream medicine (even if the histories of these clinics also necessitate contending with debates about the problems associated with civil society providing services in lieu of the state, as well as the contradictions associated with working within and against the state).[36]

The role played by already established clinics in responding to the AIDS crisis, as well as the survival of some institutions that originated as free clinics into the present, demonstrates that it is possible – and necessary – to sustain projects over long periods despite the toll it takes on the often overworked and un(der)paid people involved. If looking after other people or giving up time to help others can be draining, the solution is surely *more* care and *more* reciprocity, rather than less. The holistic understanding of health proposed by many active in the heterogeneous free clinics movement already implied an understanding of well-being that would include mental health and extend to givers of care (or refuse to distinguish neatly between givers and receivers of care at all).

Webs of care

The Black Panther Party had a holistic approach to health, foregrounding the health needs of party activists and the communities they served: 'Your body belongs to the revolution, so you have to take care of it.'[37] However, mental health care and therapeutic provision were not major components of the Black Panther Party's clinics, which is perhaps unsurprising, given the racist, carceral and pathologising tendencies of mainstream psychiatric institutions in the period and the widespread notion on the left that psychic problems could best be mitigated by solving social ones.[38] Terry Kupers, a contributor to the journal *Radical Therapist* who worked as a physician for the Alprentice 'Bunchy' Carter Black Panther Party free health clinic in LA, for instance, argued against 'practicing analysis in a ghetto'. He instead made a case in favour of challenging the theoretical bases of existing therapeutic models altogether, which, he said, encouraged people to adjust to rather than challenge existing social norms.[39] This was in line with rejections of psychiatry prevalent in liberation movements in the US at that time, as was the party's involvement in campaigns against scientific institutions that biologised violence in racially essentialising terms.[40] Yet as with the later trajectory of the St Marks Clinic, it is also possible to find subsequent examples of initiatives aimed at providing support to people experiencing both physical and mental distress with an explicitly anti-adaptive understanding of what psychic as well as physical healing might entail.

Former deputy of security for the New Orleans chapter of the Black Panther Party Malik Rahim later co-founded Common Ground Health Clinic in the city in the wake of Hurricane Katrina in 2005, a crisis that brought sharply into focus the deleterious health impact of what Ruth Wilson Gilmore calls 'organized state abandonment'.[41] Alongside offering first aid, taking people's blood pressure and testing for diabetes, Common Ground medics in the immediate aftermath of the disaster also investigated symptoms of depression and anxiety, defining themselves as motivated to offer 'solidarity, not charity'.[42] Responding in turn to the stresses and strains experienced by people involved in the response to that natural disaster, as well as addressing intergenerational and collective forms of trauma, healers with experience working in social justice contexts founded the Kindred Southern Healing Justice Collective. The collective's aim was to address

> the increased state of burnout and depression in our movements, systematic loss of our communities healing traditions, the isolation and stigmatization of healers, and the increased privatization of our land, medicine and natural resources that has caused us to rely on state or private models we do not trust and that do not serve us.[43]

Disability justice activist and writer Leah Lakshmi Piepzna-Samarasinha discusses the collective's work in their description of 'care webs' as an alternative to mainstream understandings of care provision, citing the collective's founder Cara Page as an inspiration for their realisation that 'movements themselves could and should be spaces of healing, that care didn't have to be a sideline to "the real work" but could *be* the work'.[44]

This conception of care as mutual and embedded in movements also chimes with that in Cassie Thornton's account of the Social Solidarity Health Centre in Thessaloniki, Greece. The centre was set up during the anti-austerity uprisings in 2010–11 when the public health-care system was dismantled, leaving 3 million people uninsured. As in the earlier free clinic movement in the US, expertise was questioned and 'health' was situated in relation to a person's broader living and working situation. Like the clinics set up in the aftermath of Hurricane Katrina, the solidarity clinics in Greece provided 'mutual aid in crisis', acknowledging the psychological strains that can come from caring for others by instigating a model of 'networked reciprocation' that recognised that carers also needed to be cared for.[45] These models of networked care come closer to providing an antidote to burnout than anything else I have come across – short of social transformation, and there's the rub.[46] Ameliorating burnout might rely on small-scale initiatives in the short-term, but as a means rather than an end. Rather than repeating that the only solution would involve a total social transformation, an instructive concrete example, developed within rather than against the state, could be the Cuban health-care system with its emphasis on community polyclinics and international medical solidarity (a solidarity that was refused by the US after Hurricane Katrina).[47]

Freudenberger's early work on burnout explored how initiatives created to ameliorate suffering as part of a broader social justice project could wear people out. In his identification of burnout among free clinic volunteers, he failed to make the leap to reciprocity and mutuality made by organisations like the Kindred Collective and the Social Solidarity Health Centre in Thessaloniki. Yet for all that these later initiatives articulate the value of embedding forms of healing in social movements, and for all that they recognise the support and respite needed by those who dedicate time and energy to helping others, only so much can be done in the absence of a society in which people's needs are adequately met. The next two chapters are animated by the compromises and contradictions that characterise acting in the present to achieve political goals that can only be fully realised in the future.

5

Exhaustion

'Come Unto Me All Ye That Labor and Are Heavy-Laden, And I Will Give You Rest' was written in an arc above the entrance to the church. These words touched Kopenkin, although he also remembered whose slogan it was. 'But where is my rest?', he thought, glimpsing the exhaustion in his own heart.[1]

– Andrei Platonov

For as long as I can remember, an advert has been displayed on tube platforms across London depicting a yawning woman under the slogan, 'Tired of being tired?' The product she advertises is a liquid iron supplement that promises to alleviate fatigue. Targeting commuters, the assumption seems to be that workers are exhausted and herbal extracts might help to perk them up. But the fact that the same advert has existed for so long indicates this commodity is not really a sufficient solution to the pervasive tiredness produced by contemporary working conditions. Can yawning workers of the world unite or are they simply too worn out?

Exhaustion, like burnout, is often framed as a symptom of capitalist modernity. On an overheating planet with dwindling natural resources, bodies and minds are subjected to and depleted by the ever-increasing demands of ever more precarious work. So much to do, so little time. Profits accumulate at the expense of exploited workers. New technologies and new forms of media sap attention and diminish the capacity to concentrate. Pressures build. Deadlines loom. Leisure time diminishes. Cities never sleep. Keep up or get left behind. This familiar narrative is told and retold across self-help books, newspaper articles and highfalutin philosophical tomes, but I want to explore something different: the exhaustion that comes from fighting against exhaustion's causes. Living under capitalism is certainly tiring, particularly for those who work hardest for the least reward, but struggling to overthrow the current economic system while meeting its ongoing demands can produce its own forms of exhaustion.

Militant activity can be energising, not only enervating – at least these exertions hold out the promise of a society in which rest, leisure and a good night's sleep could be available to all. In his analysis of class consciousness in the context of the July Revolution of 1830, *Proletarian Nights*, first published in French in 1981, Jacques Rancière discusses French workers who forsook sleep to dedicate themselves to their own poetic, intellectual or revolutionary pursuits by candlelight, gaining knowledge of the world and themselves in the process. In defiance of the bosses who controlled their time and stole their days, they re-appropriated the night to expend their energies in a manner of their own choosing. Yet in spite of all that their nocturnal pursuits opened up, these double lives took their toll. Not everyone survived.[2] The exhaustion caused by proletarian days is straightforward, but the political exhaustion brought about by proletarian nights is paradoxical: the very thing that prefigures life in a just and restful world can itself push the body and mind beyond their limits. This chapter will explore forms of exhaustion that emerged from periods of intense revolutionary activity and political organising. How can energy be sustained when victories remain elusive or sporadic and the urgent tasks to perform vastly outweigh the capacity to complete them (and when completing them still does not guarantee success)? Can the physical and emotional exhaustions of individuals be staved off so that movements don't exhaust themselves altogether?

Kindling a fire with ashes

In 'Emancipation and Exhaustion' (2021), Asad Haider identifies three distinct but intertwined forms of contemporary political exhaustion: the physical and mental exhaustion experienced by individual militants, the exhaustion of particular historical sequences of struggle when a lull occurs, and an epochal sense of exhaustion that results from confronting the seeming impossibility of matching the 'scale and depth' of earlier revolutionary moments.[3] Haider begins by invoking the tired militant – exhausted from building barricades in the morning, canvassing in the afternoon, reading classic texts for guidance at night – ground down by defeats and failures. Most of his essay, however, concentrates on the zoomed out exhaustions of sequences and movements. This chapter will stay with the gloomy granularity of everyday forms of tiredness and ask whether it is possible to overcome them in the absence of transformed social relations.

This chapter will examine the psychological toll of keeping going over long periods of time, experiences of engagement in different cycles of struggle across lifetimes, and efforts to sustain momentum in the face of disillusionment. How do movements sustain themselves over years or generations? How do individuals in those movements keep going, given that just surviving is difficult enough in exploitative and oppressive societies? What happens to political movements when people don't have the energy to do more than just survive?

A tension between an urgent need for political transformation and the energy-sapping qualities of life under prevailing conditions that can make fighting against them difficult are central to this chapter. This tension is articulated in a scene in Neel Mukherjee's novel *The Lives of Others*. Set in West Bengal between 1966 and 1970, the narrative explores the impact on a middle-class family when the eldest grandson becomes radicalised at university and joins the Maoist Naxalite movement. The novel's protagonist has travelled from Calcutta (now Kolkata) to the countryside and is apprehensive about meeting villagers and seeing how they live. He narrates the twists and turns of his first encounter with the peasants he has been sent to organise among. Before arriving, he imagined that it might be tricky to win them over and mobilise them:

> I had made myself exhausted thinking about the months of talks and meetings, posters and expounding. It had felt, in my imagination, like the effort that would be required to move a giant crag by pushing at its base.

Yet soon after his arrival this sense of difficulty is replaced by 'an easy, achievable optimism'. This sudden reversal is brought about not by discussions with the villagers, but by witnessing the effects of their material conditions: they are 'shrivelled by worry', hungry and unable to feed their 'bony' malnourished children, and conscious that their debts will be passed down through generations. Seeing the poverty and suffering in the village, he jumps to the assumption that its inhabitants 'would be simmering with anger and all we needed to do was a bit of stoking and there would be a giant conflagration that would bring down the bloodsuckers and burn them to cinders'. Soon, however, his attitude towards the possibility of political mobilisation reverses yet again. Mukherjee's fiery metaphors continue:

Then that hopefulness curdled: what I hadn't reckoned with was that decades and decades of this slow-burning flame of resentment and deprivation had burned *them* not the perpetrators. The embers of anger we had thought of fanning had burned down into the ashes of despair. They were already dead within their lives. They had no hope, no sense of a future, just an endless playing out of this illness of the present tense until its culmination in an early death. In other words, we had to kindle a fire with ashes. Have you ever tried doing that?[4]

In a few short pages the protagonist zigzags furiously across a wide emotional spectrum: he goes from exhaustion at contemplating the task of organising across a class divide, to an optimism based on assumptions about other people's presumed desire to change their lives, to a realisation that the difficulty of survival might make such desires, or at least the energy required to act on them, impossible. His exhaustion from organising pales into insignificance when confronted with these people's much more exhausting living conditions. Keeping a fire burning is difficult enough, but how to kindle a fire with ashes? How to create the sparks necessary to fight against material conditions that are already exhausting?

Though concerned with ongoing, sometimes mundane struggles, this chapter begins with a dramatic, ruptural event – the October Revolution of 1917, or rather, with its complex aftermath, when the rupture of the revolution settled into the routines of a post-revolutionary, actually existing socialist society. Given that the revolution was not defeated, the forms of exhaustion it provoked were ambiguous in meaning and defined in contradictory ways. Was the exhaustion that emerged from excessive revolutionary engagement in the years following the storming of the Winter Palace primarily physical (a quantitative depletion of bodily energy) or was it also tied to ideals (reflecting something more qualitative about the content of political activities and the course of the revolution)? This question remains pertinent to the chapter's ensuing discussion of psychiatric writing by Robert Coles on the relationship between exhaustion and political struggle from doing 'spade work' in the civil rights movement. (Ella Baker coined the term 'spade work' to describe the unglamorous but necessary forms of organising on which political change depends.) Coles's work confronts the problem of keeping going in the face of strategic setbacks, state repressions and interpersonal tensions.

The chapter ends by considering works by Toni Cade Bambara. Her short story 'The Apprentice' introduces a seemingly indefatigable political activist, while her novel *The Salt Eaters*, set in the fragmented aftermath of the movements of the sixties, confronts fatigue. Ultimately, I argue, Bambara proposes a model for overcoming both individual and epochal exhaustion. Bambara's novel contends with what Mukherjee describes as the 'illness of the present tense' by proposing that it is not only possible but necessary to create forms of psychological healing in a sick world. Rather than sacrificing the self for the sake of a collective future, Bambara insists on the counterintuitive possibility of turning ashes into kindling.

Revolutionary nerves

Born in the US in 1869, 'neurasthenia', colloquially known as 'nervous exhaustion', was understood as a disease of modern urban life. If today digital devices, ubiquitous screens and new forms of precarious work are blamed for draining energies and reducing attention spans, in the late nineteenth century the concern was, similarly, that in a rapidly changing society, people struggled to keep up. Everything from locomotives to cigarettes, perfume to Ibsen plays was seen as part of the damaging sensory onslaught. Industrial change and technological developments placed new pressures on people's bodies and minds, and an array of symptoms emerged, primarily of mental and physical exhaustion. Nervous energy was understood quantitively and nervous exhaustion framed in terms of depletion, understood as the sapping of an individual's finite energetic resources, frequently analogised to electrical, mechanical or economic processes.[5] Anna Katharina Schaffner's *Exhaustion: A History* devotes a chapter to neurasthenia, which, in her account, was an influential and even fashionable diagnosis in North America and Western Europe that gradually vanished after the First World War. But the pathology also had a life in Russia on either side of the 1917 October Revolution.

Although the October Revolution was not defeated and the Civil War was eventually won, years of violence, blockades, famine and epidemics took a heavy physical and mental toll, as Alexander Berkman observed in 1922: 'Long years of war, revolution, and civil struggle had bled Russia to exhaustion and brought her people to the brink of despair.'[6] In the winter of 1919, colleagues of Bolshevik Inessa Armand, the first director of the *Zhenotdel* (the party's women's section), noted that she had 'withered before our eyes'; her once elegant clothing was ragged, her appearance haggard.[7] There was no food in her unheated apartment. Eventually she caught pneumonia but returned to working as soon as she recovered.

Concerned about her exhaustion, V. I. Lenin, her friend and (it is widely assumed) sometimes lover, implored her to take a break, and eventually she agreed to spend time recuperating in a resort hotel in the Caucasus with her son. They spent several weeks in the spa town Kislovodsk in a sanatorium for Bolsheviks, one of many such spaces of respite that had been hastily set up in properties abandoned by the recently departed aristocracy.[8] Armand avoided the other guests, went on long walks and wrote in her diary that her only remaining feelings were for her son and for Lenin:

> It's as if my heart has died to all other relationships. As if having given all my strength, all my passion to V.I. and the cause of work, all the well-springs of love, of feeling for people, which were once so deep, have been drained... I am a living corpse.[9]

Having given everything to the revolution, she was too tired to access the political passions that had once motivated her. Soon after the sanatorium respite, Armand was forced to flee the region due to a White Army advance. She contracted cholera and died in September 1920 at the age of 46. When recounting Armand's difficult last months, historian Barbara Evans Clements suggests she was suffering from depression, but 'nervous exhaustion', neurasthenia and nervousness were more commonplace early Soviet diagnoses associated with feelings of physical depletion and emotional despair.

Neurasthenia and nervous illnesses, including pathological forms of exhaustion, were also diagnosed in late imperial Russia, but in the post-revolutionary 1920s their prevalence rose dramatically.[10] According to Frances Lee Bernstein, the era of the New Economic Policy (NEP, 1921–28), during which some forms of private enterprise were reintroduced into the economy, saw 'an epidemic of nervous illness that constituted an urgent social problem'.[11] Young men were particularly susceptible to nervous ailments, including many party activists and Red Army soldiers.[12] Impotence was a major symptom. Anxieties about male virility were entangled with concerns about establishing a new socialist society.[13] Sexual libido was conceptualised quantitatively, as a quota of physical energy.[14] Exhausted men were presented in medical literature as distressed and dissatisfied. This rise in exhaustion's prevalence was attributed to the specific strains of the post-revolutionary situation – 'exhaustion was deemed emblematic of the Soviet condition' – though in contradictory and confusing ways.[15]

Some psychologists emphasised the traumatic impact of the Civil War, while others drew inspiration from Friedrich Engels' *Condition of the English Working Class*, pointing to the mental and physical impact of the hardships of everyday life: overcrowded housing, poor sanitation, insufficient food.[16] Advice pamphlets gave tips on mitigating the strain of manual labour by taking a rational approach to leisure activities: 'The scientific organization of labor required a scientific organization of rest.'[17] Bolsheviks were concerned that the degradations of the bourgeois past would infect the present, an anxiety that was heightened during NEP due to its 'mixed economy'. This anxiety applied as much to individuals, formed as they were by the capitalist pre-revolutionary world, as to society as a whole. Exhaustion, some psychiatrists argued, enabled these old forms to seep back into the present, particularly among sectors of society that had failed to adapt to the new reality.[18] Others emphasised the significance of hereditary factors alongside environmental transformations, arguing that the children of the former bourgeoisie were, as Daniel Beer discusses, 'biologically defective': 'Languages of biomedical abnormality and class struggle were compatible and mutually reinforcing.'[19]

Psychologist Aron Zalkind's *Revolution and Youth* (1925) drew conclusions based on his analysis of students at the Sverdlov Communist University. He found that 40 to 50 percent of the communist students suffered from nervous disorders, but he insisted that these illnesses and the feelings of emptiness and despair that characterised them were caused not by the traumas of the war years, but by the quiescence and tedium of life that followed. For Zalkind, young people's psychic distresses were attributable to the banality of the present rather than the violence and material hardships of the past.[20] People were exhausted not from the traumas of war, he argued, but because life since the introduction of the NEP was insufficiently revolutionary. Speaking at the same university in 1925, by contrast, Aron Soltz located the causes of exhaustion in the Civil War years, but he implied that people's individual weaknesses rather than intense external pressures accounted for their problems:

> There are some young Party members who have gone through the Civil War, fought at all the fronts... and have become totally emotionally exhausted, because of the colossal self-control that has been demanded of them. The ones who lacked sufficient self-control thought that, after one last effort, they would enter the Communist paradise, but when they saw that things were more serious and required a longer period of work, they experienced a certain disappointment.[21]

Exhaustion was rife, but whether it was caused by too much continuity with pre-revolutionary society or too little, by material hardship or exposure to violence, remained contested. There was a lack of consensus over whether exhaustion was the result of fighting for the revolution or the depleting experience of living in inadequately transformed social conditions.

Armand sank into despair just two years after the October Revolution. Many Old Bolsheviks who had been active in the underground in the years before the revolution followed her into exhaustion. After years of hardship and struggle, bodies failed, but exhaustion was also psychological, prompted by political disappointments, the disorientation of shifting from insurgent opposition to ruling elite, and, for some, despair over the course the new society was taking. Exhaustion was not just physical but emotional, not only quantitative but qualitative.

In March 1921, a spontaneous uprising among sailors at the Kronstadt naval base was branded counter-revolutionary by Lenin and brutally suppressed. In a context of rigid orthodoxy and the crushing of democracy within the party, already concerning to many party members, the craven hypocrisy and stark betrayal represented by Lenin's response to a rebellion of people belonging to the class the revolution was supposed to serve had a huge emotional impact.[22] Between 1921 and 1922, over 14,000 people left the party voluntarily and there was a spate of suicides among the membership.[23] An earlier leftist tradition of martyrdom had framed suicide as an act of political resistance in the underground, meaning that death from the nervous exhaustion resulting from hard years of exile and incarceration could be venerated as an act of self-sacrifice.[24] A wave of suicides that followed the 1905 revolution was similarly narrated by Bolsheviks in political terms, as a legitimate response to the failure of the revolution. But the October Revolution had not been defeated; thus suicide as a form of political protest was deemed counter-revolutionary by the party leadership, who understood the act as the failure of an individual's will to overcome their personal problems for the sake of the collective endeavour of building the new society.[25] Forms of nervous exhaustion that led to suicide were inconvenient to acknowledge as they implied a malaise resulting from disillusionment rather than excessive commitment, but the illness was nonetheless often blamed for 'petty bickering and foul atmospheres in party collectives', suggesting that exhaustion as a medical diagnosis could equally function as a convenient means of cloaking political disagreements.[26] The discourse on nervous exhaustion was so pervasive and used in such contradictory contexts that it becomes difficult to disentangle the knotted discourses to get at what people were actually experiencing. Whatever the origins of their malaise, exhausted people did not make ideal builders of communism.

The party's response to Kronstadt prompted anarchists like Alexander Berkman and Emma Goldman to leave Russia, convinced the revolutionary project was doomed. Berkman described his mood when rifle shots of the army sent to crush the rebellion began to echo across the cold city: 'Days of anguish and cannonading. My heart is numb with despair; something has died within me. The people on the streets look bowed with grief.'[27] Goldman made of the apartment she shared with Berkman in Petrograd a refuge for devastated comrades in the aftermath: 'They came at all hours of the day and even late at night, hungry, spiritless, in black despair.' Yet she also described this turning point as a moment of psychological freedom from encroaching orthodoxy that counteracted bodily exhaustion: 'Physical pain and weariness were as nothing to our inner liberation.'[28] Goldman framed her physical exhaustion as less severe than the mental torment of political compromise.

When Lenin first demonstrated cognitive difficulties in 1921 (he would suffer his first stroke in 1922), doctors struggled to identify the cause, suggesting he was afflicted with nervous exhaustion like so many of his fellow Bolsheviks. Trotsky described Lenin between his two strokes as: 'A hopelessly tired man ... The expression of his face and of his entire figure might have been summed up in a word: tired.'[29] Lenin's death in 1924 prompted fresh waves of exhaustion and despair to wash over revolutionaries. Trotsky was absent from the funeral as he had been sent to a sanatorium in Sukhumi, Abkhazia, to recuperate. Another wave of suicides had broken out among Trotsky's supporters following a purge of those who supported the Worker's Opposition's 'New Course' in 1923, the political significance of which was the focus of a 'rhetorical struggle' between rival factions.[30] Suicides continued in the years after Lenin's death. In the first quarter of 1925, 14.1 percent of all party members who died were suicides.[31] Was suicide a counter-revolutionary 'act of indiscipline' or an act of protest against the trajectory taken by the party (as Adolf Ioffe proclaimed in a letter to Trotsky justifying his decision to end his own life)?[32] Yuri Slezkine describes Soviet sanatoria in the 1920s as sites of both 'sickness and sorrow', underlining again that post-revolutionary exhaustion was both physical and psychological: 68 percent of people who received medical treatment at the Central Executive Committee Rest Home in Tetkovo in summer 1928 were diagnosed with emotional disorders (including neurasthenia, psycho-neurasthenia, psychosis and exhaustion), while at the Lenin Rest Home in Maryino half had nervous illnesses. The Society for Old Bolsheviks received numerous requests for 'rest and therapy'.[33] By 1927, Old Bolsheviks formed a small minority of party members: 'Death, old age, purges, disillusionment and quite a few suicides had taken their toll.'[34] In contrast to the state-sanctioned vision of the New Soviet Person as strong, determined and vital, the actual revolutionaries, particularly those who had been committed to revolution for years before 1917, felt too shattered to carry on. But were rest and therapy a suitable cure for a malaise with political origins?

Victor Serge traced the disillusionments and confusions of the 1920s, describing Soviet Russia during the NEP period by way of a strange metaphor as 'a vast convalescent body, but on this body, whose flesh is our own, we see the pustules multiplying'. The body was recovering, but it was also getting sicker. Economic changes had 'worked miracles and famine was no more, but those same shifts were also a corrupting force'.[35] More tellingly, he claimed that even those who stood to benefit from the economic changes were getting sicker. Though this is a metaphor of physical rather than mental illness, it has in common with discussions of nervous exhaustion an assumption that individuals' pathologies reflected social ills. However, what people saw when they looked in the mirror depended on what they assumed Soviet society's problems to be. I want to turn now to consider theorisations of exhaustion that were not addressed to a period of revolutionary transition but to the ongoing exhaustion of a movement with no clear end in sight. In these examples, exhaustion continues to be understood as both physical and emotional, but they also pose the question of whether the scale and urgency demanded by political struggles can ever be met without exhausting the people who fight them.

Healing weariness

In 'Social Struggle and Weariness' (1964), psychiatrist Robert Coles, drawing on his observations of 'veteran activists of the civil rights movement in America', describes the 'exhaustion and despair' produced by sustained political organising and suggests ways to diminish their effects.[36] Born in 1929, Coles, a white psychiatrist from New England, had been stationed with the Air Force in Mississippi and returned to the South to work as a psychiatrist after being discharged. He spent four years primarily engaged in examining the psychological experiences of children in recently desegregated schools, and he published pieces about his research for a non-specialist readership in magazines including the *New Yorker* and the *New Republic*.[37] He had trained as a psychoanalyst in New Orleans, though some of his psychoanalytic colleagues in Boston objected to the informality and eclecticism of his methods, which included visiting people in their homes.[38] Coles also spent time living in proximity to young black student activists involved in the Student Non-Violent Coordinating Committee (SNCC) in Georgia, who participated in sit-ins and demonstrations and were also involved in the more administrative aspects of organising.[39] His methods of engagement with these young activists ranged from formal, structured interviews and consultations (including prison visits), to informal individual and group discussions. Coles describes the distrust and suspicion with which many of the student activists viewed him as a white outsider 'expert', sympathetic to but not directly participating in the movement.[40] In Coles' essay, rather than asking how activists succeeded in balancing 'inner stresses and outer trials', he instead focuses on the fact that 'an increasing number of them *don't* manage ... they grow weary and lose interest in themselves and their cause'.[41]

Coles emphasises the varied motivations and modes of engagement of young people involved in the movement, rather than presenting them as psychologically or sociologically homogenous. Despite this diversity of disposition and background, however, he notes that the experience of exhaustion was almost universal among them. The student activists exhibited a cluster of clinical symptoms after prolonged periods of political engagement: depression, 'battle fatigue', 'exhaustion, weariness, despair, frustration, and rage'.[42] For Coles, weariness was both emotional and physical, and was characterised by hopelessness and tiredness. Such feelings led many young people to abandon the movement, while those who remained became bitter and hostile. Weary activists often drank to excess, lost their appetites, withdrew from social engagements or simply disengaged from day-to-day movement work.

Coles compares the symptoms of exhaustion to war neuroses. Unlike contemporaneous studies of both social struggle and of African American social life in the US that viewed actions and behaviour through the lens of individual pathologies and cultural shortcomings, his article instead located the origins of these activists' symptoms firmly in the injustice and violence of the social world. Coles was a student of Erik Erikson, who proposed an influential theory of individual developmental stages in which adolescence and young adulthood were characterised by crisis. In this model, an individual's age was understood as a causal factor in their behaviour and disposition.[43] Youth was similarly identified as a factor in the responses of the students Coles encountered in the civil rights' movement: the young activists were 'trying to keep their courage and initiative while accepting the often sour lessons that come with growing older and living through unexpected and dismaying experiences'.[44] Yet these 'dismaying experiences' are given more weight in his analysis than youth as such.[45]

Depression among activists, Coles observes, frequently emerged only after prolonged periods of political engagement during which its effects were successfully kept at bay. This slow gestation made symptoms, when they finally emerged, difficult to treat with 'anything but the strongest of medical and psychiatric measures'. Loss of hope came with time. Coles describes people who entered the movement expecting change to come quickly but who, having engaged in similar actions again and again, had come to feel they had got no closer to victory: 'I thought we'd demonstrate and then they'd fold up before us. But it's been tougher than I ever dreamed.' The enemy began to seem impervious to attack. Resistance appeared increasingly futile and personal risk, particularly the risk of arrest and imprisonment, less worthwhile. Exhausted, an activist might also repudiate or begin to doubt their political commitments and principles, turning their anger away from the oppressive social conditions they had been fighting and onto the movement itself. Interpersonal tensions are another symptom of exhaustion. Coles quotes one of his interviewees:

> I feel I've lost those years. They've come to nothing, really. No real change. So I feel betrayed by the movement, and I guess it's easier to get angry at it than at the white world. I just want to pull out of the white world. I mean you can't hate it the way I do and live with it . . . That's it, my hate for the movement is a release or something . . . I can hate it and do something about it. You know, attack them and undermine them. But what can a Negro do to the white world without getting destroyed eventually.[46]

For Coles, hatred of a racially segregated society is rational and just, but expressing that hatred could feel self-defeating and pointless when it had no tangible effects. Failing to achieve political demands could lead to further individual psychic corrosion.

'Social Struggle and Weariness' also describes activists impatient with the slow pace of the struggle and annoyed by the increasing bureaucratisation of the movement:

> I'm tired, but so is the whole movement . . . We're becoming lifeless, just like all revolutions when they lose their first momentum . . . we

haven't won that much, and we're either holding to the little we have as an organization, or we get bitter, and want to create a new revolution.

Becoming preoccupied with internal organisational questions is, Coles claims, a core symptom of the weariness that emerges from social struggle. Frustrated by the seemingly invincible power of the enemy, people turn instead against their immediate structures and relationships. Though Coles views weariness as a clinical condition, these examples frame it as a rational response to shared social circumstances, rather than as evidence of a pathology originating in the individual sufferer. The rage, fear and despair he outlines were all grounded in concrete experiences: rage at the injustices of segregated white supremacist society, fear of punishment by cops, courts and the carceral state, despair at the slowness of progress. Indeed, Coles suggests these psychological reactions to prolonged engagement in the movement are basically inevitable:

> Weariness touches almost all the students who stay in the movement for any significant period of time – that is, long enough to taste its less than quixotic or flashy quality and its hard, grinding daily demands which are not always relieved by spectacular successes and are often encumbered with the new burden of hopes sparked but not realized.[47]

The relationship Coles identifies between 'quixotic and flashy' experiences and 'hard, grinding daily demands' lies at the core of the relationship between exhaustion and political struggle more broadly. If the trudge of day-to-day organising is not accompanied by the thrilling, ruptural rush that comes from confrontational forms of collective action (or if those kinds of actions are repeated over and over again but yield no material gains), then the scales tip and exhaustion can overpower political commitment.

Coles acknowledges the importance of recognising the external dangers faced by individuals in the movement. He recommends helping individuals to see their own difficulties in the 'larger perspective of the relationship between personal effort and social reform'. In a therapeutic context, he advocates emphasising that the resistance an individual is engaged in is objectively difficult and therefore any feelings of exhaustion should not be viewed as a subjective failing. There is, however, one key symptom that he argues a psychiatrist might help people to overcome through therapeutic engagement: guilt. He discusses the case of a twenty-three-year-old man he calls Charles, who had been arrested eighteen times for participating in sit-ins. Charles was referred to Coles by a friend who had witnessed his 'chronic fatigue'.[48] They met eight times over the course of six weeks to discuss and work through the patient's feelings of worthlessness and depression. Coles identifies guilt as Charles's prime preoccupation. Guilt exacerbated despair as Charles castigated himself relentlessly for feeling low, for being 'weak' in comparison to others. Feeling guilty, he also relativised his mental sufferings in order to delegitimise them. Coles advocates validating feelings of gloominess to help the patient see they are not self-indulgent or unwarranted. He also suggests separating limitations from possibilities as a way of enabling the patient to see that their political cause is not futile, even if many of their difficulties and frustrations are indeed real.

In some cases, the symptoms Coles observed were so severe that he recommended withdrawal from political activity altogether. But although he mentions that many people chose to leave the movement to start a family or get a job after years of exhausting work, he does not ask what psychic problems they risked experiencing in those realms. Withdrawal might alleviate the most acute symptoms of weariness, but the social problems that prompted the weary person to take action in the first place persist. Those who leave the movement before the struggle has been won must still continue to live in the racist society they had been fighting to change. The respite gained from withdrawal from the movement is therefore only ever partial.

Coles cites a dream recounted by a patient who had been 'furloughed' for 'rest and rehabilitation':

> Sometimes I wake up in a cold sweat, and I remember that I've actually dreamed that the whole movement was arrested . . . I mean all of us were taken in custody, and then I escape and a few of us get a boat and go to Africa, or we take refuge in one of the African embassies . . . I mean to get away from whites, all of them that's what the dream says; the reverse of integration, you might call it.[49]

Coles passes over the political content of the dream in silence, remarking not on its separatist, almost Garveyist vision of an escape from white persecution to safety in Africa but only on the activist's difficulty sleeping and fear of arrest. The article relies on distinguishing neatly between white society and the black movement, but work by Alvin Poussaint, a black psychiatrist from New York City who went to the South to work as southern field director of the Medical Committee for Human Rights in

Mississippi and subsequently set up a clinic for poor local residents, argued that the emergence of more militant political positions was connected to psychic problems resulting from racial tensions experienced *within* the movement.[50]

Coles focused on anxieties and frustrations that emerged in black activists as a result of exhaustion, without mentioning how racial, class and gendered dynamics exacerbated interpersonal antagonisms within the movement itself. Poussaint instead published a paper focusing on the guilt, anxiety, anger and patronising maternalism that led many white women civil rights activists to leave the movement after only short periods of engagement. In his analysis Poussaint points to underlying prejudices and hostilities that seemed more resistant to therapeutic intervention than the weariness described by Coles.[51] In 1968, Poussaint co-authored an article with sociologist and civil rights activist Joyce Ladner, arguing that psychological observations they had made in the South since the time of the 1964 Mississippi Summer Project had anticipated the philosophy of Black Power. Writing in 1964, Coles had nothing to say about a dream that envisioned 'the reverse of integration', whereas Poussaint and Ladner claimed that both black and white activists repressed their feelings of hatred and hostility towards one another, arguing that 'unresolved psychological difficulties in black-white relations within the civil rights movement' contributed to the emergence of more militant black nationalist and separatist positions.[52]

Poussaint and Ladner were not arguing that racial tensions could be understood as a psychological issue in the manner of a twenty-first century liberal advocating 'unconscious bias training' as a response to Black Lives Matter uprisings, which would be closer to taking an herbal remedy to solve the exhaustion caused by overwork under capitalism. They did not claim that racism was simply a question of individual dispositions or attitudes. Instead, they described psychic life as formed by structural and systemic issues 'developed through centuries'.[53] And the former cannot change without transforming the latter. The exhaustion that emerges from social struggle is here not only a question of immediate physical and psychological weariness but is caused by endemic social problems to which there are no therapeutic solutions.

A less despairing conclusion was drawn by Emma Jones Lapsansky, who also discussed the 'psychological clashes' between black and white activists in SNCC during Freedom Summer in 1964. She described the emergence of Black Power as a positive development that demonstrated a psychological shift in black people in the movement, enabling them to channel 'productive anger': 'The Movement fell short of social and political liberation, but it did move us as black people, a long way toward psychological liberation.' Lapansky does not equate psychological liberation with social and political change, but she presents it as a prerequisite for achieving change in the future. Indeed, rather than suggesting that psychological problems could be solved by seeking therapeutic help from experts embedded in racist institutions who worked with normative psychiatric models, she cites a woman who declares that 'Black power is my mental health.'[54] Fighting against oppression could be therapeutic in its own right.

Falling apart together

In 'The Apprentice', a short story by Toni Cade Bambara (a writer who was herself an activist scholar engaged with the Black Arts Movement in New York City, Newark and later Atlanta), veteran organiser Naomi, an archetypical committed revolutionary fully devoted to the cause (similar in self-sacrificing motivation to those described in Serge's *Memoirs of a Revolutionary*), guides her young protégé through long days spent keeping 'this committee in touch with that project in touch with thusnsuch organization in touch with the whatchmacallit league'. The unnamed apprentice-narrator is tired at the end of a 'long, long day' but knows better than to complain to Naomi, who she predicts would retort: '"We haven't earned the right to feel tired."' She knows that even if she shows physical proof of her worn out body with its bruises or blisters, Naomi would begin listing 'names of sisters and brothers who'd given their lives'.[55] Bambara described her character in 1974 as one who approached every person, every interaction, every situation 'as usherer-in of the new day'.[56] Naomi has no truck with tiredness because there's always someone more tired, there's always someone more in need of rest, there's always an urgent task demanding renewed energy. 'Naomi assumes everybody wakes up every morning plotting out exactly what to do to hasten the revolution.' She will not tolerate 'cynicism, sarcasm, smugness'. Any possible activity presented to Naomi will be met with the question, 'But how does that free the people?'[57]

Naomi's young mentee, though exhausted from long hours of waged work followed by long hours of activism, admits to feeling 'refreshed' whenever she sees Naomi. In group criticism sessions, the apprentice has been told she is too negative, insufficiently optimistic about the possibility of revolution, incapable of recognising the forms of solidarity that she's already witnessed in her daily life. She feels daunted by the struggle, incapable of matching Naomi's fervour and commitment: 'Being a revolutionary is something else . . . I'm not sure I'm up to it, and that's the truth. I'm too little, and too young, and maybe too scarified if you want to know the truth.' She feels ashamed of her tiredness, but conscious of its physical toll: 'Ain't hardly autumn and already I'm falling apart.' When out doing movement work, she is distracted by her bodily needs: her feet ache, she gets hungry or needs to use the toilet. But her mentor never seems tired: 'Naomi don't never let up.'[58] Naomi keeps coming up with new ideas for activities they could be doing, while the apprentice is ready to sit down to eat a sandwich and drink a coffee.

Sitting at a drive-in, the apprentice reflects on how exhausted the staff must be. Knowing it has been a busy shift, she thinks about how much work they must have done that day. But Naomi says that however exhausting waged work might be, there is always a source of energy left to draw on for non-alienated socially transformative activity: '"I mean you work all day, right? Dead on your feet and can't go on. But then a situation develops and you rise to the occasion, get your legs back, get your second wind. It's fantastic!"' Naomi enjoins her companion to imagine all the 'energy that would be released' if everyone worked for themselves and each other rather than for their bosses: '"Giiiiirl, it would be too much, too much. The energy, the creativity, the humanness."' Listening to Naomi, picturing this transformed world, a world in which she might grow her own vegetables rather than going to work everyday, the apprentice in turn feels energised: 'I could feel the energy coming back to my feet, waking up my legs.' Naomi cries out joyfully in anticipation of this new society. Sitting beside her the young apprentice 'can feel the new day Naomi always lecturing about, can feel it pumping through my legs'. She feels inspired to work harder for black liberation, for the revolution, for the end of exhaustion. They both say they hope they live to see it, but in that moment, it feels as though it is already there pulsing through their bodies. This seems to confirm something Naomi had told her earlier, which she couldn't really make sense of at the time: 'The revolution is here.' This contradictory temporality will, as we shall see, also be crucial to the understanding of healing proposed in *The Salt Eaters*. The experience of organising has a prefigurative energising capacity. At the end of their exhausting day, the apprentice repeats that she is tired and also repeats that there's no point saying anything to Naomi about it: 'I ain't earned the right, to hear her tell it. But hell, it'd been a long, long, long day.'[59]

At the end of the story, it remains unclear if the apprentice will learn to become more like Naomi or if the toll of tiredness will eventually be felt by Naomi too. The question of how social struggle contends with weariness remains ambiguous. Is the relationship between political necessity and personal well-being a delicate balance or an impossible trade-off? Naomi's fervour is contagious and there is little sense that her constant activity is wearing her out or wearing her down. The story also captures the renewed surge of energy that both women experience when contemplating the future that they are giving of themselves to achieve. Yet it also acknowledges that Naomis are rare and that for most people it is sometimes necessary to sit down, sleep, stop, eat a sandwich.

Salt in wounds

By the opening of Bambara's later novel *The Salt Eaters* (1980), weariness seems to have gained the upper hand. Bambara had moved to Atlanta in the mid-1970s, as part of what her biographer Linda Janet Holmes calls a 'reverse migration' among black intellectuals from the North to the South. The novel drew on her research into 'root workers, midwives, herbalists, and other healing traditions among black women in Georgia, Alabama, and Louisiana', an interest that reflected a broader shift among black radicals in the US in the period away from a more strictly Marxist-Leninist rejection of spirituality.[60]

The Salt Eaters begins with a scene of healing. Long-time activist Velma Henry goes to a healer who communes with a spirit guide embedded in her community, rather than seeking treatment from a mainstream psychiatrist. Velma has survived a suicide attempt and is sitting on a stool in the Southwest Community Infirmary where the healer Minnie Ransom asks her the portentous question that echoes as a refrain through the book: "'Are you sure, sweetheart, that you want to be well?'"[61] It takes the course of the novel to find any answers.[62] Spiritual or psychic healing, Minnie perceives, is difficult. It is also an act of volition. The wounded person must want to heal, but Velma holds fast to her woundedness. Minnie suggests that there is some consolation or comfort to be found in being wounded, angry, hurt, broken. To heal, Velma must let go of her wounds. It would be tempting to see Velma as a counterpart to Naomi, a Naomi after the exhaustion has finally taken hold, but *The Salt Eaters* implies that Velma has been struggling against exhaustion all along.

As the novel shuffles between healing in the present and scenes from Velma's politically engaged past, she is shown to have a similar determination and resoluteness to Naomi. She inhabits a world of 'staunch Marxist-Maoist-dialectical-historical-materialist[s]', a world in which the struggle came before attending to personal needs.[63] Like Naomi, Velma reproaches others for their insufficient political commitments, harbouring resentment towards her older sister Palma for choosing to pursue her art practice rather than attend a rally, for instance. Echoing Naomi's moralising comparisons, she thinks Palma 'should've been on the march, had no right to the cool solitude of her studio painting pictures of sailboats while sisters were being beaten and raped, and workers shot and children terrorized'. But it is Palma who often takes care of Velma in moments of crisis. Though Naomi's young apprentice finds Naomi's righteousness frustrating and slightly unrealistic, it is also inspirational, whereas in focusing on the difficulties Velma has encountered in attempting to pursue a fully politically committed life, *The Salt Eaters* dwells on the contradictions involved in sustaining an uncompromising position of complete dedication to a cause. At the beginning of the novel Velma has unravelled: 'The relentless logic she lived by sprung.' She must contend with the psychic toll of her years of commitment, with the weariness that has come from social struggle. As one character quips in another scene: 'The material without the spiritual and psychic does not a dialectic make.'[64]

The Salt Eaters captures the durational, ongoing nature of political struggle and the way political commitments become enmeshed with the quotidian churn of daily life. The non-linear narrative seems to take place mostly in the seventies, describing loosely intertwined groups of people of different generations engaged in multiple overlapping movements and causes, also tracing their shifts over time: black nationalist, Puerto Rican, Chicano and indigenous groups; people committed to women's liberation and gay liberation; housing, ecological and antinuclear activists; trade unions, student groups, political parties, experimental artists' collectives. Bambara also conveys the varied and relentless demands of movement spade work – 'getting out the press releases, the mailings . . . doing the canvassing, for organizing a base among campus forces, street forces, prison forces, workers, gathering the money, arranging for transportation' – underlining that it often falls to women to undertake these kinds of activities while men perform public-facing leadership roles. Velma and her women comrades express frustrations at men who seem to think that food appears by magic in the home, just as tedious administrative work gets done by magic in the movement, men who ignore 'the unmindful gap between want and done, demand and get'. The novel shows that doing and getting things is far more exhausting than simply wanting and demanding them. Minding the gap is tiring. Bambara also underscores the physically draining aspects of Velma's commitments: she 'trudged through dust, through rain, through mud'. At the social justice space called 'the Academy of the 7 Arts' which she ran with her husband Obie, Velma had done so much work that eight people are needed to replace her when she is finally unable to go on.[65]

In 'The Apprentice', Naomi's frenetic political activities draw inspiration from a trip to Cuba and she is trying to organise an event in solidarity with the Mozambique Liberation Front (FRELIMO). Like the fictional Naomi, Bambara had travelled to Cuba in 1973 and organised a screening in Atlanta of Robert van Lierop's 1972 documentary *A Luta Continua* made in solidarity with the liberation movement in Mozambique. 'The Apprentice' appears in a collection alongside the eponymous story 'The Sea Birds are Still Alive', inspired by Bambara's 1975 trip to Vietnam with a women's delegation. Laura Whitehorn, who travelled alongside Bambara as part of the delegation and later spent fourteen years in prison for her participation in militant Weather Underground actions, reflected that Bambara had been less inclined to romanticise Vietnam than the white women with whom she travelled. Whitehorn linked Bambara's rejection of an image of steadfast, ideologically pure revolutionary heroism in Vietnam, her acceptance of 'human frailty' and capacity to see that 'the essence of heroism is being imperfect but acting anyway', to her experiences in the US:[66]

> Toni saw in Vietnam more clearly than I did because she had such an appreciation for the generations of struggle Black people had already waged without 'burning out', 'moving on' or whatever those phrases are that people use to describe people who used to be active radicals and then one day stopped.[67]

By the time of *The Salt Eaters,* Bambara has the character Obie bemoan the disengagement and splinterings that have taken place in recent years. Previously the Academy had hosted events by 'Panthers, Che Lumumba Club, Young Lords', whereas in the present he is left contemplating 'factions... intrigue... old ideological splits', asking, 'Whatever happened to Third World solidarity?'[68]

Susan Willis reads the contrast between Bambara's earlier stories and *The Salt Eaters* as a contrast between epochs, a shift from the engaged sixties to the apathetic seventies.[69] Ishmael Reed similarly characterises the novel as post-revolutionary: 'It captures the despair that set in after the revolutionary fires of the 1960s had been extinguished.'[70] This temporal shift is reflected upon explicitly in the novel, but the contrast between unified past and fragmented present – between the 'flashy' ruptural moment and the daily grind that Coles identified in his 1964 essay – is blurred in Bambara's account. Struggles are ongoing and were exhausting all along. Addressing students at a lecture at Howard University in the late 1970s, Bambara refused to affirm a narrative that celebrated the active past while bemoaning the deflated present, declaring instead: 'We are now in a period of healing, study and self-development. Some see the trend as retrogressive; I find it quite interesting.'[71] While she acknowledged the ebbing of political organising in that moment, she refused to depict the period of healing as antithetical to an earlier period of more intense struggle.

The Salt Eaters' Obie describes an energetic emergence of political activism in one period followed by an enervating retreat from it at a later point, but the teeming multiplicity of the novel's non-linear narrative prevents it from giving the impression that time moves cleanly and teleologically from engagement to disillusionment. In one scene from Velma's past, she is at a rally, but far from feeling the rush of energy Naomi and her protégé felt together in the car anticipating a future liberated society, Velma is already tired. In the scene, which is framed by a discussion at a meeting in which women castigate men for doing too little, Velma is closer to the exhausted apprentice than the ever-energetic Naomi. Velma is struggling against her tired, menstruating body. She has marched 'all morning, all afternoon and most of early evening' to get to the site, while being 'shot at, spit at . . . lobbed with everything from stones to eggs', and now her shoes have worn through and her feet have swollen. 'She'd been reeking with wasted blood and rage.' By the time the sharply dressed, slick political leader pulls up in his limousine and takes to the stage in his shiny shoes, she is 'Exhausted . . . squinting through the dust and grit of her lashes . . . Her throat was splintered wood.' That evening she is left 'trembling with fatigue'. Velma goes off to find a bathroom in which to change her tampon, missing the man's main speech. Bambara focuses on Velma's physical depletion – 'nails splitting, hands swollen' – contrasting the image of Velma in the dirty bathroom stall with the image of the pristine political leader who is described as an amalgamation of various famous black male leaders, including Martin Luther King Jr, Malcolm X and Stokely Carmichael. His public confidence and ease seem to depend on Velma's hidden exhaustion and quiet dishevelment.[72]

Following his moment of lament for a lost past, Obie rebukes himself for having been overly nostalgic for an imagined history of political togetherness:

> Everyone seemed to be pulling in the same direction then. But that of course was selective memory, a chump way to excuse the self from the chaos of the moment, longing for a past and for a future as if there were no continuum, and no real thread that energized and carried one, as if time pieces ticked away in separate lockers he could open, close, lock up, climb into or fall out of.

The relationship between the self and the chaos of the moment here parallels the relationship between weariness and social struggle described by Coles. Things have become so fragmented and broken in the present: 'He wanted wholeness in his life again.'[73] But Bambara cautions against romanticising the past or sealing it off from the present, and she makes clear that withdrawing altogether is not the solution. The sense of fragmentation Obie articulates also threatens to undo Velma, but while he bemoans the fragmentation of groups and movements, she is breaking apart as a person. Velma's legs began trembling long ago. A thread connects her past exhaustion to her shattered present. Perhaps Naomi's young apprentice was right to take heed of her body's pains and limits.

The Salt Eaters is preoccupied with reinstating wholeness, but Minnie tells Velma, 'Wholeness is no trifling matter.' Velma must *want* to be well, to be whole. For Bambara, it requires effort and time to be whole in a fragmented and wounding world. But, crucially, it is not impossible, and wholeness will be necessary to keep acting to change the world. The definition of 'wholeness' implied by the novel, like its definition of 'healing', is anti-adaptive; it is certainly not analogous to a normative definition of 'mental health' that would be propounded by mainstream psychiatrists or doctors (as demonstrated by the transformation undergone by the character of Doctor Julius Meadows, who comes to acknowledge some of the racist underpinnings of mainstream medicine). Instead, the novel's definition of wholeness relies on a disjunctive temporality akin to Naomi's declaration that 'the revolution is here'. Being whole in the hole-ridden present demands a leap of faith. Wholeness is subjective, as Velma's godmother Sophie Heywood similarly perceives:

"'Have to be whole to see whole.'"[74] Seeing the whole, being whole, is the capacity to see that the revolution is here.

At the beginning of the novel, and hence at the beginning of the healing process, Minnie can tell that Velma isn't ready to let go of her pain and anger; she isn't ready to be whole. It will take time for her to relinquish the wounds that have come to define her; at the outset she is 'picking at herself as at a sore' (an image similar to the pustule-covered body invoked by Serge).[75] Healing will involve her reckoning with past experiences and encountering her ancestors.[76] *The Salt Eaters* does not describe an individual who has been pummelled passively by a hostile external world, but instead shows how the 'chaos of the moment' comes to form a part of the self. The provocation and invitation that Minnie offers to Velma, which separates the understanding of psychic life presented in the novel from Coles' assumptions about inevitable weariness, is her insistence that: "'There's nothing that stands between you and perfect health, sweetheart.'" It takes Velma a long time to declare finally: 'Health is my right.'[77] Once she can see the whole, she can become whole.

The understandings of health and healing implied by Bambara do not transcend material conditions but demand they be remade. Not only does she question mainstream health-care institutions and practices, but the literally poisonous and carcinogenic properties of the humanity-damaged earth recur as a theme in her work – a Marshall Islander in 'The Sea Birds Are Still Alive' recalls the devastation wrought by the Bikini Atoll nuclear tests, while it is implied that a character in 'Going Critical' has cancer due to her proximity to a government nuclear test in her youth. The latter story also reflects on the deleterious impact of ecological waste: 'insecticides, pesticides; industrial mining, paper, food, metallurgy, petroleum, chemical plants, municipal sewerage system, refuse disposal, swimming pool agents'.[78] Bambara's insistence on the possibility of finding wholeness does not, then, disavow the very real and material obstacles to health in the present. In *The Salt Eaters*, her affirmation of wholeness rather has implications for the seemingly fragmented political causes in the novel (whose literary form is also fragmentary, incohesive).

In one scene in *The Salt Eaters*, an old black bus driver called Fred Holt encounters a group of young activists called the Seven Sisters on their way to a local festival. He finds their politicised rhetoric alienating and their sub-cultural appearance seems to set them apart from him. But Bambara shows that his preoccupation with his friend Porter's death, which was caused by exposure to radioactivity, ties his concerns to theirs, just as the different causes the novel discusses are shown to be interlinked, as when the character Ruby is confronted by a comrade for voting down a proposal to participate in anti-nuclear or ecological actions because she thinks they will divert focus from more urgent issues facing black people: '"You think there's no connection between the power plant and Transchemical and the power configurations in this city and the quality of life in this city, region, country, world?"'[79] Reinstating wholeness, Bambara suggests, starts from the recognition of such connections and will involve joining up disparate movements, which will in turn lighten the burden taken on by individual activists. When Donna Haraway writes in 'A Manifesto for Cyborgs' (1985) of the need to act 'on the basis of conscious coalition, of affinity, of political kinship', she cites *The Salt Eaters* as a model of unity.[80] Attaining wholeness should be understood as both individual and collective, psychological and social.

Being well

In her last, exhausted days, Inessa Armand, who had lost the capacity to love and had begun to feel guilty for neglecting her children to fight for the revolution, lamented: 'There is no personal life because all time and strength are given to the general cause.'[81] Coles presented a stark distinction between withdrawal from and continuation of struggle, glossing over the difficulties of continuing to live in an unjust world, whereas *The Salt Eaters* ultimately proposes that it is possible to be well in a sick world, to be whole in a broken society, to heal in a wounded and wounding reality. The relationship between social struggle and weariness, between external pressures and internal pains, is not balanced, but weariness can – must – be overcome and social struggle need not involve giving up all time and strength. Healing is necessary and demands conviction; it is also collective. Velma's healing takes time, and it takes the care and presence of others, as well as a reckoning with the individual and ancestral past.

    The Salt Eaters opens up a conceptual space for reflection on psychic experience in a manner distinct from both mainstream psychiatric practices and liberal notions of self-help. bell hooks's *Sisters of the Yam: Black Women and Self-Recovery*, which takes its title from a group in *The Salt Eaters* and contains a dedication to Bambara, describes lessons learned through years long processes of recovery and discussion among groups of black women. Inspired by identifications and anxieties her black female students expressed after reading *The Salt Eaters*, hooks established 'a space where black women could name their pain and find ways of healing'. Unlike liberal self-help books that advocate personal change as an end in itself (a model akin to buying an herbal remedy as a treatment for exhaustion from overwork), naming pain entails identifying external causes of suffering. hooks declares her desire to 'politicize movements for self-recovery' by recognising systemic causes of psychic distress. She also acknowledges that the capacity to engage in political action depends on ongoing forms of psychic introspection and self-actualisation: 'Before many of us can effectively sustain engagement in organized resistance struggle, in black liberation movement, we need to undergo a process of self-recovery that can heal individual wounds that may prevent us from functioning fully.'[82]

Naomi's apprentice felt confused by her mentor's statement that 'the revolution is here', but Naomi's capacity to act tirelessly relied on this understanding. The paradox of revolutionary healing – the necessity for revolutionary healing to be anti-adaptive – is acknowledged by Bambara as the place from which political action must begin. As Avery Gordon perceives in her discussion of Bambara's utopianism, 'To want to be free, you have to live and act as if you are free to live, right now, right this minute, in the midst of all the life-threatening forces arrayed and ready at hand.' Likewise, to be well now does not involve denying the sickness of the world as it is, but it does require acting as if the revolution is here. According to Gordon, the relay between past and present in *The Salt Eaters*, alongside the relationship between individual and collective in the healing process, 'produces that abolitionist time of both acute patience and urgency'.[83] Sustaining an engagement in political movements demands patient urgency. For Gordon, drawing on the internationalist work of Angela Y. Davis, in order to abolish 'police power and the carceral state . . . it is necessary to eliminate the political, social and economic conditions that produce it'. Abolitionist time for Gordon is also a time of mutuality and interconnection, which are necessary for healing.

Contemporary abolitionist political organising against the carceral state is committed to 'non-reformist reform', a concept – introduced by André Gorz and elaborated by Ruth Wilson Gilmore – intended to transform the totality rather than 'tweak Armageddon'. The immediate scattered tasks implied by such organising require patience, take time and work 'from the ground up', even as their ultimate goals acknowledge the scale and scope of the systems they seek to dismantle. As Gilmore explains:

Big problems require big solutions. Nothing happens all at once; big answers are the painstaking accumulation of smaller achievements. But dividing a problem into pieces in order to solve the whole thing is altogether different from defining a problem solely in terms of the bits that seem easiest to fix.

A vision of the whole, an affirmation of attaining wholeness, is necessary because 'the structural effect of everyday political disintegration is fatal'.[84] However slow and piecemeal its gains, non-reformist reform proceeds from the assumption that abolition is possible and has that as its ultimate horizon. It begins from the whole. An analogous contradictory temporality, an analogous affirmation of possible wholeness and thus of possible healing, animates *The Salt Eaters*. Healing is urgent because healed people are needed to fight injustice, but healing, like the fight for justice itself, takes time.

Naomi's statement about the revolution existing in the present tense and the contradictory temporality Gordon identifies in Bambara's work recalls an argument made in 1958 by C. L. R. James, Grace Lee Boggs and others in *Facing Reality*. (Boggs later contributed an essay to Bambara's 1970 collection *The Black Woman* and both women had an involvement with the Institute of the Black World, which was based in Atlanta in the 1970s.)[85] Unlike many on the Western left who responded to Nikita Khrushchev's so-called 'secret speech' denouncing Stalin and to the Soviet crushing of the Hungarian uprising in 1956 by losing their faith in the revolutionary project, *Facing Reality* does not look to theoretical understandings of vanguardist parties but relates the events in Hungary to the immediate material situation of workers in the authors' own context in Detroit. They discern socialism right there on the shop floor: 'In the factories workers develop methods and forms of cooperation, of mutual help and solidarity, of organization, which *already anticipate socialist relations*.' Their searing attack on party-bound, jargon-spouting revolutionaries obsessed with class struggle in theory but detached from it in practice, describes the weariness that rigid forms of political engagement have produced and, as in Coles's essay, identifies a tendency for frustrations to turn inwards:

> Tens of thousands of devoted fighters for socialism have exhausted themselves and ended their struggles in disillusionment, often in bitterness, and not infrequently in the most savage hatred of all that they had for decades given their lives to.[86]

The conflict between social struggle and weariness is a conflict between urgency and patience. Ultimately, and paradoxically, Bambara shows that the former *requires* the latter. As she already perceived in her 1970 essay 'On the Issue of Roles':

> It may be lonely. Certainly painful. It'll take time. We've got time. That of course is an unpopular utterance these days. Instant coffee is the hallmark of current rhetoric. But we do have time. We'd better take the time to fashion revolutionary selves, revolutionary lives, revolutionary relationships.[87]

In the face of exploitation, dispossession, pervasive injustice, state violence, war and climate breakdown, time might seem like the last thing many people have. Focusing on individual well-being can seem paltry, luxurious or even decadent in the face of the dangers unevenly threatening communities around the world, but revolutionary selves are needed to make revolution. The urgency of revolution conflicts with the patience required to perform spade work or to fashion a self. It is exhausting! Bambara perceived that the urgent demands of political struggles will never be met if time isn't taken to fashion revolutionary selves. Such fashioning is not a process of creation *ex nihilo*; it requires ongoing and collective processes of reflection, care and healing. Indeed, as Akwugo Emejulu suggested in the wake of the George Floyd rebellions in 2020, exhaustion itself 'is a praxis' and can be a ground for forging solidarity: 'If you're tired of the way things are that means you understand that things can be different. Through a haze of exhaustion, you glimpse another world.'[88]

6

Bitterness

Revolutionaries must remain human throughout their struggle. Otherwise, what kind of revolution would these angry, repressed people make? Whom would it serve?[1]

– Vivian Gornick

I want to begin with three vignettes.

Japan, 1972 – Members of the United Red Army retreat to mountain bases to hide and train for future militant actions. The group engages in regular sessions that fuse *jikohihan* (self-criticism) with *sôkatsu* (collective examination of organisational problems), in which they attack one another for anything perceived as demonstrating lingering bourgeois attitudes: for seeking bodily comfort or pleasure, for pursuing romantic relationships, for expressing emotional needs or physical desires, for paying too much attention to clothing or appearances. These sessions eventually escalate to physical beatings. When the first member of the group dies as a result of a beating, it is framed as failure at self-critique. Ultimately, twelve members of the group are tortured and killed. The group's leader Tsuneo Mori proclaims: 'If one were serious about becoming a revolutionary soldier, one would not die.'[2]

England, 1974 – A group of twelve women aged between seventeen and thirty-eight meet weekly at each other's houses in South London for a consciousness-raising session. Each woman speaks in turn about her personal life, uninterrupted. After a break for tea, the group discusses general themes arising from the individual testimonies, pulling out common threads to better understand how women are systematically oppressed in a patriarchal society. Over many sessions they talk about their bodies, their friendships with other women, their emotions, their orgasms, their sexual relationships, their childhoods. Sometimes they meet socially to go to a sauna or go out dancing.[3]

People's Democratic Republic of Yemen (South Yemen), 1978 – At a school in the desert, students, teachers and other school workers gather for a 'criticism-self-criticism' session. Practical and logistical problems are raised. Teachers respond to the concerns of students and commit to addressing them. A student criticises his schoolmate for playing football while sick. The accused child stands and admits that he did this because he was feeling frustration at being stuck inside. He then offers a criticism of himself, promising not to do it again.[4]

In reminiscences about his involvement in Students for a Democratic Society (SDS) in New Orleans in the late sixties and early seventies, Eric A. Gordon recalls keeping his psychoanalytic sessions a secret from his comrades, whom he feared would see them as a 'bourgeois indulgence'. People in his activist circles expressed concerns that analysts might divulge details revealed in sessions that could endanger lives or undermine attempts to organise. He also expressed a wariness about his analyst's approach to psychic life, which he felt traced the origins of all mental problems back to some individual failing rather than locating them in society's ills. Years later he concluded that 'by leaving the collective outside and behind [psychoanalysis] was untenable and likely to fail'. He cut off the analysis when faced with a conflict between his session and a political meeting. When his analyst refused to reschedule, they argued and he quit. Gordon chose political engagement over therapy because he felt that the latter functioned by encouraging patients to adjust to and accept the society that had produced their misery in the first place: 'Really, what is there to be happy about if happiness means a healthy adaptation to the world around you?'[5] But as the three geographically disparate scenes above indicate, this kind of rejection of therapy by people involved in social movements in the sixties and seventies did not necessarily mean giving up on psychic work altogether. Instead, it often involved developing alternative sets of practices explicitly aimed at transforming subjectivity as part of a struggle to transform society.

The three vignettes with which I began have, on the surface, little in common, and in actuality they had wildly divergent intentions and outcomes, but they all share origins in communist self-criticism practices and Maoist practices of 'speaking bitterness'. This chapter does not claim that the sources of these practices were anything other than overdetermined, nor does it attempt anything as synoptic or satisfying as a genealogy of 'criticism-self-criticism'.[6] It instead begins by looking at an outsider's account of practices in one village in China in the 1940s, which influenced two distinct kinds of small group practice developed in the

US in the late 1960s. How did these different examples conceptualise the connection between personal and political change?

Unlike this book's preceding chapters, which explore concepts with particular meanings in the psy-disciplines, this chapter examines practices and theories of subjective transformation that emerged from political movements, asking how people within those milieus understood mental life and exploring conflicts that arose between their ideals and realities. The tension between urgency and patience that identified in the previous chapter's discussion of exhaustion also runs through this chapter, which explores how urgent quests for immediate subjective purity were forced to contend patiently with the often slow pace of individual transformation and deal with behaviour that did not rigidly conform with a particular revolutionary line. This tension is not unique to the historical examples discussed here but represents a familiar and recurrent conundrum: it's hard to change.

Left-wing political groups often reproduce the structural issues and prejudices – racism, sexism, ableism, homophobia, transphobia, class divisions – of the societies they want to transform. People fall out for both profound and petty reasons. Abuse and bullying are depressingly commonplace in groups, parties and organisations whose stated principles directly contradict such behaviour.[7] People formed by their experiences in this world are likely to find it difficult to act as if they were formed by a different one, but rejecting the possibility of individual transformation is tantamount to claiming that all social transformation is impossible. Can personal desires that do not directly contribute to revolutionary struggles be fulfilled within or alongside those struggles? Can political movements make space for psychic ambivalence, inconsistency and contradiction rather than viewing them as antithetical to their goals? How much and how quickly can people change? And how much advance personal change is necessary to change the world politically?

Modes of self-criticism, subjective interrogation and consciousness-raising developed as part of political struggles and social movements were not conceived as therapeutic practices – indeed, their proponents sometimes explicitly defined them in opposition to therapy – but they nonetheless situated individual transformation at the heart of political organising and made assumptions about the structure of psychic life. In theory, such methods were intended to address the question of how individuals shaped by an oppressive society could change themselves to avoid reproducing those societies' worst aspects. Their practitioners sought, moreover, to identify the social origins of individual behaviour. In contrast to the adaptative therapeutic approaches that Gordon associated with the psychoanalytic 'talking cure', these methods instead had the aim of making people 'better' in a moral or political rather than an emotional or medical sense. By rejecting existing social structures, the people that engaged in self-critical or self-reflective political practices sought to achieve a kind of dis- or anti-adaptation – widening rather than narrowing the distance between the individual and their environment – a process that would make the destruction of those structures easier for that individual to accomplish. What were the psychic consequences of attempts to embody the change people wanted to see in the world when they were still within that world? More concerned with transforming external reality than with healing internal reality, these practices sometimes increased interpersonal tensions within groups and created their own psychic wounds, impeding the struggles they had been designed to further.

Peeling artichokes

Under a grey sky, on the morning of 10 April 1948, a group of around thirty elected delegates gathered in the main street of the village of Long Bow (Zhangzhuangcun) in the Shanxi Province of Northern China to launch a campaign to 'purify' the ranks of the local Communist Party. Surrounded by a crowd of cheerful adults and children, they marched through the streets shouting slogans, until they reached a bare district office whose window frames had long since been removed for firewood. They swarmed into the building chaotically, joining the party members awaiting appraisal. After bowing three times before a poster of Chairman Mao, the communists burst into an enthusiastic, if faltering and discordant, rendition of the *Internationale*; others joined in as best they could despite not necessarily knowing the words. In this tightly packed room, as grey as the sky beyond, peasants from the village – representatives of the people, the masses – confronted Communist Party members, having been invited to participate in the self- and mutual criticism meetings that members of the party ordinarily conducted among themselves.

These events and the ensuing discussions are recounted in William Hinton's *Fanshen*, based on research conducted in 1948. *Fanshen* treated the village of Long Bow as a microcosm of a rapidly transforming society, taking its title from a word meaning 'to turn over' that took on special significance in the revolutionary context. In his preface Hinton writes that the revolutionary processes then unfolding in China 'remade not only the material life of the people, but also their consciousness'.[8] For Hinton, the longevity and strength of the revolution depended as much on this internal transformation of subjectivity as they did on dramatic external changes like land reform; the transformation of society would go hand in hand with the transformation of human consciousness.

The party's Constitution of May 1945 stipulated that party members should 'endeavour to raise the level of [their] consciousness', which meant not only mastering the key tenets of Marxist-Leninism but also uprooting the kinds of individualism or 'subjectivism' instilled by growing up in a society run in the interests of profit-driven landlords. This remoulding of subjectivity would not happen automatically or overnight; processes of public scrutiny and reflection, like self- and mutual criticism sessions or 'speak bitterness meetings', were intended to facilitate the incremental changes in the mind deemed necessary to build a communist society and instil the correct line.[9] Speaking in 1942, Mao used a medical metaphor to convey the purpose of criticising others in a manner that would ideally enable people to acknowledge, learn from and overcome their past errors:

> So long as a person who has made mistakes does not hide his sickness for fear of treatment or persist in his mistakes until he is beyond cure, so long as he honestly and sincerely wishes to be cured and to mend his ways, we should welcome him and cure his sickness so that he can become a good comrade. We can never succeed if we just let ourselves go, and lash out at him. In treating an ideological or a political malady, one must never be rough and rash but must adopt the approach of 'curing the sickness to save the patient', which is the only correct and effective method.[10]

Political maladies required delicate treatments, but they could be cured as long as the patient was willing to undergo the necessary operations. Recovery was an act of will.

Hinton described the purification meetings that he witnessed in Long Bow as dramatic and democratic, taking 'on the proportions of a truly mass movement' by enabling people from the village to voice their grievances and take on an active political role by engaging with the party. Party members were called upon to give sincere accounts of their class backgrounds, and they confessed to such social transgressions as committing violence against others (including their wives), stealing, hiding personal property and acting in their own or their families' interests. One member was severely upbraided for admitting to secretly eating a bun from a pile of buns he was supposed to deliver to workers in the fields. The explanation that he was hungry was deemed insufficient by the delegates. According to Hinton some people wept or expressed fear and guilt during these confessional sessions, but he also describes moments of laughter and jollity. This intimate process, involving individuals revealing personal infractions and imperfections in a room in a small village, was embedded in the much larger and longer process of the revolution:

> In the agony of public self-examination, they were forced to face up to their weaknesses, to ask themselves fundamental questions concerning their character and their intentions, and to make important decisions about the future. Under fire for every lapse, every weakness, they began to catch a glimpse of the Revolution as 'the hundred year task' that Chairman Mao had so often called it, rather than a great upheaval impetuously entered into and soon completed.

Hinton goes on to recount mass meetings that took place throughout spring 1948, in which dejected cadres turned from logistical problems to personal or interpersonal issues that precluded them from working well together. A long period of self-examination and internal discussion was judged worthwhile. Cadres assumed that without working to expose the group's 'inner contradictions', the contradictions structuring society could never be addressed:

> If each individual could be granted ample time to think through his own problems, make clear his own thoughts and attitudes, his own reservations, his own gripes, he might then be able to formulate, isolate, and finally lay aside the burdens that distracted him and wore down his energies.[11]

This discussion was envisaged as cathartic: through the process of self-examination, difficulties that were holding back the group could come to the surface and be dispelled.

People were asked to speak sincerely and not suppress their feelings, in an attempt to address the atmosphere of gloom that had descended upon them. The Long Bow cadre embarked on a self- and mutual criticism session that continued into the night, taking only brief breaks to eat. The meeting, in which participants often struggled to reach firm conclusions, was not only long but emotionally arduous, punctuated by sighs: 'To dig beneath the surface, to expose what one truly thought about oneself and about others was always difficult, often extremely painful; yet it had become as necessary as breathing.' The difficult process of airing grievances and collectively discussing subjective responses to shared experiences may not have immediately solved concrete problems, but, according to Hinton, the group 'began to pull together . . . It seemed as if the mere exposure of trouble had brought about a changed relationship between people.'[12] Through sharing, reflecting on and contextualising personal weaknesses, mutual sympathy arose in the place of hostility. The meeting ended by focusing on the leader, allowing people to express their frustrations with him and enabling him to respond, with the effect of dispelling feelings of bitterness being harboured towards him.

The psychic barriers that self- and mutual criticism sought to overcome are conveyed in *Fanshen* by way of a vegetal metaphor:

> The human consciousness may be compared to an artichoke. Its tender core is enclosed in layer upon layer of defences, excuses, rationalisations, approximations. These must be peeled off if one is to discover the true complex of motives driving any individual. Such a process would hardly be possible if an individual's acts, as distinct from his words, did not reveal in a multitude of unconscious ways something of the core of his thought.

Crucially for Hinton, as Mao's works also made clear, the success of the method depended on the participants' attitude towards it – their 'deep commitment' to the land reform movement led them to enter 'freely' into the process: 'This, not coercion, not curiosity, not some narcissistic self-torture made self-and-mutual criticism viable and grounded it in necessity.'[13] Hinton's artichoke metaphor is written in an almost psychoanalytic register, invoking drives and the unconscious, but in this passage the method's success is predicated on the participants' openness to undergoing it. Conscious will was needed to overcome habitual acts.

This process of self- and mutual criticism among the cadres led, in Hinton's account, to 'tolerance and understanding', but he noted that the behaviour it entailed did not come easily to the participants because it was inconsistent with their traditional cultural mores. He was impressed not only by the objectivity the process required and the openness to change it demanded but also by the ability of participants to express criticisms in such a way as to 'raise others up, not knock them down'. But in the succeeding months he also witnessed more psychologically corrosive aspects of the process, as enthusiasm gave way to exhaustion, ennui and apathy. He quotes one person reflecting in visceral language on how the exposing experience of self- and mutual criticism had made him think poorly of himself:

> Before the purification we never thought much, but now I feel as if I were a person full of scabs, scars and lumps. In the past others didn't know my faults, but now they are revealed for all to see, and it's hard to go forward.[14]

Here scabs, scars and lumps are described as having been revealed by the process, but such accounts also gesture towards the possibility that self- and mutual criticism may have also *created* scabs, scars and lumps of its own. Could a process intended to heal the wounds inflicted by an exploitative system also inflict wounds in its own right?

Hinton reflected that the scenes he had witnessed between cadres and villagers were different to the processes that took place solely among party members because the latter were well-versed in politics. As such, he attributed the psychic toll the experiences had on some peasants to their 'unskilled application' of the method rather than to the method itself; only a bad workman blames his tools. The practice of self- and mutual criticism may have been designed to participate in transforming people's consciousnesses, but this implies that it was only effective on people whose consciousnesses were already in the process of being transformed. For those new to the practice it was much more difficult. Simply participating in such sessions was only the beginning; learning to navigate them successfully required skill, which took time and patience to acquire:

> They had little or no experience with the kind of limited struggle necessary for solving problems that arose among the people. Uncompromising struggle against class and national enemies they knew well. Close unity with friends and relatives they also knew. But how to struggle and unite simultaneously, how to deepen unity through struggle and unite simultaneously, how to conquer weaknesses with criticism, how to exorcise the bad in friends and allies while developing the good – all this had to be learned.[15]

The difficult question Hinton identified – how to struggle and unite simultaneously – articulates one of *Burnout*'s animating questions: how to fight while healing? The group discussions Hinton analyses deliberately fostered interpersonal discord and encouraged self-reproach. How could solidarity grow from something that was so internally riven and had such splintering effects? In Hinton's account, the question of how to participate effectively in such sessions without acquiring scabs, scars and lumps along the way remains unanswered.

Stormy weather

Though based on observations made in one village at the end of the Chinese Civil War that preceded the foundation of the People's Republic of China in 1949, *Fanshen* was published almost twenty years later, in 1966 – the first year of the Cultural Revolution. US customs officers had seized Hinton's notes, along with his passport, at the height of the McCarthyite 'red scare', and they were only returned to him in 1958 after a protracted legal battle.[16] The book's delayed publication led to its belated reception, which coincided not only with the Cultural Revolution but also with mounting opposition to the American war in Vietnam in the West.[17] Edgar Snow's *Red Star Over China* (1937) had introduced an affable and magnetic-seeming Mao to a global audience in the aftermath of the Long March, whereas Hinton's book, which sold hundreds of thousands of copies and was translated into ten languages, introduced a distant political experiment to a new generation of young radicals in the sixties and seventies.[18] The next sections of this chapter discuss two very different self-critical practices, partly inspired by Hinton's accounts of self- and mutual criticism in Long Bow, developed within two contemporaneous milieus that emerged from the anti-war movement in the US: the criticism-self-criticism sessions undergone by members of the militant group the Weather Underground, and the consciousness-raising practices developed in the women's liberation movement.

During the Korean War a sinister image of China's methods of psychological manipulation and thought reform emerged in US discourse, described as 'brainwashing' by the American journalist Edward Hunter.[19] Anxieties about Chinese techniques for controlling people's minds came to influence US counterintelligence tactics in the Cold War though the historical realities of thought reform differed from these caricatures.[20] Similarly the small group practices adopted by Western European and US revolutionaries inspired by accounts like Hinton's were far removed from Chinese experiences and *Fanshen* was not their only source of inspiration, but they nonetheless developed practices that took on lives of their own within their own contexts.[21]

Hinton's accounts of problems encountered in daily life among peasants in Long Bow were combined with the US New Left's interest in the tactics of guerrillas in Guatemala and elsewhere. Such internationalist engagements were tied to a broader political identification with anti-imperialist struggles in the Third World and opposition to the US's ongoing war in Vietnam.[22] In a speech in 1967, SDS national secretary Greg Calvert began by describing, in terms that echoed Hinton's accounts of Long Bow, meetings between villagers and guerrilla forces in Guatemala. According to Calvert, rather than bombarding villagers with political slogans and theoretical lessons in Marxist-Leninism, the guerrillas instead gathered them together and talked to them about their own lives, describing 'how they see themselves and how they came to be who they are, about their deepest longings and the things they've striven for and hoped for, about the way in which their deepest longings were frustrated by the society in which they live'. They would then invite the villagers to share their own experiences, with the result that: 'People who thought that their deepest problems and frustrations were their individual problems discover that their problems and longings are all the same.'[23] Discussing individual issues helped identify their social underpinnings, which could then form the basis for collective political action.

In his memoir reflecting on his involvement in the Weathermen, renamed the Weather Underground in 1970, the militant anti-imperialist revolutionary group who split from SDS with the intention of dedicating themselves to supporting the black liberation movement in the US through guerrilla combat, Mark Rudd cites *Fanshen* as the major source of inspiration for the criticism-self-criticism sessions that were central to the organisation.[24] Former Weatherman Cathy Wilkerson recalled being so inspired by Mao's *Little Red Book*, which was at that time the most printed book in the world, that she enthusiastically recommended to her friends and comrades the section titled 'Criticism-Self-Criticism', in which Mao likens regular criticism to routinely cleaning dust from a room.[25] She and her comrades saw the youthful Red Guards in China as an antidote to ossified Stalinist orthodoxy (presumably unaware that criticism and self-criticism had Bolshevik origins and that Stalin himself advocated self-criticism): 'It didn't occur to any of us that the noble, youthful impulse to fight corruption would soon, for a variety of reasons, metamorphose into a degenerative zealotry.'[26] Far from the Chinese peasants and party members described by Hinton, the Weather Underground were mostly white, middle-class, university-educated young people based in cities, intent on destroying the racist society of which they were a product. Their criticism-self-criticism practices were most intense during the period between their split from the SDS in 1969 and the townhouse fire of March 1970, in which three members of the group accidentally blew themselves up while building a bomb in Greenwich Village, after which surviving members of the organisation went underground. During this period, members of the group swore to dedicate themselves to the revolution and were living in collectives, eating oats and sleeping in sleeping bags, sometimes in conditions so sparse and ascetic it made many of them physically ill.

Writing in winter 1969, Weatherman Shin'ya Ono argued that the criticism-self-criticism sessions undertaken by the organisation to transform their minds were just as important as their engagements in struggles on the streets; the latter depended on the former.[27] Bill Ayers described the sessions as a core part of their daily schedules: 'We criticized ourselves for not doing enough . . . We jogged. We marched. We drilled. More criticism. Organize, fight, practice, criticize. Criticism and self-criticism.'[28] The sessions tended to be harsh, intense, gruelling and very, very long, sometimes lasting an entire day. A selected individual would spend hours being berated mercilessly, often by their closest friends or lovers. Participants were also frequently on speed or LSD during the sessions, drugs that were understood to reduce inhibitions, adding further to their intensity.[29] Sometimes they would take place immediately after a demonstration or encounter with the cops. Susan Stern recalled being subjected to criticism-self-criticism when she was still concussed after being beaten by the police the day before.[30]

As with sessions undertaken by the United Red Army in Japan, the Weathermen's criticism-self-criticism sessions identified behaviours associated with the internalisation of oppressive social attitudes stemming from the dominant society: racism ('white skin privilege'), misogyny ('male chauvinism/supremacy'), class privilege and individualism. Tangled up with these attempts to transform consciousness was the group's campaign to 'smash monogamy', which forcibly broke up couples and encouraged casual sex with multiple partners, in an effort to overcome individualism and challenge the patriarchal norms of bourgeois society.[31] Bill Ayers recalled: 'Smashing monogamy took a lot of energy – it was part of the political line to renounce all the habits and cultural constraints of the past . . . you were supposed to fuck no matter what.'[32]

In criticism-self-criticism the person singled out for attack might be castigated for their romantic or interpersonal behaviour within the group, for showing fear of the police during demonstrations or for perceived timidity when out leafletting. Ayers, who claimed that in the sessions 'the collective assumed the stance of an eagerly policing superego', was denounced as a 'liberal creep' for admitting to liking the poem by Bertolt Brecht that forms the epigraph to this book, 'which pleaded that future generations "judge not too harshly" the necessarily harsh actions of revolutionaries'.[33] Jonathan Lerner, who was also subjected to the process, recalled that: 'Whatever you'd said would be picked apart – along with your self-esteem – and you were expected to recant, repent, and parrot back the right phraseology.'[34] At the end of the session the person being interrogated would be expected to recant and demonstrate their commitment to restructuring their thought or they would be purged.

Although the purges that resulted from the sessions were credited with ridding the organisation of FBI informants, first-hand accounts of criticism-self-criticism sessions unanimously suggest that they inflicted serious psychological damage on participants, rather than transforming people's consciousnesses in more positive ways.[35] But former Weather Underground members' memoirs, in which these sessions are inveighed against, could be read as continuations of the process of self-criticism rather than its abnegation. The genre conventions of self-criticism texts in the organisation's pamphlets, position papers or communiques demanded a strident and polemical rhetorical tone, but though the memoirs abandon stridency and allow for equivocation, they nonetheless evince a similar urge to reassess past actions, to assign guilt, to identify forks in the road, to confess mistakes.[36] The memoirists do not reflect explicitly on this irony: the very act of writing an individual account of the group seems to perform a function that criticism-self-criticism sessions might have fulfilled had they been capable of addressing perceived infractions or imperfections with less uncompromising harshness. The memoirs denounce a denunciatory practice while practicing a non-collective version of it, enacting in print the kind of empathetic self-criticism the organisation failed to practice at the time but for which many former members retrospectively expressed a desire.

If Hinton's artichoke metaphor pictured self- and mutual criticism in Long Bow as facilitating a process that peeled back psychic defences in order to reveal a person's hidden core, the Weather Underground instead demanded the overcoming of perceived weaknesses and timidity, particularly in relation to violence, with the aim of psychically hardening participants. But they didn't just create hard shells; they tried to replace their vulnerable, organic flesh with hard metal. They wanted to become tools of the revolution – 'a saw, a rasp, a clawbar, a hammer' – and tools have no psychic lives. Far from encouraging mutual understanding, the sessions seemed designed to push people to castigate themselves for weaknesses assumed to have arisen from their upbringings and class positions, with the intention of toughening them up to commit selfless acts on behalf of the revolution:

> We had to be stronger, we told ourselves, more selfless, uncompromising. We had to combat liberalism with a revolutionary political line, oppose idealistic foolishness and sentimentalism with hard materialist reality. We had to stomp out anything that might cloud our steely-eyed judgment in combat. We had to toughen up, and quick.[37]

But isn't materialist reality also soft? Can the harshness and violence of life under capitalism only be destroyed by matching them? Can anyone really become completely hammer-like and unfeeling? What kind of society does this valorisation of hardness portend?

Criticism-self-criticism became the psychic equivalent of the groups' karate and weapons training activities that focused on developing physical strength, endurance and skill. Historian Jeremy Varon characterises the events as 'part political trial, part hazing, part shock therapy', with the effect of increasing hostility, fear and suspicion between people in the group, as well as heightening their senses of self-doubt.[38] David Gilbert remarked on the gap between the theoretical ideas and historical precedents that had inspired the process and its practical application, which, even years later, he still attributed to the participants having been psychologically shaped by an individualistic and competitive society which made them incapable of entering into the sessions in a caring and constructive manner. Like Hinton, he did not identify anything inherently cruel in the method itself.[39] But if the point of the process was to help people cast off habits of thought and behaviour instilled by the society they had grown up in, then this observation is a contradiction in terms.

In *The Hundred Day War: The Cultural Revolution at Tsinghua University*, based on observations made twenty years after *Fanshen*, Hinton traces the bitter disputes between warring factions at a Chinese university that played out in summer 1968. In the book's introduction he warns US radicals about the allure of ultraleftism, which he distinguishes from Mao Zedong Thought and from the actions of workers, cautioning against '"I am the core" thinking, which maintains that I and my group are the real revolutionaries while people with other ideas, or people who have come to the same ideas at a later date, really don't deserve consideration as comrades'.[40] Following the disaster of the townhouse fire, members of the Weather Underground reflected on their commitment to armed struggle and came to similar conclusions regarding their dogmatic inflexibility and asceticism. At a retreat in a coastal hippie town in northern California to discuss strategy in April 1970, they agreed to shift their focus to 'armed propaganda', targeting property rather than people, expelling John Jacobs, who continued to advocate for 'armed squads'.[41] The tone and length of their criticism-self-criticism sessions changed as a result and collectives placed more emphasis on supporting one another as the organisation went underground.

Hinton describes the tendency of ultra-leftists to isolate themselves from others, but the problem of the 'later date' he identifies, the fact that it takes time to acquire political ideas and to cast off habits of behaviour, could also describe the issue that arose *within* criticism-self-criticism sessions, narrowing the core still further. The problem the Weathermen encountered during their most militant phase was that people were always lagging behind revolutionary ideals, dooming any form of political change from the start. It was always already too late to be a perfect revolutionary.

Consciousness sinking

The phrase 'the personal is political' is now so familiar that it has the ring of platitude, but like a fraying, well-worn garment it was once crisp and new. In her 1969 paper, which was given the title 'The Personal Is Political' by editors Shulamith Firestone and Anne Koedt when it was published in *Notes from the Second Year: Women's Liberation* the following year, Carol Hanisch argued that the consciousness-raising undertaken in feminist groups was distinct from conventional therapy because it proceeded from the assumption that the only possible 'cure' to the problems identified in their discussions would be a total social transformation.[42] Unlike therapy, she contended, consciousness-raising was not concerned with helping participants to adjust so they could function within the existing structures of society. Instead, the personal experiences discussed in consciousness-raising groups allowed participants to identify shared forms of oppression, which could become the basis for future action.

Hanisch presented consciousness-raising as part of the means of women's liberation, not as an end in itself. She was clear that recognising that women's personal experiences were tied to common social structures was only the beginning. Acting together to change those conditions was what distinguished these discussions from conventional therapy: 'One of the first things we discover in these groups is that personal problems are political problems. There are no personal solutions at this time. There is only collective action for a collective solution.'[43] Though the phrase 'the personal is political' retains a certain ambiguity that lends itself to liberal readings, Hanisch did not argue that a personal transformation constituted a political transformation in and of itself.

Anne Forer Pyne recalled that the practice of consciousness-raising began in 1967 at a meeting of a group that would become New York Radical Women; the term 'consciousness' came from the Old Left and was connected to the notion of class consciousness and the emerging understanding of women as a distinct oppressed group. Hanisch later claimed that *Fanshen*, introduced to New York Radical Women by Kathie Sarachild, also provided a model for consciousness-raising.[44] Sarachild had been active in the civil rights movement in Mississippi and cited the practice of 'telling it like it is' as another key source of inspiration.[45] On the wall of their meetings in the late sixties hung a poster emblazoned with the slogans 'Tell It Like It Is' and 'Speak Pains to Recall Pains', as Hanisch recalled:

> It was our way of acknowledging and uniting with those who taught and inspired us. It was also our response to those who called our meetings petty and unpolitical and group therapy. Like the peasants of Long Bow, we "spoke pains to recall pains" to examine our lives—to get at the truth of who was oppressing us and how—so we could better figure out what to do about it.[46]

Irene Peslikis, a member of Redstockings, a group which formed after the breakup of New York Radical Women in early 1969, blamed 'anti-woman sentiment' for leading people to dismiss consciousness-raising as therapy and to overlook its similarities to small group practices undertaken in other contexts: 'When women get together to study and analyze their own experience it means they are sick but when Chinese peasants or Guatemalan guerillas get together and use the identical method they are revolutionary.'[47]

Such was the influence of Hinton's book on the movement in the US that a collective in Seattle even gave themselves the name 'Fanshen Women'.[48] *Fanshen* was also cited as an influence by people involved in the women's liberation movements in Britain, France and West Germany.⁴⁹ In *Women's Estate* (1971), British feminist Juliet Mitchell described consciousness-raising as a 'reinterpretation of a Chinese revolutionary practice of "speaking bitterness"' and argued that articulating problems collectively enabled the identification of forms of oppression and injustice that had previously seemed 'natural':

> The first symptom of oppression is the repression of words; the state of suffering is so total and so assumed that it is not known to be there. 'Speaking bitterness' is the bringing to consciousness of the virtually unconscious oppression.⁵⁰

Hinton's descriptions of 'speaking pains to recall pains' occur in passages of *Fanshen* dedicated to the Women's Association in Long Bow in which peasant women 'voice[d] their own bitterness' and encouraged others to do the same, revealing cruel treatment at the hands of their husbands in the process and encountering hostility from men who opposed the meetings that strengthened their solidarity. In *Fanshen,* the verbal sharing of experiences was a preface to action: 'Words soon led to deeds.' Identifying and sharing grievances prompted peasant women to act together to resist male violence. As a group they confronted a violent husband who was angry that his wife attended meetings with the Women's Association. When he expressed no regret, they beat him up. After this protest he promised never to hurt his wife again and this served as a lesson to other men in the village: 'Having once shown their power the women did not have to beat every man in order to make progress on this question.'⁵¹

I have no intention of attempting to gloss or relitigate the vast and complex literature on feminist consciousness-raising here – how groups spread, how the practice morphed, how some rejected consciousness-raising as apolitical while others went on to develop distinctly feminist therapeutic practices, how splits emerged in the movement over time and so on. I will simply note that many first-hand retrospective accounts of the movement take a similar shape: they describe initial encounters with consciousness-raising groups as euphoric, uplifting and transformative before reflecting on the emergence of interpersonal antagonisms, splits and increasingly dogmatic behaviour that arose between women in the movement.⁵² The tension between emancipatory euphoria and corrosive dogmatism, as with that between solidarity and suspicion, is often narrated as a linear trajectory, even if many friendships outlasted the movement to endure over decades.

In 'TRASHING: The Dark Side of Sisterhood', first published in *Ms.* magazine in 1976, Jo Freeman – whose 'Tyranny of Structurelessness' (first delivered as a paper in 1970) remains a touchstone for understanding how toxicity and hierarchies can emerge in supposedly anti-hierarchical political groups – reflected on the animosity she experienced in the Chicago Westside Group that led her to drop out of the movement in 1969.[53] She recounted the 'numb despair' and sense of isolation that followed: 'I felt psychologically mangled to the point where I knew I couldn't go on.' Though she initially understood her experiences in individual terms, she gradually came to see trashing as a widespread phenomenon within the movement, one that had shared causes and specific targets. She encountered other women who had had similar experiences: 'With each new story, my conviction grew that trashing was not an individual problem brought on by individual actions; nor was it a result of political conflicts between those of differing ideas: It was a social disease.'[54]

Consciousness-raising sessions allowed women to discover that experiences assumed to be personal were shared and grounded in systemic forms of oppression. Freeman's analysis of trashing claims that it too was animated by a relationship between the individual and the social but, emerging from within the very groups that had come together to organise collectively against the patriarchy, its structural causes were disavowed rather than acknowledged, and the societal forces that underpinned it as a phenomenon, ignored.[55] Women who could not remould themselves quickly enough were often trashed.

Freeman takes trashing as evidence of a failure of women in the movement to overcome the social norms they attacked. She defines the practice as a 'traditional' form that, far from practising the revolutionary rhetoric it preached, fell back on conventional understandings of women's social roles:

> There is nothing new about discouraging women from stepping out of place by the use of psychological manipulation. This is one of the things that have kept women down for years; it is one thing that feminism was supposed to liberate us from. Yet, instead of an alternative culture with alternative values, we have created alternative means of enforcing the traditional culture and values.[56]

Freeman argues that the movement's emphasis on the personal as a political realm ironically enabled trashing to take hold as if it were a legitimate feminist praxis that sought to transform both people and the world, when in reality it encouraged dogmatism, made individual women feel terrible about themselves and tore apart a collective movement. She identifies an impatience with the pace of social transformation as one of the causes of trashing: women were criticised for not having already become their ideal feminist selves, as if they could immediately undo years of patriarchal oppression through an act of will.[57]

Embodied gaps

Vivian Gornick, who reported for the *Village Voice* on early meetings of New York Radical Women (attended by both Kate Millett and Shulamith Firestone) and soon became swept up in the movement, described the emotions associated with those early years of collective discovery as not primarily personal but interpersonal:

> I stood in the middle of my own experience, turning and turning. In every direction I saw a roomful of women, also turning and turning. That is a moment of joy, when a sufficiently large number of people are galvanized by a social explanation of how their lives have taken shape, and are gathered together in the same place at the same time, speaking the same language, making the same analysis, meeting again and again . . . It is the joy of revolutionary politics, and it was ours. To be a feminist in the early seventies – bliss was it in that dawn to be alive.[58]

But Gornick also identified a disavowed conflict that emerged 'between the ardor of our revolutionary rhetoric and the dictates of flesh-and-blood reality . . . nearly every one of us became a walking embodiment of the gap between theory and practice'.[59] The strangeness of this metaphor – how can anyone embody a gap? – articulates the problem that recurs through Weather Underground memoirs recounting experiences of criticism-self-criticism. The activists had a clear and rigid vision of how the world should be and of how they needed to think and behave in order to achieve that world. They created groups that were in some ways prefigurative, organised in ways that differed from the societies in which they were formed, but personal transformation could not happen fast enough. They could not tolerate the fact their desires sometimes contradicted their precepts. They not only enacted their theoretical positions but strove to become fully identical to them, as if they could undo their own previous experiences, as if they could un-live in society. They could not tolerate a gap between theory and practice; they could not tolerate their embodied selves.

In a new introduction to the reissue of her 1977 book *The Romance of American Communism*, based on oral history interviews conducted in the mid-1970s with former members of the Communist Party USA, Gornick recalled that witnessing the emergence of dogmatic behaviour at a feminist meeting at which she was accused of being 'an intellectual and a revisionist' prompted her to revisit the communist milieu of her youth so as to examine the contradictory ways people lived their intensely felt political commitments within ideological constraints.[60] Greeted with disdain by contemporary reviewers who mocked Gornick's florid emotive style and accused her of trivialising Stalinism, *The Romance of American Communism* approached the history of the CPUSA by focusing on affective attachments and passionate feelings. Countering stereotypical representations of communists as soulless grey automatons, she turned instead to examine the 'impulse, need, fear, doubt, and longing' that she associated with the political discussions she had witnessed around her family's kitchen table in the Bronx in her childhood.[61]

Gornick's prose is sometimes overblown, but the metaphors of light and flame that stud her sentences are echoed by her interviewees. Membership in the party and belief in the revolutionary cause, they tell her, made things seem higher and deeper, brighter and larger. A man who worked for the party as a doctor says: '"The relation for me between the personal and the historical was intense, deeply felt, fully realised . . . The world is smaller, colder, darker by far for me than it was when I was a Communist."' Commitment to the party and faith in communism provided a grand context in which to live, imbuing daily life with meaning and intensity. Everything was lit up in red. Communists glowed from within. The sense of a life suddenly infused with a larger meaning, of an individual finding a connection to a collective project and to a totalising vision for social transformation, echoes Gornick's own account of first encountering the women's liberation movement. An actor who left the party after twelve years described the '"powerful bond"' she found among her comrades, but she also reflected on her eventual decision to leave after seeing dogmatic rhetoric trample over personal feeling. She nonetheless recalled the many kind and idealistic people who were drawn into the party: '"Good people, people who were marked by the deepest of human longings. Genuinely tender people who felt intensely for the suffering and deprived of the world."'[62] How could tender people motivated by injustice, who found joyful solidarity in the party and who were sympathetic to the exploitation of others, become so cruel?

A contrast between loneliness and togetherness runs through the conversations Gornick recounts. The party is presented as an antidote to both literal and existential loneliness. Without the grand vision of the world communism provided, and without the routines and rhythms provided by life in the party, intense loneliness also characterised many former member's experiences of life after they left. Gornick not only contrasts collectivity with isolation, however; she also discusses the tensions that arose between party members. Weather Underground self-criticism sessions could result in denunciation and expulsion, but within the context of the CPUSA Gornick discusses less formalised interpersonal dynamics and minor infractions that could result in people being cast out or treated with contempt for failing to live according to the party line (though forms of self-criticism were also practiced in the CPUSA and an intensive period of self-criticism followed Khrushchev's 'secret speech' in 1956, which prompted an exodus from the party).[63] Many of the former communists Gornick encountered expressed bemusement or hostility towards the politics of the younger generation to which Gornick belonged. They resisted the emphasis placed on personal transformation as a political act by second wave feminism and the New Left, but they nonetheless constantly articulated themselves in emotional terms and discussed how their psychological investment in communism shaped their engagements with others and gave their lives meaning. Meanwhile, many people on the New Left distanced themselves from the party form, vanguardism, the USSR and Stalinism, but they did not thereby avoid dogmatism.

One man whom Gornick interviewed admitted trying to discuss personal psychological problems with a comrade who talked to him 'as though I were counterrevolutionary vermin'. Gornick describes denunciations and expulsions as intimate affairs playing out among people who had been close friends for years yet spied and reported on one another. Her interviewees also discuss the sudden invisible border that would arise to separate people expelled from the party from those still in it: '"We were on the other side of some kind of wall inside his mind."' A woman describes how, after she quit the party, friends of many years would suddenly ignore her in the street or at the supermarket: '"I had become – literally overnight – nonexistent."' Such behaviour, which the interviewee had participated in as a member, and the kinds of rigid psychological barriers it involved constructing, in retrospect struck her as almost unbelievably callous: '"My God, how came we to do such things to each other?"'[64] Another man Gornick meets breaks down in tears recalling how he cut himself off from a close friend who spoke out against the party at a union meeting. These regretful recollections recall the tone of Weather Underground memoirs, which similarly express bafflement about past behaviour and confusion at the way dynamics within a group dedicated to ending oppression and exploitation could become so inward-looking and spiteful, as Bill Ayers observed: 'I cannot reproduce the stifling atmosphere that overpowered us.'[65]

In Gornick's interviews the same contradictions repeat again and again: people who felt so deeply driven they devoted themselves to a moral cause on behalf of strangers nonetheless bullied their closest friends, people committed to humanity behaved inhumanely, people intellectually opposed to discussions of psychic life were overpowered by their emotions. '"We who were fighting capitalism because it dehumanized people had dehumanized ourselves in this way, and had lost the only thing that counts between people: the ability to see ourselves in each other."' Gornick expresses regret in her self-critical 2019 introduction that her romantic attitude to the people about whom she was writing led her to omit some of their 'complexity', which seems like a euphemism for cruelty:

> There would be no presentation of the branch leader who loved humanity yet ruthlessly sacrificed one comrade after another to party rigidities; or, equally, the section head who could quote Marx reverentially by the hour, then call for the expulsion of a CP member who had served watermelon at a party.[66]

Gornick presents the appeal of communism in universal terms, as answering a generalised human need to find meaning in a meaningless universe, but she suggests that the cruelties and antagonisms that arose between people within both the CPUSA and the women's liberation movement in the US were specific to those political contexts. The grandiose explanations of the world that infused communist and feminist lives with meaning, that were the source of expansive elation and transformative solidarity, were, for Gornick, also the origins of dogmas that caused people to demand impossible standards of behaviour from themselves and others: 'I saw daily the fear, rage and frustration of women beginning to grasp the political meaning of their lives. I knew that a subjected people didn't emerge into clarity with proportion and generosity.' She summarises the attitude of former communist Arthur Koestler to his previous commitments thus: "'I can taste the ashes but I cannot recall the flame.'"[67] Indeed, in a strange aside in his contribution to *The God that Failed: Six Studies in Communism* (1949), Koestler admits in his typically grandiose prose that he was unable to reproduce the mood that accompanied his original faith in the party: 'Irony, anger and shame keep intruding; the passions of that time seem transformed into perversions . . . the shadow of barbed wire lies across the condemned playground of memory.'[68] For a communist turned anti-communist author like Koestler, who left the Communist Party in 1938 in the aftermath of the purges and Moscow trials, the ultimate trajectory of Stalinism, encounters with dogmatism and deadly denunciations allowed him to retroactively dismiss all his earlier positive experiences and idealism as misplaced and wrongheaded. Although Gornick's work vividly conveys the warmth of the original flames, her fatalistic arguments about dogmatism and antagonism nonetheless suggest that the ashes were somehow inevitable.

Though by no means identical to or as extreme in its implications, the teleological structure of Gornick's claim that dogmatism inevitably emerged from idealism has a similar shape to accounts of the Stalinist purges that narrate them as an inevitable outcome of the 1917 October Revolution – and weren't the Bolsheviks themselves obsessed with the French Revolution's Thermidor? Likewise, Gornick's claim recalls accounts that depict poorly conceived, violent direct action as the natural apotheosis of the diverse radical movements of the sixties, a tendency in the historiography that Max Elbaum's *Revolution in the Air* seeks to redress.[69] Such narratives not only fail to admit the possibility of other outcomes but also seal off the violent extremes from proper scrutiny by casting their participants as pathological or the ideals that drove them as tending inevitably towards indiscriminate violence and intolerance.[70] After all, unlike the US military in Vietnam or cops on the streets of cities in the US, most left-wing groups who bombed targets in the seventies explicitly sought to avoid harming people. The emergence of dogmatism and the turn to violence at the end of the sixties in the US were indeed, according to Elbaum, confrontational, 'bitter', 'difficult', 'abrasive': 'Many activists felt a deep sense of loss, even trauma.'[71] Nonetheless, reducing diverse movements to decontextualised bomb blasts not only shifts attention away from the brutal state repression of militant groups in this period, repressions that were far more severe for black revolutionaries than for their white comrades, but it also fails to apprehend that some people also continued to struggle and sought to work through the interpersonal difficulties they ran into along the way.

A lifetime of work

In 'A Black Feminist Statement' (1977), Combahee River Collective (CRC) members reflected that the group's consciousness-raising sessions were able to expand on white women's insights because they discussed race and class alongside sex, delving into the specificities of black women's experiences and addressing the 'psychological toll of being a Black woman and the difficulties this presents in reaching political consciousness'.[72] But they also noted that some members of the group were concerned that consciousness-raising functioned primarily as 'emotional support', and these members rejected it to focus on more directly political work.

Former CRC member Barbara Smith recalls her first encounter with the term 'women's liberation': in 1968 she invited Mark Rudd to speak at Mount Holyoke where she was studying. (Rudd was prominent in SDS before he joined the Weathermen.) The young white woman who accompanied him described herself as involved in women's liberation, and Smith initially found the notion baffling and slightly absurd: 'I could not even understand—what the hell is she talking about? I could not—this is '68, right? . . . my perspective then was like, "What do white women have to complain about?"' Prior to the formation of the CRC in Boston in the mid-1970s, Smith had been involved in the Civil Action group, anti-Vietnam War organising and women's groups. Reflecting on the statement's composition and lasting significance, Smith notes that the group were not only coming together as black women, but that they were also mostly lesbians, were all anti-capitalist and were, moreover, committed internationalists:

> We were third world women. We considered ourselves to be third world women. We saw ourselves in solidarity and in struggle with all third world people around the globe. And we also saw ourselves as being internally colonized. We were internally colonized within the United States.[73]

The genealogy of the term 'identity politics' can be traced back to the CRC statement. In the CRC's definition, identity politics facilitated the articulation of interlocking oppressions – race, class, gender, sexuality and so on.[74] Colleen Lye discusses how the concept came to be treated as synonymous with the theory of intersectionality later articulated by Kimberlé Crenshaw in 1989, a conflation which, Lye argues, risks masking internal differences and historical shifts within the radical black feminist tradition. While the CRC's goal was 'the quest for a revolutionary anticapitalist subject to which Black women might belong and, in belonging, transform and advance', Crenshaw's theory demonstrates the impossibility of representing such a subject. Lye reads this distinction as reflecting a historical shift away from 'the emancipatory promise of a politics of subjectivity'.[75] A concern with subjectivity was retroactively reduced to a concern with individualism, but by insisting on a historically contextualised reading Lye shows that subjectivity was seen by the CRC as a crucial site in the struggle for collective social transformation. The inescapably circular logic that also undergirded the Weather Underground's self-criticism practices returns here: socially formed psyches need to transform in order to transform society, which formed the psyches, which need to transform and so on and so on. Yet the CRC statement expressed far more patience for processes of both social and psychological transformation than the Weather Underground's self-destructive self-criticism practices.

Lye proposes reading the CRC statement as a 'document of US Maoism'.[76] Prising the CRC statement apart from its subsequent reception, Lye plunges it back into the immediate internationalist political context of its composition, reading Mao's dialectical understanding of contradiction, in which particularity and universality coexist, into the CRC's definition of 'identity'.[77] Identity for Mao does not signal the splintering of a whole into discrete fragments; instead, he sees parts as linked to a totality. Lye notes that the CRC statement's concluding emphasis on subjective transformation could seem strangely disappointing and deflating, its revolutionary bombast undercut by humble proposals for future endeavours. The CRC writes:

> As feminists we do not want to mess over people in the name of politics. We believe in collective process and a nonhierarchical distribution of power within our own group and in our vision of a revolutionary society. We are committed to a continual examination of our politics as they develop through criticism and self-criticism as an essential aspect of our practice ... As Black feminists and Lesbians we know that we have a very definite revolutionary task to perform and we are ready for the lifetime of work and struggle before us.[78]

Lye underlines how diffuse and dispersed their concept of a 'very definite revolutionary task' seems here – the multiple oppressions they identify are matched by the plethora of concrete political causes with which they were engaged. She also draws attention to the Maoist origins of the practice of 'criticism and self-criticism' they invoke and the pervasive interest in Maoist precepts within feminist, black and Third World movements in the US that would have made the term recognisable as a Maoist allusion (although, as I've noted already, the practice had earlier Bolshevik origins).[79] As Robin D. G. Kelley and Betsy Esch discuss in their analysis of Maoist influences on black liberation struggles and organisations in the US, '"consciousness raising" in the Maoist style of criticism/self-criticism... was more than propaganda work; it was intellectual labor in the context of revolutionary practice'.[80] Read as an engagement with Maoist theory, Lye argues, the CRC statement's closing lines seem less like a retreat into individualism than a commitment to revolution as a 'protracted and unceasing process, centrally involving the construction and reconstruction of political subjectivity'.[81] This notion of a long and arduous commitment that acknowledges the difficulties that can accompany political and personal change and proposes methods for group reflection, provides an alternative to Gornick's fatalistic claims about the emergence of dogmatism and animosity within political movements.

In an article on the West German women's liberation movement's engagements with accounts of women's experiences in China and Vietnam, Quinn Slobodian discusses how perceptions of China were marked by a de-idealising shift following the end of the Cultural Revolution and Mao's death in 1976, the moment of the CRC statement's composition and a time after which Kelley and Esch also claim 'the heyday of black [US] Maoism had passed'.[82] A delegation of West German women who visited China in 1977, for instance, expressed bemusement at discovering that Chinese women they encountered often spoke in a jargon-laden manner and only 'recounted bitterness in the past tense'.[83] They did not believe that Chinese women's problems had genuinely ceased, that liberation had arrived. Indeed, they assumed that the capacity to speak bitterness represented freedom, which was defined as a continual process of self-realisation and group reflection, rather than a final destination. Similar reservations were expressed by members of the New York–based Redstockings, in response to an account of a trip to China that suggested that women's collectives were disappearing as they were no longer deemed necessary.[84] Despite the proclaimed influence of Chinese small group practices on Western feminists, Slobodian identifies a major difference between the two understandings of their function: 'Whereas Western feminists used group speech to locate the cracks and points of tension in everyday life, Chinese cadres used it, at least ideal typically, to create a more seamless melding of the individual to the whole.'[85] The CRC statement is similarly attentive to cracks and tensions, and although it evinces an understanding of identity grounded in totality, it does not aim for a final unity when the need for all criticism and self-criticism will come to an end.

Not in our lifetime

Refusing to read the CRC statement through the lens of a later, depoliticised historical moment, as Lye proposes, is illuminating but it does not change the history that subsequently unfolded. In 1990, in the brief interregnum between the fall of the Berlin Wall and the collapse of the Soviet Union, that 'end of history' period contemporaneous with the publication of Crenshaw's essay, Carol Hanisch looked back on her life of political engagement and asked if it had all been a waste of time. In excerpts from a letter to a friend written the previous year in the wake of the Supreme Court's Webster decision that allowed states to restrict state funds relating to abortion, she reflects on her 'bouts of depression and burnout', on the 'debilitating loneliness' she felt in the 1980s when 'Me-ism' triumphed and the movement had ceased to move. With no partner, children or secure job, she asked herself why she had given up the chance of a 'normal' life, but more than this, echoing many of Gornick's interviewees, she mourned 'the lack of a Movement with its forward thrust, community, sense of purpose, excitement of new discoveries and fruits'. These listless feelings shifted when the Supreme Court decision was met with anger and protests that included younger women, lifting Hanisch's sense of cynicism, hopelessness and despair and making her determined not to fall into nostalgia. She acknowledged the sixties slogan 'Liberation in our lifetime' would not come to pass, that battles won once might not be won forever – as the overturning of *Roe v. Wade* in June 2022 has starkly underlined – but she also reflected on what had been achieved and vowed to keep fighting. Hanisch's recent embrace of transphobia is a bleak reminder that fights for liberation must be fought on all fronts and that history does not move inexorably in any direction. The lines of attack are constantly being redrawn and noone's solidarity can be taken for granted.[86]

Lye imagines readers of the CRC statement today finding its closing lines strangely anticlimactic in their modesty, but I was struck by their similarity to the concluding remarks of reviews of the 2020 reissue of Gornick's *The Romance of American Communism*. By the time of the book's republication, the original edition had already gained cult status among left-wing millennials in the UK and US, with PDFs and heavily annotated second-hand copies circulating among Corbyn supporters and DSA members; the book was republished immediately after the defeats of Corbyn and Sanders. Ari Brostoff's closing image of Bernie Sanders in old age celebrating the recent resurgence of the left while reflecting on how much remains to be done, like Alyssa Battistoni's affirmation of sustained organising over intense flurries of activity, chimes with the CRC statement's reference to 'a lifetime of work and struggle before us'.[87] It would be possible to dismiss these rhetorical moves as strained, hopeful platitudes appropriate to times when flames have turned to ashes, just as it would be possible to characterise the temporality they invoke as reformist capitulation, but they envisage continuing to fight for ideals against the odds, while accepting cracks and tensions. Gaps between ideal theories and lived practices cannot be completely closed, but such gaps should not represent dark holes into which both perfect theories and imperfect practices disappear. (Probably the theories were imperfect, hole-ridden and in need of constant revision anyway.) As Hinton discusses in *The Thousand Year War*, rigid dogmatism can have a totalising rhetoric that can become so uncompromising that it leads to myopia, sect formation and a detachment from struggles on the ground. The exclamatory tone of William Wordsworth's paean to pure revolutionary enthusiasm – 'bliss was it in that dawn to be alive' – invoked by Gornick can obscure as well as illuminate, just as staring directly into the sun can damage the eyes.[88]

The question of how to sustain movements without messing over or messing up the people involved in them remains open, but the conclusion of the CRC statement stays with the troubles of collective organising and the sticky difficulties of small group interaction. The CRC statement exhibits forbearance with psychic transformations that might fail to keep pace with political convictions, acknowledging that engaging in long-term struggle will depend on devising ways of continually reassessing and working on immediate relationships within movements, constantly modifying strategies and not just leaping to transform the totality.

Continuing to struggle for a better world will require a patient attitude to ourselves and to one another. As the previous chapter showed with respect to *The Salt Eaters*, this demands patient urgency, a sense of urgency for social transformation that can tolerate difficulties, differences, delays, subjective gaps and interpersonal strains. In an interview conducted in 2023, more than four decades after the CRC statement appeared, Barbara Smith noted that immediate social conditions demand responses that cannot wait until a perfect political vocabulary has been developed; urgency requires patience:

We're always in the process of trying to build, and get to better places politically, and that includes our own individual consciousness. In the meantime, there are people who are in dire situations because of how the system works... Can we wait until somebody has the perfect vocabulary for how we talk across differences? Or do we try to get work done in the meantime?[89]

All we have is the meantime. As Hinton observed in the concluding pages of *Fanshen*:

No person could break free of the past all at once. The spectrum of man's [sic] consciousness could not be refocused in one night no matter how earnestly he might desire such a shift. Change had to come in one area, then spread to others. It had to dissolve old contradictions only to set up new ones. It had to expand the struggle between the new and old until the entire personality was involved in painful conflict. No-one going through such inner strife exhibited a character that was all of one piece. Habits, superstitions, and prejudices left over from the past marred and undermined efforts to act on the enlightened motives of the present.[90]

It's hard to change, but change, understood as an ongoing process rather than a completable project, need not result in hardness.

PART III

Concepts Transformed: Anti-Adaptive Healing

7

Trauma

> *Traumatic events cannot be banished from consciousness when they are not banished from communal reality. Acknowledging this reality is a social process, beyond the bounds of individual psychotherapy.*[1]
> – Samah Jabr

On 12 October 2002, three bombs were detonated in Kuta, a tourist district on the island of Bali in Indonesia, killing 202 people. Members of the Islamist group Jemaah Islamiyah were convicted of terrorism for their involvement in the attack, which had been framed as retaliation for the US role in the War on Terror. In the aftermath of these bombings in Bali, a year after 9/11, there was an influx of international aid to the island, with an emphasis on treating and raising awareness of post-traumatic stress disorder (PTSD).

The growth of a 'trauma industry' that saw international aid organisations increasing their spending on 'off the shelf' PTSD programmes in response to a range of events began in the late 1980s.[2] Global humanitarian and relief work organised around PTSD proliferated in the 1990s and 2000s: in war zones, in the wake of a slew of natural disasters, and, as in Bali, in the aftermath of terrorist attacks (as the War on Terror began to wreak its own violence and Department of Defense spending on PTSD also began to shoot up). Didier Fassin and Richard Rechtman argue that the period witnessed a profound discursive shift that originated in psychiatry but had much further-reaching implications for understandings of historical events and past experience, establishing what they call a 'new condition of victimhood'.[3] By unpicking the imbrication of the medical with the moral in dominant trauma discourses in the decades around the millennium, they further demonstrate how PTSD as a diagnostic category broadly indifferent to the political contexts in which traumatic events occur was suited to a 'post-political' historical moment.[4] They cite the response of international humanitarian organisations to the

1988 Armenian earthquake just before the collapse of the Soviet Union as a key turning point in this history, tracing the origins of 'humanitarian psychiatry' to an international conference entitled 'Trauma: Care and Cure', held at the Maison de la Mutualité in Paris in March 2002. Fassin and Rechtman note that the same building had played host to international conferences on conflicts and forms of state repression for decades but that twenty or thirty years earlier the audience would have been made up of activists whose discussions of Palestine or dictatorships in Latin America would have been framed in completely different terms to those at the 2002 meeting:

> The focus was not so much on trauma as on violence. The talk was of the resistance of fighters rather than the resilience of patients. Those who were being defended were always oppressed, often heroes, never victims. The focus was on understanding not the experience of people suffering, but the nature of social movements. No one thought in terms of psychological care; they campaigned for national liberation movements.[5]

By pointing out that it was not always taken for granted that psy-professionals would be involved in humanitarian responses to wars (or that responses to wars would be discussed alongside responses to natural disasters and terrorist attacks), Fassin and Rechtman denaturalise the concept of PTSD.

The word 'trauma' entered Indonesian from English and was not widely used until after the fall of Suharto's New Order regime in 1998. Similarly, PTSD as a diagnostic category was rarely used in psychiatric contexts under the New Order.[6] Major General Suharto had come to power after six generals of the Indonesian army were killed in a coup attempt on 30 September 1965. Although the circumstances of the coup remain contested, the generals' murders were blamed on the Communist Party of Indonesia (PKI) and used as a pretext for a brutal purge. Members of the PKI and trade unions, as well as ethnic Chinese people and many with tenuous, rumoured connections to the left (or the family members of people rumoured to have such connections) were killed in massacres carried out in 1965–6 by the military, with the participation of various youth militia groups and backed by the US. Approximately 1 million people were killed. Many more were brutally tortured and incarcerated without trial in prisons and camps.[7] A vivid, fabricated counter-narrative of the coup circulated in propaganda and schools, while discussions of the massacres that deviated from official state-sanctioned accounts were forbidden.[8] The killers were celebrated as heroes. The threat of re-emergent communism was kept discursively alive long after most actual communists were killed.[9] Even after Suharto's fall in 1998, the Indonesian state did not officially acknowledge the atrocities.[10] For decades a gulf existed between people's direct experiences of the massacres and the state's official version of events.

Leslie Dwyer and Degung Santikarma observe that NGOs and international aid organisations who arrived in Bali in 2002 to treat PTSD framed 'the terrorist bombings as an event of extraordinary, unprecedented horror – as an exemplary site of trauma'.[11] Contesting this characterisation, their article 'Posttraumatic Politics: Violence, Memory, and Biomedical Discourse in Bali' contrasts the site of the 2002 blasts with a nearby field in which a similar number of people accused of being communists were slaughtered in 1965. The site of the Kuta bombings was almost immediately at the centre of discussions around both public memorialisation and psychiatric treatment, while the site of the 1965 killings remained anonymous, its graves unmarked, and the experiences of its survivors erased from collective historical memory.[12] The new attentiveness to PTSD in Bali that emerged in 2002 stood in stark contrast to the long silence surrounding the massacres of 1965–66 in which 5 to 8 percent of the island's population are estimated to have been killed in total.[13] The comparison of these two violent incidents in Bali's history underlines the institutional, political and social circumstances that contribute to the formal recognition of events as traumatic, which has implications for people's ability to access clinical treatment. Rather than understanding PTSD as a universal somatic response to extreme experiences, the example demonstrates that traumatic events should always be situated culturally and historically: 'Trauma is always more than a biological state.'[14]

Dwyer and Santikarma identify tensions between PTSD as a universalising concept and local 'taxonomies of mental illness' in Bali but claim that their Balinese interviewees expressed more anger about 'inattention to the presence of long-term structures of violence and inequality' that caused them psychic distress than they did about Western biomedical approaches to mental illness.[15] Outreach materials produced by PTSD programmes in Bali spread ideas about 'the intrusion of history into the mind as a troubling symptom and the importance of gaining control over the past in order to move beyond it'.[16] But Dwyer and Santikarma contend that even if treatment had been made available to survivors or witnesses of the 1965–66 massacres, a therapeutic approach focused on the individual mastery of painful memories would have been impossible in relation to those events given the length of the silence, the pervasiveness of the state-sanctioned counter-narrative, the fact that victims and perpetrators continued to live side by side, continuing fears of state repression, and the events' enduring material legacies, which caused mental distress in their own right (in relation to the housing or work situations of those with perceived associations to PKI members, for example).

Palestinian psychiatrists and psychologists have criticised PTSD as a diagnostic category in similar terms, as their clinical work has shown that the mental suffering experienced by many of their patients derives from the ongoing brutalities of the Israeli occupation 'that has controlled all aspects of life for generations', rather than being confined to a discrete, overwhelming past event that disrupted the rhythms of the everyday. Psychiatrist Samah Jabr argued in the wake of the 2014 Gaza War that the psychosocial damage inflicted during the war, while profound, was just the 'tip of an iceberg', noting that individual psychotherapeutic treatment could not proceed effectively without acknowledging a broader social context in which violence and injustice were routine: 'Treatment that ignores the political reality can do more harm than good.'[17]

German psychotherapist David Becker, who worked extensively with victims of political repression in Chile during and in the aftermath of Augusto Pinochet's dictatorship, has described PTSD as 'the Coca-Cola of psychiatry', characterising it as a diagnosis exported as part of a broader project of cultural imperialism.[18] Becker's scepticism towards PTSD emerged from his clinical work in Chile and drew on psychoanalytically informed work with Holocaust survivors conducted in the immediate aftermath of the Second World War. Becker and his Chilean colleagues not only identified the limits of PTSD and rejected the notion that traumatic symptoms could be measured, but they also developed an alternative, context-bound theory of trauma attentive to the specific psychic effects of political persecution in an environment in which social reparation was foreclosed.[19]

Before exploring this re-conceptualisation of trauma alongside a trilogy of documentary films by Patricio Guzmán that meditate on the psychological and social legacies of the dictatorship in a less individualised register, this chapter will first gloss the psychiatric origins of PTSD in the aftermath of another anti-communist conflict in Southeast Asia: the American war in Vietnam. Trauma is part of the collective histories of the left, histories filled with brutal repressions, torture and mass death.

PTSD as a diagnostic category, as we shall see, while acknowledging a trigger in the outside world, can downplay the sociopolitical conditions in which extreme and distressing events occur, as well as failing to take into account the politicised environments in which traumatised subjects continue to live, a limitation evident in the examples considered here. Though traumatic experience ties the traumatised subject to the past, the alternative understandings of trauma explored in this chapter are oriented to a transformed future.

From guilty perpetrators to passive victims

A descendent of hysteria, shell shock and war neurosis, PTSD entered the third volume of the *Diagnostic and Statistical Manual of Mental Disorders (DSM-III)* in 1980, the 'standardized psychiatric nosology', whose publication represented a 'paradigm shift' in the definition of mental illness.[20] Rather than focusing on the underlying causes of mental experience as previous editions of the *DSM* had done, the new edition placed an emphasis on overt symptoms and introduced a standardised set of diagnostic categories. A small group of psychiatrists associated with the American Psychiatric Association, headed by Robert Spitzer, were responsible for the *DSM-III*'s new approach to classification. They were inspired by an approach indebted to the German psychiatrist Emil Kraeplin, who proposed that mental illnesses were analogous to physical diseases, that their definition should be based on observable phenomena, and that research would ultimately prove their origins to be organic or biochemical.[21]

Creating categorical definitions of mental illnesses 'legitimized claims to be treating real diseases', bolstering the medical legitimacy of psychiatry as a field at a time its authority was waning as it faced attacks both from the medical establishment and the antipsychiatry movement.[22] Moreover, the shift away from psychoanalytic understandings of the unconscious to symptom-based diagnostic categories made it easier to apply for reimbursement from insurers, enabled researchers to apply for state funding to investigate specific conditions, and facilitated a broader shift from talking therapies to drug treatments in the wake of deinstitutionalisation. Though the previous editions of the manual had remained relatively marginal, the *DSM-III* attained the status of a 'biblical textbook', central to a 'historic shift from a psychosocial to a symptom-based view of mental health'.[23] Not only did this shift have implications for treatment, it also had broader political implications: rather than mental illnesses being understood primarily in relation to a person's environment and life experiences, they were understood as biological in origin.

Though most definitions in the new *DSM-III* emphasised symptoms over causes, distinguishing PTSD's symptoms from those of other diagnoses, such as depression, required acknowledging 'etiological agency' – that is, an external cause (a fact which made some psychiatrists on the *DSM* committees hostile to the idea of including PTSD at all). A proposal to distinguish between catastrophes of human origin and natural disasters failed to make it into the *DSM-III*. The *DSM-III* defined the external event as 'a recognizable stressor that would evoke significant symptoms of distress in almost anyone', while the revised *DSM-III-R*, published in 1987, defined it as something 'outside the range of usual human experience' that would be 'markedly distressing to almost anyone'. But what is 'usual human experience'? Who is 'almost anyone'? Are extreme events that are commonplace in some contexts less traumatic than in contexts in which they are rare? The definition relied on normative assumptions about experience that were not made explicit.[24]

PTSD came into existence as the result of activism to recognise the ongoing mental suffering of US veterans who had fought in the American war in Vietnam and who were seeking state-funded treatment for a cluster of shared symptoms. Jewish Holocaust survivors who had been seeking financial compensation from the resistant and antisemitic West German legal system in the 1960s and 1970s benefitted from a strategic alliance with campaigners advocating for Vietnam veterans. Identifying commonalities of experience, including the delayed onset of symptoms, helped lead to the recognition of PTSD in the *DSM-III*, which Dagmar Herzog frames as a broadly positive outcome for people involved in those specific struggles for recognition and recompense. But she also acknowledges that there were unforeseen consequences when the PTSD diagnosis was later applied to an ever more disparate range of contexts as part of the emerging trauma industry, which 'mixed perpetrators together with victims and depoliticized the experiences of both'.[25]

The Vietnam vet eventually became a 'trauma icon' in the US.[26] Joseph Darda describes how the liberal anti-war movement and the hawkish right converged in recognising the figure of the 'trauma hero'. He identifies a paradox in contemporary 'trauma culture' which has provided a language for acknowledging 'silenced and delegitimized knowledge' among marginalised groups, while the origins of PTSD enabled a victim narrative that centred white men to emerge in the immediate aftermath of the liberation movements of the sixties and seventies. In Darda's account, the archetypical PTSD sufferer was a white veteran experiencing nightmares and flashbacks about the My Lai massacre (known as the Sơn Mỹ massacre in contemporary Vietnam), where US soldiers infamously killed up to 500 unarmed Vietnamese civilians on 16 March 1968. Perpetrators of the massacre were perversely situated as victims, Darda claims, while the experiences of Vietnamese people were elided, leading to the creation of 'a dehistoricized trauma culture in which all could claim the status of survivor'.[27]

Nadia Abu El-Haj complicates the 'widely accepted history' of PTSD that ties the emergence of the figure of the passive traumatised subject suffering as a result of a decontextualised and hence depoliticised external event to psychiatric responses to the experiences of US veterans of the American war in Vietnam. She discusses how 'post-Vietnam syndrome', as it was originally formulated in the 1970s by anti-war psychiatrists who were involved in *DSM-III* Working Group and committee discussions, acknowledged that veterans were disturbed by their role in perpetrating atrocities they could not politically justify and for which they felt morally responsible: 'For them no American veteran was innocent. The war itself was the crime.' Rap groups organised by Vietnam Veterans Against the War (VVAW) emphasised that psychological healing was as much about social reparation as it was about individual therapy. Abu El-Haj claims the shift towards passive victimhood occurred during the Reagan years in response to feminist campaigns to recognise sexual violence perpetrated by men, on the one hand, and the demands of the victims of crime movement, on the other. These changes in definition were enshrined in the *DSM-III-R*, in which guilt was deemed 'non-critical' and the question of moral transgression removed, which retroactively recast the experiences of US veterans and fit with rightward shifting narratives of the war. By the time the *DSM-IV* was published in 1994, guilt had completely disappeared from the definition of PTSD.[28]

Ghosts of the My Lai massacre

Psychiatrist Robert Jay Lifton, as Abu El-Haj discusses, was central to the development of 'post-Vietnam syndrome'. Lifton's *Home from the War: Vietnam Veterans: Neither Victims nor Executioners* (1973) discusses his work with VVAW rap groups in New York, which were filled with 'anti-war warriors'. He describes the veterans he encountered as preoccupied with the 'evil' and absurdity of the war. Critical of military psychiatrists whose role was to help 'men adjust to their own atrocities', the rap groups instead enabled veterans to confront their experiences of both witnessing and perpetrating violence.[29] He claims the men, who often referred to themselves as 'monsters', were not only troubled by particular instances of brutality but also plagued by their sense of complicity with an imperial war they now believed to have been unjustified.

Lifton departs from Freud, who argued in *Totem and Taboo* (1913) that the origins of guilt could be traced to prehistoric parricide, claiming instead that guilt emerged from a more general feeling of responsibility for any form of killing or destruction, literal or symbolic. Lifton identifies two distinct forms of guilt: static and animating. Static guilt traps the individual in a closed world in which they cannot fully confront their past actions yet continuously anticipate punishment, while animating guilt, propelled by the 'anxiety of responsibility', emanates from 'a formative dissatisfaction with the self and the world' that makes it possible to criticise past actions and so imagine a life beyond them. For Lifton, animating guilt among veterans further allowed them to situate their psychological sufferings in a broader social context: 'Changes in the self required an altered relationship to the external world.' Antiwar veterans were not seeking to displace their feelings of guilt from inside to outside as a form of exculpation, but transforming their guilt involved, 'confronting the responsibility of society as a whole, and of its leaders in particular, for the killing and the dying'. He credits the rap group participants with perceiving that politics could not be separated from 'personal growth and well-being': 'Indeed for antiwar veterans a believable critique of society lived out in some form of political protest, became crucial to psychological health.'[30]

In the opening pages of *Home from the War* Lifton notes that when he began working on the project, 'despite all of the American writing on Vietnam, very little was understood about what either GIs or Vietnamese really experienced there'.[31] His book is dedicated to twenty-four people (presumably rap group participants), plus 'Hoang', who is described as a child survivor of My Lai, but though *Home from the War* includes disturbing self-reflective testimonies from GIs about their role in the My Lai massacre, Vietnamese perspectives remain largely absent from its pages.

So vast is the psychiatric and historical literature on PTSD and US veterans of the American war in Vietnam that attempting to search library or academic journal databases for English-language materials that discuss the mental impact of the war on Vietnamese people is difficult. Among the huge volume of publications on US veterans, it is possible to find studies by psychiatrists based in the US and Australia that discuss PTSD in Vietnamese refugee communities (focusing on the trauma of fleeing and relocating). One can also find a 2012 paper on the long-term health impact of the war on people in northern Vietnam that concluded that both veterans and civilians may have been shielded from trauma by 'moral certainty (that the war was justified), common purpose (fighting for independence), and victorious outcome', which 'can lend resilience that heals and buffers from physical and psychological ills in the long run'.[32] Though the latter paper acknowledges differences in context between the US and northern Vietnam, it does not frame the differences of experience in terms of culturally distinct vocabularies and practices for working through extreme experiences. It also fails to consider how much more devastating the war was for people in Vietnam, affecting the entire population rather than a small subsection of it; their home *was* the site of the war.

Anthropologist Heonik Kwon takes the 'simple fact' that however difficult and damaging the war was for some US veterans, it was self-evidently more violent and devastating for people in Vietnam where everything and everybody was impacted, as his starting point for asking if Vietnam therefore saw a similar surge of interest in the psychic impact of the war in its aftermath.[33] After the unification of Vietnam following victory over the US in 1975, official commemorations encouraged by the socialist political authorities focused on celebrating revolutionary heroism. Memorials and cemeteries dedicated to revolutionary martyrs proliferated but the state rhetoric emphasised the bright and prosperous future over the dark and violent past. Public expressions of grief and sadness were discouraged and the lines demarcating mournable from unmournable deaths were sharply drawn.[34] Kwon identifies a shift that came about as a result of liberalisation in the 1990s, when people living in rural communities in central Vietnam began to rebuild traditional ancestral temples and domestic shrines where they practiced their own commemorative rituals that related to war deaths in a manner that departed from the state-sanctioned image of heroic sacrifice.[35]

At the same historical moment that humanitarian PTSD programmes were proliferating globally, residents of My Lai spoke of their experiences of violent conflict in a very different register. They described living alongside 'grievous ghosts', 'invisible neighbours' and 'the spirits of the dead in pain'.[36] They described hearing lamentations coming from the site of the killings. They reported seeing old women ghosts sucking the limbs of ghostly children as if to soothe them and young women ghosts carrying the limp bodies of small children in their arms. People killed at My Lai did not receive proper burials but were thrown into mass graves without funeral attire. Without coffins, their bodies became entangled and unidentifiable, making funeral rites impossible and severing genealogical lineages. Villagers in My Lai performed rituals and gave offerings to these ghosts, whose existence they explained through the concept of 'grievous death' or 'unjust death' [*chet oan*]. The dead continued to suffer their traumatic experiences, 'captivated by the memory of injustice', and the living had an obligation to intervene to help free them from their incarceration in an eternal present of historical pain.[37]

Kwon claims that understandings of commemoration and grieving in My Lai evince a 'culturally specific conception of human rights, the right of the dead to be liberated from the violent history of death'. This process of liberation that sets the dead soul free from repeating pain is called 'disentangling the grievance' [*giai oan*]. The process of working through the violent past does not take the form of individualised therapy in this context but of a collective ritual practice; traumatic memory is not located in the individual brains of the living but in the ghosts of the dead generations who continue to exist as part of the social world. Kwon is clear that this relationship to the traumatic past should not be understood as a metaphor, nor can it be translated into the medicalised register of PTSD:

> In this milieu of interaction with the past, the apparitions in My Lai are more than history's ruins or uncanny traces. Rather, these ghosts are vital historical witnesses, testifying to the war's unjust destruction of human life, with broken lives but unbreakable spirits. The sufferings endured by My Lai's ghosts are not the same as those we gloss over as traumatic memory. However, we can imagine that their collective existence is a reflection of the historical trauma this community as a whole suffered.[38]

While the state favoured a triumphant celebration of revolutionary victors that emphasised the future over the past, the persistent presence of ghosts in My Lai suggests that moving away too swiftly from the experience of historic injustice and the horrors of violence, even when the enemy had been defeated, caused wounds to fester.

There are certain similarities that can be identified between PTSD as defined by the *DSM* and the ghosts of My Lai that Kwon describes – the re-experiencing of the traumatic event, for example, or the inclusion of people from both sides of the conflict among the traumatised.[39] Despite describing haunting and trauma as 'kin', however, Avery Gordon identifies important distinctions between the two experiences: both may involve 'unresolved social violence', but unlike a traumatic memory, the ghost, she claims, is not 'constitutively unknowable'. Ghosts make demands and produce a 'something-to-be-done', which opens up possibilities for the future, whereas trauma is regressive, fatally binding an individual or a collective to an original scene of horror and to its repression; trauma is a past moment from which the future cannot fully escape. Substituting haunting for trauma, she argues, can establish a more transformative relationship to past injustice, making it possible to explore 'how to live otherwise than in the putatively inevitable repetition of the degradations and depredations that injure us'.[40] In My Lai, the souls of the 'grievous dead' who were violently and unjustly killed could ultimately be liberated from incarceration in their pain by the interventions of the living. Rather than being read as an abandonment of the psychiatric in favour of the supernatural, Gordon's conceptual distinction between trauma and haunting could perhaps instead be understood as distinguishing two modes of relating to traumatic experience, recalling Lifton's distinction between static and animating guilt. Popular understandings of PTSD may indeed conform to Gordon's definition of trauma as unknowable and inescapable, but the understanding of trauma Lifton developed with anti-war veterans also included the possibility for future transformations grounded in social change.

Cumulative, continuous and chronic trauma

In *The Jakarta Method*, Vincent Bevins demonstrates how the brutal suppression of the left in Indonesia, which was approved of and quietly facilitated by the CIA, came to serve as a model for regimes elsewhere. Evidence gathered for the Truth Commission in Brazil revealed the existence of an extermination plan that was given the name 'The Jakarta Operation', while in Santiago, Chile, in the early 1970s the words 'Jakarta is Coming' or 'Jakarta' appeared pasted on city walls. Postcards bearing the same message were sent to Communist Party members and members of Salvador Allende's Popular Unity coalition government, which had come to power in 1970 and ended in a brutal military coup on 11 September 1973.

Between 1973 and 1990, the years of General Augusto Pinochet's dictatorship, the Chilean Psychoanalytic Association continued to operate.[41]

Despite the widespread persecution experienced across Chilean society as a result of the dictatorship, the association maintained a detachment from politics, interpreting psychological distress in intrapsychic terms rather than in relation to any broader social context; the significance of patients' inner worlds was magnified, while their experiences of the external world were obscured, the intertwinement of external and psychic reality downplayed: 'During this period, whenever clinical material was discussed or papers were presented, the ever present climate of fear and persecution was ignored.'[42] In her discussion of this history, Carla Fischer Canessa reflects on the paradox of a discipline which had elaborated sophisticated definitions of denial and disavowal in theory, but nonetheless denied and disavowed in practice the immediate social environment that was impacting the lives of both analysts and analysands. Canessa discusses a graduate of the Chilean Psychoanalytic Association whose subversive actions and speeches led to arrest, the details of whose imprisonment and presumed death remain unconfirmed. This man's fate was narrated by one psychoanalyst at the association in terms of individual insanity, rather than being understood as a rational if dangerous act of political commitment, while other analysts seemed incapable of acknowledging the disappearance at all.

It was left to psychotherapists working beyond the auspices of the Psychoanalytic Association to develop forms of therapeutic care and theories of trauma that acknowledged and sought to address the specific psychic effects of political repression under Pinochet and in the dictatorship's aftermath, including experiences of torture, 'disappearance', murder and exile. Canessa mentions the organisation the Latin American Institute of Mental Health and Human Rights (ILAS), which was set up in 1988 to provide psychotherapeutic support to victims of political repression, claiming that their work was seen as 'quite alien' to the Chilean Psychoanalytic Association.[43] This was the organisation with which David Becker was involved, having previously offered psychotherapeutic support to victims of the regime through various organisations that operated partly under the auspices of the church.

Becker argues that his clinical experiences in Chile working with victims of political repression from the mid-1970s to the late 1990s led him to conclude that PTSD is not 'an adequate diagnostic instrument'.[44] Though he expressed concern that the ubiquity of current discourses around trauma threatened to hollow out its meaning, he nonetheless insisted that the concept remained clinically indispensable for describing catastrophic subjective discontinuities that can result from extreme experiences. However, his reconceptualisation of trauma dispensed with the other letters in the acronym PTSD.[45] Becker claimed that the term 'post' gave a misleading impression about the temporality and duration of traumatic experience, failing to capture the experiences of many victims of political repression for whom trauma is often 'cumulative and continuous'. 'Stress', he argued, is 'qualitatively different' from trauma as it does not imply an 'irreparable tear of self and reality' but leaves the 'structure of the person ... basically intact', while the word 'disorder' risked mimicking the language of persecutors who employ pseudoscientific language to dehumanise particular social groups perceived as an internal threat.[46]

Though many patients who sought therapeutic help through ILAS exhibited severe symptoms, it was important to approach them as people 'suffering the consequences of a disturbed society', rather than as people whose psychic disturbances were strictly individual:

> In our own definition, we intend to transcend the individual level, without denying it, and to include the social reality. Or said in another way, extreme traumatization is never only individual destruction or only a sociopolitical process. It is always both.[47]

Central to Becker's and his collaborator's writings on trauma is the idea that traumatic experience can be sequential; in this they were influenced by psychoanalyst Hans Keilson's work with Jewish children in the Netherlands. These children had survived the Holocaust but were orphaned. They had experienced successive traumas, which Keilson saw as belonging to three distinct sequences or phases. In Keilson's view, as Dagmar Herzog explains, trauma should be understood as a process rather than an event.[48] His work showed that trauma could be cumulative and therefore chronic, and that it could persist long after persecution had ended.[49] Becker discusses clinical cases in which symptoms were delayed, as well as those in which traumatic experience was dispersed and pervasive, effecting entire families or communities, not only those who had directly experienced violent persecution.

Becker and his collaborators advocated for adopting an 'ethically non-neutral' form of therapeutic relationship or 'bond of commitment' that departed from the neutrality conventionally demanded of psycho-analysts by explicitly acknowledging the socio-political origins of psychic distress: 'Amid the harsh political repression of the dictatorship, it was necessary to make explicit the political, social, and psychological alliance established between patients and the therapists who chose to work with victims of the regime.'[50] The issues of political and clinical neutrality were also central to debates and schisms within the psychoanalytic community in Argentina in the period immediately preceding Pinochet's coup. The Argentinian Psychoanalytic Association (APA) was officially politically neutral after the 1966 coup that established a dictatorship by military junta. But Argentinian analysts on the left challenged the notion that psychoanalysis should be understood as adaptive rather than transformative, insisting it could be compatible with a project to reject the status quo rather than seeking to enable people to function more smoothly within it. Freud, they maintained, should be read alongside Marx. In the context of rising political repression that was impacting patients and analysts alike, these dissident analysts eventually split from the APA in 1971. Alongside the flourishing of efforts to democratise psychoanalysis in order to make it accessible to people from all class backgrounds, the abandonment of political neutrality went hand in hand with a rejection of clinical neutrality in the consulting room. As with ILAS in Chile, a less detached, more empathic therapeutic approach was encouraged, one that acknowledged the social origins of patients' fears and shared experiences of 'living in the midst of state terror'.[51]

In their group therapeutic work with the family of a thirteen-year-old boy who was killed by the military regime at a protest in 1984, ILAS therapists describe how giving the family food at the end of a session functioned as a symbolic intervention that demonstrated care and helped to establish a 'deep affective bond'.[52] They also insisted on distinguishing between accidental and deliberately inflicted traumatic experiences, between those resulting from natural disasters or car crashes and those with socio-political origins. They used the term 'extreme traumatization', introduced by Bruno Bettelheim in his writings about his experience in a Nazi concentration camp, to signal this difference: 'Unlike notions linked to "post-traumatic stress disorder", use of the term *extreme traumatization* put the emphasis on the traumatic situation as an explicative factor.'[53] A person's trauma was not interpreted as the result of a generic shock from the external world, but was seen as a response to a specific politically motivated and unjust form of violence. Becker and Díaz articulated the motivation for abandoning neutrality very clearly:

> If the destruction we are dealing with is not only individual but also social, then our research cannot be exterior to the reality with which it deals. We are thus not neutral investigators intending to understand

an alien reality, but are active participants in therapy and research, operating within the political process.[54]

This challenge to clinical neutrality had implications not only for how psychotherapists interacted with their patients but also for how traumatic experiences were defined. These authors acknowledged that external reality was not alien but comprehensible. The wounding forces that structured external reality were not neutral but political. And the persistence of those forces into the present obstructed mental healing.

Testimony was central to this model of treating trauma: 'The idea is to bring together the bits and pieces of a life history that is full of terror and fear, losses and black holes.'[55] The psychoanalyst Margarita Díaz discusses the case of a patient she worked with at ILAS who had returned to Chile in 1990 at the age of nineteen, following a fourteen-year exile. The patient's father had been a left-wing political leader who went underground following the coup, which took place when the patient was just two. Then she was kidnapped as a young child in a failed attempt to lure her father out of hiding. Upon her return to Chile, she felt like an outsider and remained ignorant of many details of her childhood. Díaz describes her patient's history as being 'full of voids'. The patient reported a recurring dream of falling into an abyss and claimed to feel empty, to feel nothing. The inability to remember or represent experience is typical of trauma, according to Díaz, which only surfaces through symptoms that 'bear witness [to] a "hole" in the mind'.[56]

According to the 'antimimetic' understanding of traumatic memory discussed by Ruth Leys in *Trauma: A Genealogy*, it is axiomatic to speak of trauma as unrepresentable. Definitions of PTSD, she argues, conform to this model, which treats perpetrators and victims of violence alike as 'casualties of an external trauma that causes objective changes in the brain in ways that tend to eliminate the issue of moral meaning and ethical assessment'.[57] In antimimetic definitions of trauma, she claims, a 'rigid dichotomy' separates internal from external, 'such that violence is imagined as coming to the subject entirely from the outside'.[58] The traumatic event is unavailable to the traumatised subject. The event's impact is belated, delayed, deferred. The traumatic event is not remembered in any conventional sense, but it leaves a permanent imprint on the brain. It cannot be integrated, comprehended or cognised. It cannot be spoken or narrated. The intensity and extremity of the traumatic event are too much for the subject to process and so the event returns only in the form of a literal flashback. Díaz's example of a patient who cannot remember, who talks of voids, abysses and black holes, seems at first glance to conform to this aporetic antimimetic understanding of trauma. Yet in her case history the traumatic event did not return in a flashback or a nightmare like an intrusive image experienced in the present tense that literally replays the original experience and thus evades the kinds of distortions or mediations ordinarily associated with representation and recollection. And, as the therapeutic process progressed and the transference was established, the patient's dreams began to change: 'She falls into the void, but this time, unlike in the dreams where she fell endlessly, [she] falls into the water and comes up explosively to the surface.'[59]

The distinction between the endless void and the finite void in the case history is analogous to a distinction between absence and loss articulated by Dominick LaCapra, in an argument that could in turn be mapped onto Avery Gordon's distinction between trauma and haunting or Lifton's between static and animating guilt. Absence is general, transhistorical, timeless, whereas loss is particular, historical, open to transformation. Conflating loss with absence, according to LaCapra, removes experience from history, leading to a 'melancholic paralysis'.[60] The lure of the aporia, of a hermeneutics of absence, is the lure of a fatalism that blocks all possibility of mourning and hence of social transformation. Through the therapeutic process, Díaz's patient moved from absence to loss. The losses she experienced were always historical and political, but it took her time and therapeutic care to recognise them as such. Eventually she began 'to negate the damage' and by articulating the socio-political origins of her wounds came to recognise that 'the possibility to heal... could exist'.[61] Ghosts could be exorcised.

Bones and stars

In 1996 the filmmaker Patricio Guzmán returned to Chile after over two decades in exile, with the intention of screening his epic three-part documentary *The Battle of Chile* (1975, 1976, 1979), which had been smuggled out of the country by boat and was banned during the Pinochet era. The three films that comprise *The Battle of Chile* document the last months of the Popular Unity government led by Salvador Allende, who was elected to power in 1970, and the violent counter-revolution that led to his overthrow in 1973. After completing the films in exile in the late 1970s, Guzmán experienced a long depression and period of emotional paralysis, which he only began to emerge from a decade later. Reflecting on that period in 2012, he remarked on its being an experience that many other exiled Chileans shared and also suggested that it was necessary for his later works on history and memory:

> I feel I've lost a lot of time, but on the other hand that's not strictly true because memory needs that time to reflect. It's not something that can be produced on the spot. It's a long and profound reflection, and I'm actually happy that I went through that process. It's the best way to resolve a stain—a wound that has marked my life, and the lives of another five million in Chile.[62]

Guzmán's *Chile, Obstinate Memory* (1997) saw him return to the country of his birth to talk to people who appeared in his earlier films. The film also documents screenings of *The Battle of Chile* to audiences of mostly younger Chileans. Guzmán films the often emotional reactions to the documentary, as well as capturing dialogues between young people and those who lived through the dictatorship. Survivors reflect on memory and forgetting. In *Chile, Obstinate Memory*, a doctor compares psychic pain to a wound that, if not properly tended, can become infected and never heal.

The emergence of psychiatric trauma programmes in the 1990s also coincided with the development of an influential body of work on trauma in literary and cultural theory by thinkers including Cathy Caruth, Shoshana Felman and Dori Laub. Influenced by psychoanalysis and by Frankfurt School critical theorists' writings on the Holocaust, this body of work emerged from the Yale School's engagements with Jacques Derrida's philosophy of deconstruction.[63] Ruth Leys has forcefully argued that despite being expressed in different registers, the dominant contemporary neurobiological understanding of psychic trauma enshrined in PTSD as a diagnostic category from 1980, and later epitomised in the work of popular neuroscientist Bessel van der Kolk, has much in common with the aporetic definition of trauma propounded by these poststructuralist thinkers.[64] For van der Kolk trauma is understood as a wound caused by an external event so extreme it cannot be registered at the moment it happens; it is then physically reexperienced or replayed in the form of literal flashbacks. In both cases, traumatic memory is held to be distinct from other kinds of memory and, as such, resists representation.

Guzmán's reflections on memory and wounding – both individual and collective – respond to a shared traumatic historical event. His return to Chile in the 1990s coincided with the peak influence of the Yale School work on trauma. Yet the aesthetic approach of Guzmán's films that reflect retrospectively on the coup cannot be neatly aligned with an aporetic understanding of trauma, the aesthetic counterpart of which tends to be characterised by fragmentation, discordance, fracture, disjunction and non-linearity, formally reflecting the rupture in subjectivity and the delayed onset of symptoms produced by the traumatic event. From the perspective of such an approach, one indebted to Jean-Francois Lyotard's writings on art and the sublime, exemplary post-traumatic artworks are understood as responses to a past that cannot be represented, that take the traumatic aporia itself as their subject, that formally convey the paradoxical presence-absence of the traumatising past event.[65] This chapter closes by moving away from psychiatric understandings of trauma to a discussion of Guzmán's later trilogy of films – *Nostalgia for the Light* (2010), *The Pearl Button* (2015) and *The Cordillera of Dreams* (2019) – which I propose offers an alternative model for approaching shared historical trauma arising from political repression.

By returning again and again in film after film to the subject of the coup d'état, Guzmán's filmmaking demonstrates something like the 'compulsion to repeat' that Sigmund Freud associated with the death drive. Freud had previously assumed that repetition was tied to pleasure and that every dream was the fulfilment of a wish, but his encounter with soldiers who had fought in the First World War could not be fit into this schema. They reported that their wartime experiences returned as nightmares. In his strange speculative essay *Beyond the Pleasure Principle* (1920), in an attempt to make sense of this form of unpleasurable repetition, he first introduced the concept of the death drive. The death drive is backward-looking; it seeks to return the organism to an inorganic state prior to life. It exists in a constant tussle with the life instincts or Eros, seeking to pull apart what Eros unites; the death drive destroys, Eros assimilates. Yet the goal of the death drive is not anguish or pain: it came into existence to protect the fragile organism from the onslaughts of the external world and it seeks to reinstate the quiescent state that preceded life.

Following Rebecca Comay, who treats trauma not as a psychological experience but as 'a modal, temporal, and above all a historical category' defined by anachronism, dissonance, untimeliness and belatedness, the death drive can be understood as a desire to start over: 'It is the desire to return to a time before the beginning—to go back not for the sake of regressing but in order to take it over again, to do it otherwise.'[66] In *The*

Cordillera of Dreams, Guzmán returns to his childhood home to find it still standing but in ruins. The camera moves up above the building to look down into the roofless, rubble-strewn rooms. Guzmán's voiceover reflects on the loneliness he has experienced since the coup. The ruins of his childhood home become a metonym for the destruction of a socialist dream in Chile:

> I've never spoken of the loneliness that has stayed with me since that 11th of September, 1973. It is like a hidden anxiety beneath my feet that something has collapsed, like an earthquake... I never stopped feeling alone, working in isolation in the midst of everyday life. In my soul, the smoke never cleared from the ashes of my home. I would like, if it were possible, to reconstruct it, to begin again.

Guzmán wants to return again to the beginning, to start over, to go back to a time before the ruins and ashes. At the end of the film he declares: 'My wish is that Chile recovers its childhood and joy.' This impossibly utopian yearning for a time before trauma, for an individual and national childhood naively pictured as innocent and pure, is combined in the films with an engagement with physical space and distant times so that trauma becomes not only a historical category but something geographical, astronomical, archaeological, geological. It is not, ultimately, through the expression of a desire to return to a time before but through moving outwards from individual memory and recent history that Guzmán, somewhat counterintuitively, succeeds in developing a distinctly political aesthetic of trauma.

Despite returning to the same ruptural event, Guzmán does not return obsessively to the literal site of the coup in this trilogy of films. Santiago is not at their centre, nor (unlike in some of his other documentaries) do these later films centre prominent political figures involved in those political events. Instead, the films focus on the natural world: desert, sky, sea, mountains. His camera caresses the textures of a world that seems remote from political action: ice, rock, leaves, sand, bark, moss, shells, waves. This spatial emphasis, this emphasis on the non-human, on the materiality of Chile as a physical place, alongside a stress on the *longue durée* of history, is key to how the films relate to the traumatic memory of the coup and dictatorship. These spaces are not external to history for Guzmán but provide a counterpoint to the supressed memories of 11 September 1973 and its aftermath; they register what the state brutally repressed.

In *The Pearl Button*, whose theme is water, Guzmán shows divers excavating pieces of railway track from the sea floor, the camera zooming in on corroded lumps of barnacle-encrusted metal; the bodies of the 'disappeared' had been lashed to these segments of railway track and thrown into the sea from helicopters. *The Cordillera of Dreams* ponders the mountains overlooking Santiago. Guzmán's camera pans across paving stones made from mountain rock which, he points out, would have felt terror march into the city. Now memorials to the dead are scattered among them. If they could speak, he says, they would speak of the blood that ran over them. His insistence that deserts, oceans and mountains witnessed historic violence should not be understood as sentimentality or mystical animism. It rather functions as a reminder that the material world retains traces of a past disavowed by the state. The repressed was right there. A counter-history exists that contradicts the history that was written by the victors, and it not only lies in the memories of individual victims (many of whom were forced to leave Chile) but remains embedded in the sand, the sea-bed, the city's streets.

Guzmán's 2010 documentary *Nostalgia for the Light* begins by reflecting on his childhood, a time when he was obsessed with astronomy. After the opening shots of a giant telescope, the camera cuts from an image of the surface of the moon in the vastness of the cosmos to a sun-baked domestic interior. Dappled light plays on a wall. Leaves rustle outside a window. Old household objects sit in a quiet room, reminding Guzmán of his peaceful childhood, when Chile seemed isolated from the forces of history and detached from the world beyond. He would gaze at a map of the stars whose names he committed to memory. He lived as if only the present existed. Guzmán's present-tense childhood, the film informs us, did not last. Something happened. Chile was swept into history by revolutionary forces. Allende's victory, Guzmán reflects, awakened his generation from their peaceful slumber and thrust them into an eventful world. The film explores what survives after their hopes were violently extinguished.

At the same moment that Allende came to power in 1970, Guzmán points out, astronomers in the Atacama Desert were exploring the skies through giant telescopes. After the coup in 1973, these scientific endeavours were cut short along with 'dreams and democracy', but Chilean astronomers continued to work as best they could. In the desert, nothing grows and nothing moves, but if the North American desert symbolised timelessness and the absence of history for Jean Baudrillard, for Guzmán the Atacama desert is a haunted and historical place filled with ghosts, memories and bones. Despite being mostly uninhabited, barren, salt-encrusted, alien-looking and vast, the desert is not a void or an aporia; it is the site of history. And so too, in a different sense, is the sky.

Astronomers, the film explains, are not only concerned with figuring out the distant origins of things, but because the light of the stars takes time to reach the earth, everything astronomers observe is in some sense already historical. Astronomy, like trauma, is anachronistic. The stars shine in the present from a before-time, recalling the image of happy childhood with which Guzmán begins the film. An archaeologist he interviews acknowledges his discipline's affinity with astronomy. *Nostalgia for the Light* surveys the ancient past of the skies and of the earth, to penetrate the more recent past of collective memory and of individual psyches. Guzmán speaks to those studying the ancient pasts of galaxies and civilizations, asking what the significance of these forms of backward-looking analysis might be in the context of a country seemingly incapable of examining its most immediate history. Guzmán's film may not be strictly therapeutic but it could be understood as socially reparative, placing the coup in a longer history of pre-colonial civilizations and a natural history of distant galaxies, obliquely showing that things could have been otherwise.

The film goes on to introduce women who wander the desert searching for the remains of their loved ones, people 'disappeared' by the regime during the dictatorship. It is impossible for these women to find peace while the fate of their loved ones remains uncertain. According to Becker and his ILAS colleagues, the disappeared acquired a peculiar 'living-dead' status for their surviving relatives, a status that blocked processes of mourning:

> If family members choose to accept the death of the loved one, they 'kill' him or her. If they choose to maintain hope, they deny their everyday experience of the loved one's absence. The long-range consequences of this double bind situation are profoundly altered processes of grief and related depressive symptomatologies.[67]

Tiny pieces of bone are discovered by women scouring the desert in the film, not identifiable remains but shards, fragments and slivers whitened by the sun. A seventy-year-old woman searching for her husband's remains sifts through the sand, propelled by so many still unanswered questions. 'Hope gives you strength,' she says. Searching for material evidence of the dead is a form of hope because it represents a refusal to forget or to accept. It aims to replace absence with loss. It aims to close the void.

While astronomers seek celestial bodies in the skies, women search for the lost bodies of their loved ones in the desert below. Guzmán's film makes a further analogy between these two searches through the past. He interviews the scientist George Preston, who declares that his lectures begin by telling a story about how the calcium in human bones was created as a result of the Big Bang. The calcium was there from the very beginning; the universe is part of us. The stardust in the skies is materially no different from the fragments of bone scattered across the desert. *Nostalgia for the Light* concludes by interviewing Valentina, an astronomer. As a small child she and her grandparents were detained by Pinochet's police, who threatened them in order to find out the location of her parents, who were subsequently disappeared. Astronomy became a way for Valentina 'to give another dimension to the pain'. She found she could mitigate her own personal pain by looking into the galaxies which gave her a different sense of time and cycles of existence. Stars also die, she reflects, but other planets are born. Studying the stars reassured her that nothing really comes to an end. Like Adi, the brother of a man murdered in the 1965–66 massacres in Indonesia who quietly confronts a series of perpetrators of violence in Joshua Oppenheimer's documentary *The Look of Silence* (2014), Valentina is shown with her child. Both Adi and Valentina express the wish to confront the past so that further trauma is not passed down to the next generation.

Close to the observatories in Guzmán's *Nostalgia for the Light* are the ruins of the concentration camp Chacabuco, built on the site of miners' housing. In the camp a group of political prisoners formed to observe the stars, learning to recognise constellations in the clear sky above. Gazing up at the skies gave them a feeling of freedom, one former prisoner recalls in the film, but they were soon forbidden to stargaze by the guards, who thought they might follow the stars to escape. They did not escape the camp, but the sky provided a kind of 'inner freedom', a psychic galaxy within, unconstrained by the barbed wire of their immediate surroundings.

As in Guzmán's trilogy of films, Raúl Zurita's poetic work *INRI*, written in response to President Ricardo Lagos' 2001 televised acknowledgement that the bodies of the disappeared had been dumped from helicopters into the ocean and scattered in the desert, turns to those locations to provide a testimony of the silenced. The earth cries out for the silenced and blinded dead anonymously scattered across it. Landscapes of water and stone registered events that went unremarked upon by those responsible for them. Stars weep, deserts and stones cry out, fields of flowers bend in the wind. In 'The Desert of Atacama VI', Zurita writes that 'Arid plains do not dream' and yet, haunted by the ghosts of the dead and literally scattered with their bones, perhaps they do. 'If water has memory, it will also remember this,' Zurita says in an interview in Guzmán's *The Pearl Button*.

In both Oppenheimer's documentaries about the massacres in Indonesia, *The Act of Killing* and *The Look of Silence*, it is remarked that people living in areas in Indonesia in which killings of accused communists took place did not eat the fish because fish were known to have devoured the mutilated corpses dumped into rivers. Carnivorous fish also appear in Zurita's book-length poem *INRI*. They consume the human bait that has dropped from the sky:

> I heard millions of fish which are tombs with
> pieces of sky inside, with hundreds of words that
> were never said, with hundreds of flowers of red
> flesh and pieces of sky in the eyes . . .[68]

This gruesome detail is transformed into an image of the world bearing witness to murders that were committed with impunity. Somewhere the historical trauma was registered, metabolised. Blue hydrangeas and white magnolias sprout defiantly from the eye sockets of the dead.

Forever engraved

In their account of therapeutic work with children of victims of repression, Becker and Díaz stressed that overcoming transgenerational trauma was dependent on the possibility for social reparation without which 'historical truth can only appear as individual craziness'.[69] In January 2023, Indonesia's President Joko Widodo issued a statement expressing regret for 'gross human rights violations' that took place in Indonesia between 1965 and 2003. Despite acknowledging the significance of the statement, many activists and human rights organisations in Indonesia also underlined that this was no substitute for concrete actions that would bring about justice for victims or accountability for perpetrators. The end of the dictatorship in Chile did not immediately bring about forms of recognition either. As Tomás Moulian noted in 1998:

It is incongruous to grieve for the dead and celebrate the memory of Salvador Allende and at the same time be the administrators of a society that exploits its workers, concentrates property into a few hands, sells off assets to foreign capital and restricts democracy.[70]

Guzmán contrasts his experience as an exile with the lives of people who stayed, interviewing a filmmaker in *The Cordillera of Dreams* who relentlessly took to the streets to capture resistance to the dictatorship on camera for posterity and remarks on the injustice that continued in the aftermath of the dictatorship. *The Pearl Button* also reflects on continuities between the violence of colonialism in Chile and the violence of the Pinochet regime, depicting Allende's regime, which committed to agrarian reforms that responded to the needs of indigenous people, as a brief crack of light between two long stretches of darkness.

When protests erupted in Chile in October 2019 over a 3 percent rise in subway fares, their meaning soon expanded. Sergio Villalobos-Ruminott observed that this thirty-peso increase 'came to represent thirty years of post-dictatorial governments . . . it has become evident that people are not only protesting a rise of the subway fare, they are protesting *everything* that has happened during the last three decades.'[71] In *My Imaginary Country* (2022), Guzmán's camera follows the enormous, percussive demonstrations through the streets, lingering on dislodged rocks strewn across the ground. In October 2020 Chileans voted to overturn the constitution that dated back to the dictatorship. A slogan spray-painted on walls and painted on banners in Santiago during the protests read: 'Neoliberalism was born and will die in Chile,' a phrase repeated by left-wing former student movement activist Gabriel Boric after he won the presidential election in December 2021. Such a death might help bring an end to the post-dictatorship sequence of trauma identified by Becker and Díaz, enabling a process of social healing to begin but even more modest social reforms that would not depend on global economic shifts are far from guaranteed; a proposal for a redrafted constitution was rejected in a national plebiscite in September 2022.

Guzmán described his films from the 1990s as attempts to tend to shared wounds, to resolve the psychic 'stains' of history, but as the ILAS psychotherapists perceived, socially inflicted wounds cannot fully heal in the absence of changed social conditions. William Rowe, the translator of Zurita's *INRI* into English, writes that the poem offers no redemption because 'the wound to our common human existence persists, the disappeared dead are still dead'. Instead, the poem 'seeks a place where the wound can be included inside the making of a different reality'.[72]

Though his method is artistic rather than scientific – he trains a camera on vast landscapes rather than performing an fMRI scan of an individual brain – Guzmán's films suggest that positive memories, memories of the euphoria of social transformation, also leave permanent traces in the mind that transform forever the people who experienced them. Memories of revolutionary possibility survive the brutal destruction of revolutionary movements and can be reactivated. In *The Cordillera of Dreams*, Guzmán remarks that he and his peers 'were marked by the same utopia', while in *Nostalgia for the Light* he opines: 'This time of hope is forever engraved in my soul.' Such experiences cannot undo traumatic pasts, but the notion that they too can change people irrevocably offers a counterpoint to a concept of trauma as aporia: in place of an aporia is the knowledge, based on a past experience of collective political transformation, that a different, less wounding reality might one day exist.

8

Mourning

> *There are no stories in the riots, only the ghosts of other stories.*
> – *Handsworth Songs*, Black Audio Film Collective (1986)

On 14 June 2017 a fire broke out in a tower block in North Kensington, West London. It quickly spread. The residents' organisation based in the Grenfell Tower had frequently raised safety concerns about the building's upkeep and maintenance, and they had expressed anxieties about the poor quality of renovations undertaken there. Their concerns were routinely ignored. The cheap combustible cladding covering the exterior of the building caused the fire to spread rapidly. The local authority's emergency response to the blaze was also insufficient. Seventy-two people died in the fire. Years later many survivors remained in hotels or temporary accommodation.[1] This was an atrocity that could have been avoided and that could be classed as having resulted from 'organised state abandonment', as Brenna Bhandar has argued.[2] Though the residents of the building were mostly working-class people of colour, living in social housing provided by the council, the tower was located in the Royal Borough of Kensington and Chelsea, one of the richest in the country. The fire starkly and tragically revealed deep structural inequalities in austerity Britain.[3] It was an extreme, though by no means isolated, example of the human consequences of a callous, profit-driven system.

Photos taken at a silent march held on 14 October 2017, marking four months since the fire and protesting the failure of the local council to provide adequate permanent housing to survivors (and many other failures besides) show a memorial wall on which the following Biblical verse had been painted: 'Blessed are they that mourn, for they shall be comforted' (Matthew 5:4). But the inadequate political response to the crisis and the gross negligence that enabled such a catastrophe to occur in the first place obstruct the process of mourning. Handwritten notes pasted on the walls beneath the sign attest to the difficulty of finding any comfort. How is it possible to mourn, which implies the possibility of moving on from the original loss, in the face of such glaring social injustice? How is it possible to continue the struggle for justice while grieving? How is it possible to fight while healing?

Before his execution by firing squad in November 1915 at Sugar House Prison in Utah, union organiser and militant song writer Joe Hill wrote a letter to International Workers of the World (IWW) leader Bill Haywood. It began: 'Goodbye Bill: I die like a true rebel. Don't waste any time mourning – organise!'[4] These parting words were subsequently transformed into a slogan that could soon be found emblazoned on the walls of IWW offices and painted on banners: 'Don't mourn: organise!'[5] Though Hill was referring to his own life rather than the life of an ongoing collective political struggle, the words attributed to him have often been appropriated to refer to less individualised forms of mourning.[6] The call is to affirm the hopeful future over the defeats of the past, to keep fighting for the living, rather than wasting energy in weeping over what has been lost. A wish for vengeance in the face of injustice is understandable – and the desire to rid the world of social forces responsible for inflicting loss is urgent – but what are the psychic costs of not mourning? Rather than alleviating mourning, seeking immediate redress can take its own toll, as David Wojnarowicz writes: 'A lot of people say that after they punch a wall they feel a lot better, but their hand is broken.'[7] Rather than turning to organising as a substitute for or sublimation of mourning, would it be possible to mourn *and* organise?

Mourning interminable

Jacqueline Rose notes that the canonical definition of 'mourning' given by Sigmund Freud in *Mourning and Melancholia* (1917) is surprising. For Freud, in contrast to melancholia, which is pathological and continuous, 'normal' mourning ends. Rose observes that it seems uncharacteristic of Freud to define mourning as 'something to be worked at, completed, got over', 'strange for a psychoanalysis which maintains that nothing ever goes away'. She reads this strangeness psychoanalytically, as a disavowal on Freud's part, as an 'attempt to drive mourning away (or at least to provide a narrative for mourning with a beginning, middle and an end)'. She also reads it historically, situating Freud's essay in the 'moment of cultural dismay' in which it was written, a time of war when all beginnings and middles seemed to collapse into the rubble of a terrifying and unanticipated end without end.[8]

Rose contends that in *Mourning and Melancholia*, Freud was attempting to 'preserve' or cling to an understanding of civilization that seemed increasingly untenable. (In Freud's essay, she reminds us, he claims in passing that it is also possible to mourn an ideal or an abstraction.) For Rose, 'mourning shifts her colours and her terms' if it is no longer defined as a completable process. Gradually severing psychic connections to the lost object in the manner proposed by Freud does not seem to provide the basis for a 'viable psychic or political future'. Instead she proposes a form of mourning that refuses 'to let go of the dead while also refusing to identify with what Freud . . . was able to refer to without self-consciousness as the "riches" of Western civilization'.[9] Mourning, like the process of psychoanalysis itself, could then be thought of as potentially interminable, especially in the context of a social world in which scars are prevented from healing and new wounds are constantly being inflicted.

In her oft-cited essay 'Paranoid Reading and Reparative Reading' (1997), Eve Kosofsky Sedgwick stresses the importance of finding a vocabulary that can 'do justice to a wide affective range'. According to Sedgwick, 'A disturbingly large amount of theory seems explicitly to undertake the proliferation of only one affect, or maybe two, of whatever kind—whether ecstasy, sublimity, self-shattering, *jouissance*, suspicion, abjection, knowingness, horror, grim satisfaction, or righteous indignation.' Her theoretical approach, she contends, is instead capable of attending to multiple, contradictory, or overdetermined affective states. But before outlining her solution, she caricatures – with her characteristically lacerating wit – various reductive approaches to affect:

> It's like the old joke: 'Comes the revolution comrade, everyone gets to eat roast beef every day.' 'But Comrade, I don't like roast beef.' "Comes the revolution, Comrade, you'll like roast beef.' Comes the revolution, Comrade, you'll be tickled pink by those deconstructive jokes; you'll faint with ennui every minute you're not smashing the state apparatus; you'll definitely want hot sex twenty to thirty times a day. You'll be mournful *and* militant. You'll never want to tell Deleuze and Guattari, 'Not tonight, dears, I have a headache.'[10]

Assuming I'm not just being paranoid, among this avalanche of pithy dismissals is a jibe at Douglas Crimp's now canonical essay 'Mourning and Militancy' (1989), a text I found myself returning to again and again in my attempts to think about how revolutionaries, activists and political organisers have responded to psychological damage and developed forms of psychological care within their milieus. Contra Sedgwick's satirical characterisation of his understanding of emotion as straight-jacketed by a reductive binary, Crimp explicitly claims that a wide range of emotional states accompany political movements and their aftermaths. He is not concerned simply with the seemingly contradictory coupling of mournfulness with militancy but with attending to 'frustration, anger, rage, and outrage, anxiety, fear and terror, shame and guilt, sadness and despair'.[11] Being a mournful militant consists precisely in acknowledging this litany of conflicting negative emotions.

In the essay, Crimp recalls that following the unexpected death of his father, with whom he'd had a difficult relationship, he expressed no sorrow and soon resumed his regular routines. Weeks later, however, he developed a large abscess in his left tear duct which eventually burst, spilling 'poison tears' down his face, a symptom he interpreted as a physical manifestation of his repressed grief: 'I have never since doubted the force of the unconscious. Nor can I doubt that mourning is a psychic process that must be honored.' This personal anecdote attesting to the psychic tenacity of unprocessed loss is recounted in the opening pages of his essay, in which Crimp confronts the seemingly oxymoronic relationship between his two eponymous concepts. Writing in the context of the AIDS crisis in the US, and addressing his community of fellow AIDS activists (he was involved with ACT UP New York), Crimp describes how mourning processes and rituals like candlelit vigils were frequently decried as anathema to militant political struggle – 'indulgent, sentimental, defeatist' – by those involved in the movement. As people lost lovers and friends to the ravages of AIDS-related illnesses, the call was to fight for the living rather than to weep for the dead. But Crimp insists on the necessity of mourning within radical political communities and, more importantly, he cautions against the dangers of not mourning: 'It is because our impatience with mourning is burdensome for the movement that I am seeking to understand it.'[12]

Crimp acknowledges that mourning, as defined by Freud in *Mourning and Melancholia*, does indeed seem incompatible with political activism. For Freud, though a finite process, mourning is all consuming; it 'leaves nothing over for other purposes or other interests'.[13] Crimp frames his argument in relation to Freud's outline of the concept of mourning, but he nonetheless acknowledges that 'normal' mourning in Freud's sense is impossible within the context he is describing.[14]

According to Crimp, Freud's theory says very little about communal grieving rituals, nor does it address the possibility that such rituals could be socially obstructed. Central to Freud's discussion of mourning is 'reality-testing', through which the subject comes to acknowledge and eventually accept the loss of the loved object, consequently withdrawing or detaching their libido from it. 'Reality', however, was not a neutral empirical backdrop in the context of the AIDS crisis because of the homophobic US state's 'ruthless interference with bereavement' and because loss was not a fact of the past to come to terms with and move on from but part of an uncertain future: 'Whether we share this fate is so unsure.' In the face of 'social and political barbarism' and the enforced silencing of grief within a hostile and homophobic society, Crimp declares that 'mourning *becomes* militancy'.[15] Except his argument doesn't end there. Though sympathetic to the transformation of sorrow into rage, he claims that because this process only takes place on a conscious level it leaves unconscious antagonisms unresolved. Militancy cannot function as a substitute for mourning but instead results from the socially enforced disavowal of grief; poison tears remain unwept. In this sense, militancy *represses* mourning.

Crimp complicates and reconceptualises Freud's definition of mourning by calling into question the notion that mourning can be accomplished by deferring to or accepting reality. Instead, he insists that the subject must attempt to survive within the structures of the violent external world without accepting them, while also being attentive to the damaging qualities of internal unconscious processes. In this (re)definition, mourning no longer entails a 'respect for reality' as Freud outlined, and certainly not for the 'riches' of 'Western civilization'; it instead involves reconfiguring both external and internal realities. Crimp also implicitly challenges Freud's statement that in mourning 'there is nothing about the loss that is unconscious', but though he identifies a certain melancholic self-doubting disposition in the AIDS activist community, he refuses to follow Freud in defining melancholia as pathological, nor does he claim that this emotional state results from a melancholic (and hence fully unconscious) relationship to the lost object.[16] Crimp's understanding of militant mourning is thus distinct both from (normal) mourning and (pathological) melancholia as defined by Freud.

Sarah Schulman's *Gentrification of the Mind* (2012) seeks to redress the absence of a public conversation about the consequences of AIDS in the US, with the intention of overcoming the pervasive social amnesia that persists about the scale and impact of mass death. Schulman writes that 'every gay person walking around who lived in New York or San Francisco in the 1980s and early 1990s is a survivor of devastation and carries with them the faces, fading names, and corpses of the otherwise forgotten dead.' She contrasts the 'barely mentioned' 81,542 people known to have died of AIDS in New York City as of August 2008 with the 2,742 people killed on 9/11 whose deaths have been officially memorialised through national mourning rituals and commemorative sites. Her fury is not only directed at the forgetting of the dead but, moreover, at the forgetting of the politicians who have never been held accountable for their actions which enabled the crisis to reach such a devastating scale: 'The names of our friends whom Ronald Reagan murdered are not engraved in a tower of black marble.'[17] Crimp similarly discusses the 'gross political negligence' that exacerbated the AIDS epidemic, and he addresses the psychic damage inflicted by a homophobic society which delegitimised experiences of bereavement and 'blamed, belittled, excluded, derided' people who died of AIDS-related illnesses and those who mourned them rather than offering empathy, support or adequate health care (here a parallel with the aftermath of the Grenfell Tower fire is apparent).[18]

Yet despite identifying brutal governmental policies and negligent social practices, Crimp nonetheless warns against carving too neat a dichotomy between the external and the internal, the social and the psychological. Yes, he says, the world is violent and unjust and this must be combated. However, violence is not only located outside the subject in a hostile society; it also operates on an internal, unconscious level. No single line can be plotted that moves inexorably from external violence (cause) to internal misery (effect). Instead, suffering might better be understood as resulting from ongoing conflicts between and within the social and the psychological, conflicts which are always mutually constituted and whose origins are never located in a single time or place: 'Violence is also self-inflicted.'[19] For Crimp, focusing solely on transforming the external world through militant action does nothing to resolve the corrosive effects of unconscious processes. After all, whatever activism might succeed in achieving, nothing can ever undo the original traumatic events. Here he cites Jacqueline Rose's discussion of a disagreement between Freud and Wilhelm Reich concerning the origins of misery, which echoes a passage in *Sexuality in the Field of Vision* (1986) in which she identifies a long-standing tendency for left-wing theorists seeking to politicise psychoanalysis to imagine that a clean distinction can be made between psychic and social processes:

Historically, whenever the political argument is made for psychoanalysis, this dynamic is polarized into a crude opposition between inside and outside—a radical Freudianism always having to argue that the social produces the misery of the psychic in a one-way process, which utterly divests the psychic of its own mechanisms and drives.[20]

Following Rose's insights, Crimp insists that locating all negative feelings in the external world only serves to *compound* psychological antagonisms and experiences of suffering: 'By making all violence external, we fail to confront ourselves, to acknowledge our ambivalence, to comprehend that our misery is also self-inflicted.' As such, Crimp insists that activists should be able to acknowledge feelings of 'frustration, anger, rage, and outrage, anxiety, fear, and terror, shame and guilt, sadness and despair' (to repeat the list cited above) and also attend to the experiences of those 'who feel only a deadening numbness or constant depression . . . who are paralyzed with fear, filled with remorse, or overcome with guilt', those for whom coherent expressions of anger in the form of explicit political action may be impossible.[21] This, however, entails an expansive understanding of militancy rather than a rejection of it.

Caring for remorseful and withdrawn friends and comrades is a political practice that can accompany other more public or combative forms of resistance. Committed to direct action, ACT UP additionally formed networks of care, with affinity groups transitioning into care teams. In *Let the Record Show* (2020), her panoramic history of ACT UP New York based on extensive oral history interviews, Schulman also describes celebratory nightlife and group experiences as forms of care – sex, love, companionship and forms of collective joy existed alongside proximity to sickness and death. Joe Ferrari reflects on how the coexistence of grief and conviviality provided emotional support within the movement, meaning carers were also cared for: 'We had the deep pain of watching people die, we had the extraordinary joy of being together, and we built a community.'[22]

Crimp concludes his essay with a demand for a militancy that acknowledges the necessity of mourning:

> The fact that our militancy may be a means of dangerous denial in no way suggests that activism is unwarranted. There is no question but that we must fight the unspeakable violence we incur from the society in which we find ourselves. But if we understand that violence is able to reap its horrible rewards through the very psychic mechanisms that

make us part of this society, then we may also be able to recognize—
along with our rage—our terror, our guilt, and our profound sadness.
Militancy, of course, then, but mourning too: mourning and militancy.[23]

Crimp's use of the conjunction 'and' in the essay's title and in this closing line risks suggesting that mourning and militancy remain distinct but parallel processes, whereas the essay 'Mourning and Militancy' redefines both terms. Crimp concludes by advocating for mournful militancy, a militancy that can be expressed in numerous affective registers – grief and anger, care and sadness, collectivity and withdrawal – and allows people to tend to psychic wounds while simultaneously attempting to radically transform society.

Mourning as militancy

Following the assassination of Patrice Lumumba, the first Prime Minister of the independent Democratic Republic of the Congo, in a plot orchestrated by the US and Belgian governments in 1960, his widow Pauline Opango Lumumba led a procession through the streets of Kinshasa (then Leopoldville) on Valentine's Day 1961, demanding that his body be returned. In the march she led through the streets, which was both a funeral procession and a protest, she walked stripped to the waist and bare-footed. Photographs of the event in the US press described it as representing a reversion to traditional African mourning rituals, but, as Tamar Garb argues, this reading depoliticises the gesture, which mixed grief with rage: 'In the context of the street and the crowd, the bared chest and feet suggest an insubordinate act in which grief is overlaid with defiance and mourning comes laced with anger.'[24] This was an act of mournful militancy.

Crimp addressed a political movement in which he feared militancy acted as a substitute for mourning, leaving loss unprocessed. He suggested that mourning could form part of political struggles, implying a more expansive definition of militancy, but would it be possible to conceive of militant collective action as a form of mourning in its own right? Schulman discusses the 'political funerals' of the early 1990s, among them a procession for David Wojnarowicz, who died in July 1992. Eventually actual corpses were brought to the streets, memorial services held in public spaces, open caskets laid out in parks. As in the funeral procession led by Pauline Opango Lumumba, anger at injustice and mourning were brought together; the dead could not be ignored.[25]

For Freud, 'when the work of mourning is completed the ego becomes free and uninhibited again,' but, as Rose underlines, the notion that mourning comes to a neat end seems uncharacteristically naive and optimistic.[26] The possibility of defining mourning as a process of closure is particularly troubling when loss is inflicted by social and political forces that continue. How could every ego become free in an unfree world? Mournful militancy is oriented to both the past and the future: calling for an acknowledgement of loss and demanding a world in which the same injustices cannot be repeated.

In *Working-through Collective Wounds: Trauma, Denial, Recognition in the Brazilian Uprising* (2018), psychoanalyst and social theorist Raluca Soreanu analyses the protests that erupted in Brazil in 2013 that have come to be known as the June Journeys or June Days, proposing that those collective gatherings in streets and squares could be understood as sites of collective mourning. What is being mourned in such situations and how is mourning enacted? Could her analysis be extended to other historical moments or movements?

In Soreanu's account, the streets and squares of Brazilian cities throbbing with joyful and enraged masses of people in protest created a site or 'frame' for mourning. These events, described by Sean Purdy as 'the most important political struggles in the country since the great working-class and popular mobilizations of the late 1970s and early 1980s that eventually ousted the military dictatorship in 1985', saw as many as 2 million people take to the streets.[27] Originating as demonstrations against increases to the price of public transportation, as the protests grew so did their broader social significance and their demands, which soon encompassed issues of health care, education, policing and government corruption. Soreanu is less interested in the manifest demands made by the protests than in their latent significance as therapeutic sites for tending the wounds of collective memory.[28]

Soreanu describes her own participation in these events in phenomenological terms and discusses the powerful psychic effect of physically moving with a crowd of people marching and chanting, breathing and pulsating together. She examines 'socialities of radical mutuality, socialities of psychic resonance, socialities of corporeal connection' and euphoric experiences of affinity conventionally assumed to be remote from or even antithetical to experiences of trauma and mourning. Embodied experience is a significant aspect of the psychic life of the crowd. Soreanu explores 'how collectives create meaning, via rhythmic entanglements', and asks: 'Is it possible to come to speak of the rhythm of solidarity?'[29] She describes herself moving back and forth between her psychoanalytic consulting room and the protests, with this movement from the couch to the streets acting as a counterpart to the theoretical relationship between the psychic life of the individual and the psychic life of the collective with which her book grapples.

The atmosphere and emotions generated by a protest provide a potent, uplifting and embodied experience of connection and togetherness, but they are also marked by antagonism and violent confrontation. Soreanu captures the enveloping sense of 'political love' on the streets in terms that resonated with my own experiences of being caught up in the surging crowds of a political gathering. She also reflects on the 'hatred, violence and destructiveness' that accompany the rush of solidarity when, for example, a crowd clashes with the police. She examines both 'the sociability of traversing clouds of tear gas with others' and the solidarity enacted when vinegar is shared among a group as its antidote. Yet for Soreanu the act of demonstrating in the streets is not only about an exuberant mutuality and collective antagonism in the present moment but bears a relationship to the past that enables it to become a site for social healing: 'We were never as close to the brink of mourning as when we were protesting, on the streets, and in the squares.' Her book asks whether and how trauma can be worked through collectively; to do this, she identifies moments in which crowds reference historical moments or figures, make intergenerational connections, or transform shared experiences of wounding into collective symbols.[30]

Like Crimp's, Soreanu's theoretical approach to these questions is psychoanalytic, but her main frameworks come not from Freud but from the Hungarian psychoanalyst Sándor Ferenczi, whose 'radically politicisable' concepts she transposes from the domain of the individual into that of the social.[31] Traditionally psychoanalysis has conceptualised masses as regressive rather than emancipatory. In 'Group Psychology and the Analysis of the Ego' (1921), Freud canonically characterised the group as 'impulsive, changeable and irritable'. Unlike in individuals, repression lifts in group situations so that the group is then led by the unconscious, unleashing primal destructive instincts. Groups for Freud are overly trusting, gullible, uncritical, easily swayed by irrational claims and prone to extremes. There are explicit political implications to Freud's definition of the group: 'Fundamentally it is entirely conservative, and it has a deep aversion to all innovations and advances and an unbounded respect for tradition.'[32] Freud's discussions of group or mass psychology, which emphasise the significance of leaders for groups, influenced subsequent theorisations of the psychic appeal of fascism, which cemented an association of groups with regression, cruelty and intolerance.[33] Soreanu pushes against this characterisation by refusing to view the protesting crowd as a site of irrational regression. And unlike the groups discussed by Freud, such crowds have no leaders. If for Freud groups have a tendency to simplify, to homogenise the heterogeneous, for Soreanu they can also retain a capacity for subtlety. She notes the crowd's remarkable capacity for 'sophisticated symbolic activity' that creates connections with the past, through generations and across history.[34]

Urban spaces are haunted; the past is always entangled with the present. The rhythms that emerge in protest are also ghostly:

> The rhythms of past losses, traumas, injustices, conflicts, dispossessions, or exclusions have been imprinted in materialities and in memories of movement. But ghosts can also be reparatory and transformative: to walk with them is also to walk the path from unmourned loss to mourned loss.[35]

In this context, haunting should not be understood as a metaphor for psychic repression, which would assume that an exorcism could be achieved solely through an individualised process of reflection on the past. Instead, a collective engagement with the social conditions of the present is required. Hauntings are manifestations of material historical processes and can only be addressed by acknowledging how the past has shaped both contemporary reality and the struggles to change it. Stephen Frosh, whose work Soreanu engages with, articulates this in the following terms: 'Ghosts cannot be removed by being spoken about; they can only be set free by some kind of action to bring them the justice they deserve.'[36] Haunting is connected to retribution, mourning to redress. Mourning in this definition comes closer to Crimp's discussions of the need to carve out spaces for grieving within a hostile society than it does to Freud's emphasis on the process of coming to terms with external reality as it already is.

Soreanu not only refutes Freud's assumptions about mass psychology but also challenges psychoanalytic understandings of repetition's relationship to trauma. In *Beyond the Pleasure Principle* (1920), Freud revised his own previous assumptions about the relationship between repetition and pleasure. In the wake of the First World War, confronted with soldiers beset by traumatic dreams, Freud was forced to acknowledge a painful and

Mourning

compulsive form of repetition that led him to posit the existence of the death drive. Just as Freud's connection between regression and groups ossified into the dominant psychoanalytic understanding of mass psychology, so the association of repetition with trauma, Soreanu argues, has become fixed. She suggests that the kinds of reenactments and connections with the past that she witnessed in protest could instead be understood as forms of 'creative' repetition. The crowd in protest may be engaging with collective traumatic experience – 'traumatic residues operate as a force that organises the scene' – but trauma should not be understood as 'inescapable and irrevocable', nor as 'non-symbolisable or non-representable'. In addition to the two forms of repetition outlined by Freud (pleasurable and unpleasurable), Soreanu proposes a 'reparative and restorative' mode of repetition that she elaborates by drawing on Ferenczi's notion of 'reliving'. Scenes of protest are characterised by 'complicated forms of re-living' and unleash what she identifies as *the capacity for analogies*, which provide the grounds for working through.[37] Crowds in protest can be understood as engaging with a traumatic past in a manner which, far from signalling their incapacity to move on, instead tends towards healing. In this sense, protest can become an act of mourning. Demonstrations can function as sites in which ambivalence can be worked through rather than disavowed.

Soreanu describes a scene from the 2013 protests in Brazil that exemplifies how an analogy between the violence of the past and the violence of the present was enacted on the streets. An old man stepped out of the crowd to angrily address a line of cops guarding a municipal building:

> Last night at the Palácio Guanabara, why did you shoot at these youngsters? Why did you chase them down the streets with your guns? Why did you beat them? Why did you humiliate them? Don't you see? This is just like the times of the military dictatorship?

Here the elderly protester stood before the young masses and articulated a connection to history that clarified continuities and identified forms of intergenerational inheritance. In an argument that recalls the approach to Chilean history taken in Patricio Guzmán's documentary *The Pearl Button* (discussed in the previous chapter), Soreanu argues that in Brazil collective trauma cannot be understood as solely connected to the brutalities of the military dictatorship; rather it is located in disavowed connection between dictatorship and democracy, as well as having deeper roots in histories of slavery and colonialism. The logic of torture had been inherited but forms of ongoing violence were disavowed.[38]

Situating injustice in the *longue durée* is also crucial in the case of the Grenfell Tower fire. The Grenfell Tower was named after Francis Grenfell, a military officer who commanded armies that waged war on colonial populations in South Africa and Sudan, before becoming Governor of Malta and Commander-in-Chief of Ireland. The histories of migration that led residents of the tower to London and the histories of urban development that led to the building's neglect are also linked to long histories of racial capitalism.[39] The difficulty of those who mourn to find comfort – to return to the Biblical verse written on the wall near the Grenfell Tower – is connected to the way those histories continue to shape the present. In Steve McQueen's 2020 TV film *Mangrove*, the scaffolding-covered Grenfell Tower is shown being constructed in the background of scenes of British Black Panthers in the 1970s addressing protesting crowds in West London. It is a ghostly presence, but the ghost comes from both the past and the future. The inclusion of the tower in the film is not a gesture of historical fidelity as the events depicted predate its existence.[40] Instead, the building is a deliberate, haunting reminder of the history that was yet to unfold, connected to histories that had happened long before, whose afterlives and effects the Black Panthers were seeking to interrupt.

Emphasising protest as a site or frame for mourning in Soreanu's account also complicates discussions of collective mourning in Latin America that tend to focus on official institutionalised forms of memorialisation as ways of acknowledging the brutalities of life under military dictatorship. She points to the therapeutic limits of official forms of civic commemoration like memorials and truth commissions, which, unlike protests, do not involve the synchronised 'vocalisations and movements' of a collective or its 'material-corporeal mesh'. She instead makes the case for a pluralised understanding of both sites and acts of mourning that would encompass 'semi-spontaneous mourning' rituals like the political demonstration.[41] State-sanctioned forms of memorialisation in Brazil suppressed connections and continuities between past and present, enacting a disavowal that could be compared to the overly neat distinction between internal and external realities identified by Crimp. In the streets, by contrast, these links leapt into view. The protests formed part of a struggle to acknowledge the still unhealed wounds of the past, both psychological and social, alongside an acknowledgement of continuing injustice, oppression and exploitation.

Crimp's experiences led him to rework Freud's definition of mourning in a social context in which politically exacerbated mass death was still ongoing. In Brazil, the state's violent suppression of the protests indicated an ambivalence towards mourning: the state may have organised truth commissions and built monuments to victims of the dictatorship, but it could not tolerate spontaneous invocations of the past enacted on the streets, which threatened to link past violence to the continuing oppressions of the present. Mourning is obstructed in a society that seems to acknowledge and atone for the violence of history, while continuing to enact violence in a still structurally unequal and racist society.[42] Though the left was in power in 2013, neoliberal policies alongside pragmatic compromise with and capitulation to the centre and right continued, as did police brutality against black people and people involved in social movements.[43]

The protests unleashed a collective mourning process that was prematurely cut off and swiftly erased from public memory, an erasure that risked causing re-traumatisation. Soreanu addresses the suppression of the memory of the June Days in their immediate aftermath and hints at a link between this suppression and subsequent events in Brazil, but she does not explicitly discuss the impeachment of Dilma Rousseff or the subsequent election of Jair Bolsonaro in 2018. Bolsonaro had served as a member of the armed forces during the military dictatorship, and in 2019 he instructed the army to commemorate the fifty-fifth anniversary of the March 1964 coup which imposed the brutal military regime that controlled the country until 1985. The oppressions of both past and present were celebrated, new wounds inflicted while salt was rubbed into the old ones. After Luiz Inácio Lula da Silva's narrow defeat of Bolsonaro in the October 2022 election, militancy in the present seemed more urgent than mourning past events but as Rodrigo Nunes cautioned, although political concessions would be necessary, the danger of capitulation must be staved off: 'The decision to work within existing constraints, without striving to change them, will only prove disastrous.'[44] Soreanu's work suggests that such discussions are not as remote from psychological concerns as they might seem.

Ghosts in the riots

The case of Amarildo de Souza, a bricklayer from a favela who vanished after being taken into police custody on 14 July 2013, took on a special significance within the Brazilian movement. The masses on the streets would shout, 'Where is Amarildo?', and an individual's death became a catalyst for a broader movement, as in Iran in 2022 when the death of Mahsa Amini sparked the movement of feminist resistance to the Islamic Republic. Outrage and anger at one individual's treatment by the police, Soreanu posits, were linked to events in the present but also to a history of anonymous and still unresolved disappearances that happened throughout the years of the military dictatorship. This connection across time opened up a 'passage from unmournable loss to loss that can be mourned ... The symbolisations around Amarildo bring an escape from an endless trail of unidentified bodies – bodies in black rubbish bags, bodies buried without ceremony.'[45] In Soreanu's reading, the name 'Amarildo' was evoked to enunciate an analogy between past and present that enabled the commencement of a collective mourning process for multiple lives lost at the hands of the state.

In an interview reflecting on the continuities between the uprisings in Ferguson in 2014–15 after the police killing of Michael Brown and those that shook the US and world after the murder of George Floyd in Minneapolis in 2020, Hannah Black discusses events in which one person's death can become 'an object of collective grief and anger' in protests that instantiate an 'interweaving of present and past'. Individual deaths of black people at the hands of the police are linked through history as crowds on the streets repeat a long litany of names, signalling the continuity of injustice:

> There is a huge archive of the dead and it gets activated every few years across time. It's like some massive activation. The wide circulation of these really distressing last words of people being murdered by police, for example Elijah McClain. I don't like to listen, but I read the transcripts. So, the dead literally speak. The dead speak and people riot as a kind of revolutionary mourning practice, and this happens unpredictably.[46]

Protests and riots can be acts of mourning; they are also acts that testify to mourning's impossibility in the current state of things. Revolutionary mourning breaks out when reality is tested (in Freud's terms) and found wanting. When mourning is obstructed, mournful militancy smashes through the poisonous complacency of the murderous present.

In the aftermath of police killings of black people in the US, candlelit vigils and burnt out cop cars are often rhetorically treated by mainstream media pundits as antithetical responses to the events, as two irreconcilable poles. Legitimate mourning rituals and peaceful forms of protest are contrasted to illegitimate property damage and looting. The candles, the cars and the Third Precinct police station in Minneapolis burnt with the same fire, but only some flames could not be contained. In 2020 the flames were so widespread and blazed so brightly that the usual rhetoric of condemnation briefly ceased. Mourning *and* militancy. Freud's definition of 'normal' mourning relies on a neutral definition of reality, but no such mourning is possible when reality remains unlivable. The uprisings in 2020 which saw people burst onto the streets after months of quarantine during the Covid-19 pandemic, Tobi Haslett observed, 'breached the surface of social life'.[47] The riots tore through 'normal' reality, momentarily shattering its seeming inevitability and permanence. If left melancholia reifies past losses, militant mourning erupts and interrupts.

Reflecting on the protests that followed the killings of Trayvon Martin and Michael Brown, Angela Davis stated that 'the major challenge of this period is to infuse a consciousness of the structural character of state violence into the movements that spontaneously arise'.[48] Davis invoked a Leninist shift from spontaneity to consciousness which would see outrage at individual deaths transform into an emphasis on the shared underpinnings that connect violent incidents perpetrated by the state across time and space. She emphasised the insufficiency or indeed impossibility of individual legal solutions when the so-called justice system is founded on and grounded in racial injustice, as the acquittal of Martin's killer George Zimmerman in 2013 and the failure to indict Brown's murderer Darren Wilson in 2014 underlined. When people took to the streets in 2020 and shouted George Floyd's dying words, 'I can't breathe', they invoked his individual memory, but those words took on a broader resonance when shouted collectively in cities across the US and across the world. The words were reproduced on walls and placards in Kenya, India, Syria, Argentina, Palestine. The words are also ghosts of other stories, as they were also the last words of Jimmy Mubenga (who was killed by G4S security guards on a deportation flight from the UK to Angola in 2010) and Eric Garner (killed by a cop on Staten Island in 2014). The scale of the George Floyd uprisings in 2020 could be taken as evidence of the shift in consciousness Davis describes, and they could also be interpreted as semi-spontaneous mourning rituals of the kind described by Soreanu, though it is not easy to discern what the legacy of those now extinguished flames will be. When an individual death links to collective experiences, when a murdering cop is identified as being part of a murderous system, when 'normal' mourning is impossible because 'normal' reality remains lethal – this is when mournful militancy emerges.[49]

Mournful militancy is not just about vengeance but about justice; it is not just about honouring the past but about transforming the present for the sake of the future. The dead will be safe from the enemy only when it is defeated.[50] And justice cannot be achieved through existing laws, systems or institutions but only through their abolition, through the demonstration of their foundational injustice. Mourn, organise. Mournful organisers must also heed Crimp's warnings and provide space for respite, paying attention to self-inflicted wounds and accepting that not everyone can always join the crowds on the streets. Mournful militancy is not intended to strip mourning of ambivalence; it instead evinces the hope of opening up space and time to sit with ambivalent feelings.[51] As Israeli bombs killed civilians in Gaza in October 2023, Saree Makdisi observed that the 'scale of the death and destruction is so massive, so unrelenting, there's often no time to mourn'. It is imperative to organise globally for Palestinian liberation to stop the killing, to end the occupation and to make mourning a possibility.[52] As Abdaljawad Omar argues in 'Can the Palestinian Mourn?', 'The very attempt to break Israel's militarism, is an active yearning to mourn without interruption, to construct a chronal refuge where tears do not have to be defiant.'[53] Mournful militancy is not a lament but a demand. Mournful militants do not look melancholically at the past but intervene with rage and with care in the present for the sake of the living. Without a social reckoning mourning is impeded, which is another way of saying: no justice, no peace.

Afterword

Now there are no maps and no magicians.[1]

— Muriel Rukeyser

We argue endlessly about whether it was us who died or them, but the one thing we all agree on is the barbed line that separates us. Sometimes we pluck that line. It makes a high and barely audible electric screech, like some useless old record. It puts immense pressure on the inside of our skulls, like boiling bleach, like the abolition of all memory. It speaks of heartbreak, of denial, of new advances in somnambulism. Of revenge fantasies and drug addiction. It has nothing to say about where to go from here, about the day we crawl out from under our scattered rocks, and burn their border controls to the ground.[2]

— Sean Bonney

Some time in the middle of a long pandemic winter in lockdown, I lost all sense of why I was writing this book. That is to say, I lost all sense of hope. I wondered why I had thought there might be any value in excavating experiences of defeat, in collaging loss, in cataloguing despair.

During the UK student movement over a decade ago I remember people enthusiastically passing around copies of philosopher Gillian Rose's *Love's Work* with its epigraph from the Eastern Orthodox monk Staretz Silouan: 'Keep you mind in hell and despair not.'[3] While writing this book I would sometimes think of those words. But I felt so angry. If people have to live in the hellish world while seeking to transform it, can't they at least feel despair? What if it isn't possible to believe in salvation, in redemption? What if it's all too hard to bear?

I wondered what I thought I'd find when I started writing about burnout. Maybe I thought that by tracing emotional histories and confronting the difficulties of keeping going while attempting to overturn immiserating systems and oppressive structures I could show how things might have been different or declare confidently that they could still be better. I wanted to get to the end and have some kind of an answer. I wanted to be able to say maybe it will be OK and actually believe it. I wanted to say here are some small things that people could do that might make it easier. I wanted to make practical suggestions that didn't just sound like feeble self-help platitudes. I wanted to pretend that psychological pain could be somehow generative. I wanted to present some neat little theories that might help make sense of painful emotions as they arise. Look, I wanted to say, this person did this thing and they felt a bit better and then they carried on. I wanted to say that they won. I wanted to believe that these small things could work, could mean something, could all add up to something bigger, could at least help in the meantime. I wanted to believe all these past strivings weren't for nothing.

Instead, sitting alone in my room, I ended up thinking that it was no fucking wonder that people lost their minds. No wonder people couldn't carry on, gave up, fell out. No wonder they had nightmares, stayed in bed, ended their lives. I didn't think that the many losses and repressions were inevitable, that people weren't right to have tried, that there couldn't have been other outcomes, but once situations passed a certain point, the psychic responses to them seemed hard to imagine otherwise.

I came across this autobiographical passage by the poet Anna Mendelssohn and copied it out long hand:

> I found joy in sharing my questioning with others, giving validity to that questioning, to diving into unmapped, untrodden territory. We lost our way many times – in a world full of answers it's hard to hold a question, when all you know is what feels wrong. Friendships suffered, we all expected of ourself and each other to have the answer, and we fell into despair and mistrust. The joy turned sour. There was no nourishment for us in the world we were born to, and the initial fuel we had found in each other was burning out. It was a lonely time. And I blamed the State for our alienation – though by that time I was numb from the harm we do to each other.
>
> It hit me that our political activities arose out of despair – that I never really believed that the revolution was possible anyway, let alone inevitable. Everything out there was all too big, too complicated, to take on; too anarchic to make any logical sense of. I'd slowly progressed from world politics to city (London) politics to local politics, till finally I was left with the smallest unit – myself.[4]

Afterword

Mendelssohn was active in far-left politics from the late sixties and incarcerated in Holloway Prison in London after being charged with conspiracy for her alleged involvement in planning Angry Brigade bombings. The passage captures so much of what I had spent the previous months thinking about: an original feeling of joy followed by the curdling of hope, animosity emerging between comrades, the emotional numbness produced by prolonged political engagement, the shrinking of possibility. If milk turns sour it cannot be made fresh again. Is it possible to move from the smallest unit back to the largest?

Again and again, I kept coming to the same conclusion, which provides no consolation at all: psychological experiences require patience while so much in the world demands urgency.

The problem with anti-adaptive healing is that it is necessarily asynchronous: to get better in the present it is necessary to change so many things in the world. And the problem with that is that by the time it's done it will already be too late.

I wrote the word 'hope' and it clanged on the page.

I thought of a line in a poem by Muriel Rukeyser written in the aftermath of the Spanish Civil War, and it suddenly seemed to make sense to me:

the terrible time when everyone writes 'hope.'[5]

Having written all these words about despair and defeat, failure and loss, I suddenly imagined what it would have been like if I'd written a completely different book. What if I'd written a book about the future, about imagination, about prefigurative possibility, about fresh growth, about love, about overcoming past sufferings, about building a less pain-inflicting society? What if I had pictured a world in which pain-inflicting political struggle was no longer necessary? What if I had written a book about people stirred and moved and elated? What if I had written a book where even milk didn't turn sour? What if I had written a book about solidarity, about victory, about feeling really alive? What if I had written a book about abolishing the family, private property and the state, about tearing down prisons, about societies without police? What if I had written a book about what it feels like to pour forth on to the streets, what it feels like to win, what it could feel like to live otherwise? Perhaps I no longer believed that such a book, let alone such a world, was really possible.

Sometimes I would read polemical books by my peers whose political arguments I broadly agreed with and I would wonder why I couldn't just write like that too. I felt guilty for finding their tone tiring and stifling. I worried that it betrayed something reactionary or resigned that I found myself admitting ambivalence, equivocating, lacking assurance. But something about my subject – not just political defeat, but psychic life – resisted such treatment. I didn't want to ignore emotional difficulties, which meant I couldn't reach any pat conclusions. After all, even in the extremely unlikely event of a global revolution, psychological distress will not simply disappear.

In Hannah Black's beautiful reimagining of the recent past of social democratic campaigns, pandemic and anti-racist uprisings that is also a vision of an alternative near future, *Tuesday or September or The End* (2021), the characters Dog and Bird, who are in a romantic relationship, embody a tension between reform and revolution. These two positions could in turn be mapped onto the tension between patience and urgency that I have found myself crashing into over and over again. Black narrates the two modes as interdependent, mutually reinforcing:

> Dog wanted Bird to be a hopeless insurrectionist so that he could feel his own secret fidelity to sudden transformation still alive under layers of pragmatism and policy; Bird wanted Dog to believe in incremental progress in the abattoir of capitalism so that her inner sense of abyss could acquire walls and a floor. Bird searched in Dog for ground, and Dog searched in Bird for lightness and fire. Their difference was binding and animated their love, which was sometimes exhausting and mundane, with the five fingered chords of world history.

Even the ultimate lightness and fire of love can be tiring and mundane. And love requires work. At the end of the novel riots erupt. In the crowds of people emerging from pandemic-induced isolation onto the streets Bird briefly forgets to dwell on her past and experiences the rush of riot as 'medicinal and magical':

> The losses themselves were healed by the novelty of being with others, and not only that, but seeing police cars burn, and not only that. Her soul rushed towards the riot. She had no opinion about her fate. The wheel of fortune spun wildly; the future was infinitely open.[6]

As the riots become revolution – as prisons open, as the police are abolished, as commodities are liberated from the value form, as the revolution becomes the ground of a new reality – the open future acquires walls and a floor. Spontaneity settles into consciousness and opens a space for the unconscious. The healing process continues but its medicine is not magical or instantaneous like the riot; it requires effort, time and care. Black describes psychoanalytic groups meeting in empty lots and small groups of people gathering in the streets to talk about their past lives: 'The buried wounds of the past came up for air.'[7] A similar acknowledgment that past pains will not be instantly overcome even if the world is transformed by revolution underpins M. E. O'Brien and Eman Abdelhadi's *Everything for Everyone: An Oral History of the New York Commune, 2052–2072* (2022), in which the imagined interviewees of the liberated future who are building communism in the ruins of the damaged and flooded world often reflect on their participation in communally organised, innovative forms of lay therapy, group reflection and trauma processing.

These books imagine utopian post-revolutionary futures, but the futures they envisage are not hermetically sealed worlds that leave all scars behind. Reading them reassured me that attempting to write about psychic suffering was not antithetical to revolutionary political commitments, however disconsolate and demoralised doing so has sometimes left me feeling. People who have lived through political struggles and the social changes they bring about will have psychological issues to continuously work through even if they succeed. Finding ways – methods, institutions, practices, infrastructures, concepts and treatments – capable of attending to those issues is itself a vital political question. The revolutions imagined by these two utopian books usher in the beginning of a process of healing rather than marking its end: 'Fertilized by the new abundance of time, past pain unfurled leaves on which were written a glowing scripture of new life.'[8]

For a long time I have collected revolutionary dreams.

Revolutionary dreams tend to be envisioned as dreams of the future: daydreams, prophetic dreams, dreams that provide an image of a wildly different reality. Euphoric, expansive, utopian – revolutionary dreaming is usually conceived as an imaginative act that reaches beyond the constricting parameters of the present. Lenin famously declared, 'We must dream!' in *What Is to Be Done?* (1901–2), by which he meant something like 'revolutionaries must imagine a better society and work to make it a reality.' Revolutionary dreaming is, as Jackie Wang writes, a 'vision of an elsewhere'.[9]

I gathered dreams dreamt by revolutionaries, but these were not dreams of revolution or visions of the future in the sense implied by Lenin. Dreams dreamt at night, at least according to the canonical Freudian definition, might represent the fulfilment of wishes, but their contents – both latent and manifest – come from the past. They certainly don't provide political blueprints. Of course, it is no substitute for strategy or analysis or actually doing things, but I nonetheless found something consoling about approaching recounted or fictional dreams as weird poetic texts detached from individual dreamers. They seemed to signal, however obliquely, a desire for another world.

In Muriel Rukeyser's novel *Savage Coast*, set during the Spanish Civil War and written in 1936 immediately after her time in Spain, the protagonist dreams of the sea:

> A green streaked sea, with black tremendous currents. And headlong, plunging through the stream, a force rushing, which carried her along; until she ceded her will to it in a huge gesture. In that moment, she revived, she drew will from the enormous source, and thought, even in the dream: O Parable.[10]

Audre Lorde dreams of a sexual encounter in a utopian counter-Moscow:

> I was making love to a woman behind a stack of clothing in Gumm's Department Store in Moscow. She was ill, and we went upstairs, where I said to a matron, 'We have to get her to the hospital.' . . . And I realized I was in Russia, and medicine and doctor bills and all the rest of that were free . . . For a while, in my dreams, Russia became a mythic representation of that socialism which does not yet exist anywhere I have been.[11]

Agnes Smedley, in her autobiographical novel *Daughter of Earth* (1929), dreams of infinity, which, like the sea described by Rukeyser's character, opens out from the material constraints of the present to vibrate with possibility:

> I stood on the outer verge of the world. The earth lay back and below me. I was suspended in the air by my own weight. About me was the universe – deep blue, shot through with grey. Unchanging, never-ending. Before

me, above me, below me, stretched nothing but this colour. This was Infinity, I thought.

Then I stood gazing slightly upward, and from the vastness teardrops were falling. They fell just before my face, a row of large, dark, grey drops, and by their side, a row of small rose-hued drops. I listened ... they fell into nothingness below me, without a sound ... there was nothing to make a sound. I neither heard them come nor go. How slowly and endlessly they fell!

The large grey drops were tears of pain, I recalled with unquestioning finality, and the small rose-hued ones that came so slowly were tears of joy.

Above me stretched Infinity, soundless, unbounded in immensity. A dim humming came ... the dim, never-ceasing humming of the cosmic universe. The uncomprehending vastness of it filled my being.

I turned restlessly and awoke. Infinity hung over my spirit.[12]

Reading this vision of vastness, of a humming universe, of rose-hued colours felt like opening a window out from the gloomy images of defeat I had been contemplating.

I thought of C. L. R. James writing about *Moby Dick* while incarcerated on Ellis Island. I thought of Rosa Luxemburg looking through her prison bars at sparrows, blackbirds and birch catkins. I thought of Victor Serge in exile in Mexico, writing in his notebook in 1944, less than a decade after he escaped the Stalinist purges and soon after fleeing encroaching fascism in Western Europe. Serge knew that he would die soon and that 'tyranny' would outlive him. He thought of the past, of his many dead comrades, of the war he had been spared, but he also tenderly described the soft textures and sonic tremors of the world around him:

> At night, more distinctly than during the day, the garden full of mango, lemon, orange, and banana trees and flowering oleander produces a symphony of rustling, whispering, whistling, buzzing and vibrations.[13]

He wrote no platitudes about hope but remained committed to a cause whose victory he knew he would not live to see.

While I was in the process of finishing this book, I came across accounts by women involved in the UK Miners' Strike of 1984–5 in Yorkshire. In contrast to my earlier experiences of reading similar material in my attempt to conceptualise an alternative to 'left melancholy', I was struck less by their descriptions of the negative emotions associated with defeat than by their emphasis on positive and lasting subjective transformations. A woman from Castleford characterised her involvement in the strike as having an almost therapeutic effect, but one that conventional psychiatric treatments had failed to accomplish:

> I suffer from agoraphobia, and I'd been virtually housebound for thirteen years before the strike started. I couldn't even go to the shop on my own. My husband and son are both miners, so when the kitchen started up in the Church Hall at Hightown they persuaded me to volunteer. I was a bit nervous about the idea, but I came down and did a bit of washing up and got talking to the other women, and it did me a world of good.
>
> Since then I've hardly missed a day and I really enjoy it. It's a marvellous atmosphere, everyone is so friendly. Whenever anyone's got to go to the shops I'd always volunteer – at first people who didn't know me couldn't understand why. I've been to psychologists and psychiatrists and even spent money trying to find a cure, but this strike is the only thing that done it. The only way I can explain it is – it's like being reborn. I know that I've got to keep active after the strike.[14]

I started this book with the conviction that it was important to acknowledge the emotional toll of political defeat. I wrote this book because I felt suspicious of rhetorical appeals to hope that failed to account for the difficult emotional realities of political defeat. I finished this book reminded that experiences of political struggle can also change people positively and in lasting ways.

As winter turned into spring, I received a message saying there was an immigration raid happening near my flat in Glasgow. I went with my flatmate to Kenmure Street where people were milling around an immigration enforcement van surrounded by cops. Someone was underneath the van to stop it driving off, we were told, with the two detainees inside. Over the course of the next few hours the crowds grew. I emailed to cancel my psychoanalysis session and stayed on the street. I saw people I hadn't seen for months due to Covid-19 lockdowns and met others for the first time. Strangers shared water and snacks. Someone let me into their flat to use their bathroom. It seemed as if the cops were about to kettle the crowd or charge into it at any minute. Rumours and photos of the cops' activity on neighbouring streets circulated. As more and more people arrived, the atmosphere grew thick. We waited. We remained together. We gossiped. We shouted: 'These are our neighbours, let them go!' After hours on the street, the rumour rippled around that the people in the van would be released. Shortly afterwards, they were. They emerged waving. In that moment, when the crowd erupted and the row of cops shrunk back, it was as if the darkness of all the previous months spent in isolation had suddenly lifted. Three days later we took to the streets again to protest Israeli air raids on Gaza City.

Another couple of years later, having emerged from lockdown, I was in a museum in Glasgow where I saw a painting of fruit in a bowl by Gustave Courbet. It is part of a series of still life paintings completed by the socialist artist between 1871 and 1872, while he was in prison for his involvement in the Paris Commune. It is a small, unassuming, brown-hued work. Had I not read its accompanying sign I might not even have noticed it. I stared at the small round pears and thought about the Commune's brutal defeat. Why had a political prisoner been compelled to paint this humble, dull-coloured fruit in a bourgeois domestic interior?

Art historian Jeannene M. Przyblyski proposes the following reading of Courbet's post-Commune still lifes:

> They engineer the encounter between the snugly privatized frame of a genre deeply bound to the bourgeois love of property and the officially imposed (de)privation of state suppression and incarceration. By superimposing such axes of power and powerlessness, Courbet's paintings invoke the terms by which the nineteenth-century cult of interiority was intimately connected to the invention of a modern discourse of the carceral, even as they suggest the ways in which the Commune itself might be seen as the suppressed other side of classic modernity, largely written out of French history and the history of French visual culture.[15]

But I wanted to see something different in the painting. Ignorant about artistic genre conventions, I thought about the fruit rather than its setting. I thought of Courbet imagining the taste of apples and pears. I thought of the image Hannah Black conjures of a post-revolutionary New York City in which fruit can be plucked directly from trees lining the city streets. I thought also of the closing pages of Bruno Jasieński's novel *I Burn Paris*, first serialised in the communist newspaper *L'Humanité* in 1928, which describes a plague breaking out in Paris. In response the city enters a lockdown. Some time later incarcerated members of the proletariat spared from the illness and death that have swept the city emerge from the prisons to build a new society (a fictional plot very different from the actual experiences of incarcerated populations during the Covid-19 pandemic). At the end of the novel, war and toxic fog engulf the rest of Europe. Paris is believed to lie in ruins, but a curious pilot flies above the fortified city and glimpses the new Paris Commune with its crop-filled streets:

> Where once the Place de la Concorde had stretched with a measureless sheet of polished asphalt, from La Madeleine to the Chambre des Députés, from Champs-Elysées to the Tuileries, a meadow of ripe grain now rippled in the gentle southerly wind. This grain was being gathered by mechanized harvesters driven by brawny, tanned men in white undershirts. Men and women dressed in the same light harvesting clothes were nimbly piling the ready sheaves onto a waiting truck... Where the Luxembourg Gardens had once sprawled were now rows of cauliflower growing white in the sun in a chessboard of colorful plots, a gigantic vegetable garden.[16]

Our minds (and bodies) may be in hellish conditions, but they're nevertheless on the earth, where things can still be organised differently.

Asked in a 2016 interview to respond to Raymond Williams' dictum that 'to be truly radical is to make hope possible, rather than despair convincing', Mike Davis rejected the premise that it is necessary to have hope in order to fight to overthrow capitalism. In this book I have tried to make the case that the damaging psychological consequences of engaging in that fight should be acknowledged and can be mitigated. But the fight will not be painless, requiring something like despair of the intellect, hope of the will. Davis can have the final word:

> 'Hope' is not a scientific category. Nor is it a necessary obligation in polemical writing... I manifestly do believe that we have arrived at a

'final conflict' that will decide the survival of a large part of poor humanity over the next half century. Against this future we must fight like the Red Army in the rubble of Stalingrad. Fight with hope, fight without hope, but fight absolutely.[17]

Acknowledgements

This book does not have a chapter devoted to 'anxiety', but it does have this. I obsessively read other people's acknowledgments, but I kept putting off writing my own. The temporality of thinking and writing is so strange. It's so hard to know where to begin and where to end.

I'm enormously grateful to the people who read and discussed draft chapters with me at various stages: Victoria Browne, Helen Charman, Eve Dickson, Sam Dolbear, Larne Abse Gogarty, Aurelia Guo, Danny Hayward, Lizzie Homersham and especially Benjamin Morgan for going through the whole manuscript so carefully.

I began the research for what eventually became this book while I was a postdoctoral research fellow at the ICI Berlin and am grateful to Christoph Holzhey, Manuele Gragnolati, Claudia Peppel, Arnd Wedemeyer and my fellow fellows.

My parents Marilyn and Neil Proctor have not only supported me in general but also let me stay in their house at various times to write, which I very much appreciated. There's a road in Cumbria that I have now walked along so many times I could do it in my sleep.

In Glasgow, thanks to Helen Charman, Lucy Duncan (who I'm pretending never left), Caspar Heinemann, Chris Law, Hussein Mitha, Akshi Singh (who I'm pretending was here all along), Holly White and Tom White. Love and solidarity to friends and comrades involved in the Red Sunday School – it has been a real antidote to the kinds of things this book is about. I wrote a lot in the margins of my time as a Wellcome Trust fellow at the University of Strathclyde. I'm grateful to Laura Kelly, Matt Smith and others at the Centre for the Social History of Health and Healthcare for being such supportive colleagues. I was also grateful to meet so many colleagues in the Strathclyde UCU branch on the picket lines over the years – hopefully one day universities will cease to be such hotbeds of workplace burnout. Thanks to staff in libraries across Glasgow and to the 'Save our Libraries' campaigners who fought for libraries on the Southside to reopen after lockdown. No thanks, however, are due to Glasgow City Council/Glasgow Life for shortening the opening hours of the Mitchell Library.

Thanks to the distant friends whose support, encouragement and advice I relied on at various points over the years I was working on this: Larne Abse Gogarty, Sarah Crane Brewer, Eve Dickson, Sam Dolbear, Aurelia Guo, Sam Goff, Owen Hatherley, Lizzie Homersham, Pete Mitchell, Benjamin Morgan, Branwyn Poleykett, Daniel Reeve, Michael Runyan, M. Ty and many others who I'll no doubt lose sleep over accidentally leaving out.

Though it feels extremely gauche to include this, I am also grateful to friends and strangers on social media who answered my questions so generously and suggested things to read.

Way back in 2015, I co-organised an event at MayDay Rooms with Sophie Jones and Amy Tobin as part of a seminar series we ran called 'Under the Moon', which discussed the Red Therapy pamphlet alongside Marge Piercy's *Woman on the Edge of Time* (1976). Former members of the Red Therapy collective joined our discussion. Some seeds were sown in my mind that evening, as well as through discussions with Amy and Sophie, even if it took them a long time to sprout.

Larne Abse Gogarty and I co-wrote a piece called 'Communist Feelings' together, which was first presented as a paper at Historical Materialism Beirut in 2017 before being published in *New Socialist* in 2019. Around the same time we also co-wrote two presentations on the politics of dreaming, the first in conjunction with Hannah Black's exhibition 'Some Context' at Chisenhale Gallery in London and a second for 'diffrakt' in Berlin. Our conversations nourished and inspired this project in its early stages, and I missed working on something so genuinely collaborative when I was stuck inside with my own thoughts. (Thank you to Hannah Black as well, who I recall sending me reading recommendations back when I was first starting to think about these themes in Berlin and whose book *Tuesday or September or the End* made me feel less hopeless when I was trying to write a conclusion.)

I've learned a lot from being involved with the *Radical Philosophy* editorial collective over the years. The two articles and two reviews that I published in the journal between 2016 and 2022 all fed into this book in various ways. Thanks to Tom Kuhn for granting permission to use his translation of Brecht's 'To Those Born After' and to Liveright Publishing Corporation. My chapter on 'Mourning' began as a paper I delivered at the National Museum of Modern and Contemporary Art, Korea in Seoul

Acknowledgements

in October 2017. Thanks to Nick Axel for editing the subsequent publication that appeared in the eflux collection *Superhumanity: Post-Labor, Psychopathology, Plasticity*. Some of the passages on Shulamith Firestone's *Airless Spaces* were originally written for an event at the KunstWerke Berlin organised by Dorine van Meel and Caspar Heinemann in November 2017. Thanks to Victoria Browne for inviting me to present some work-in-progress to a seminar at Oxford Brookes University in autumn 2022. Thanks to Henry Bell and the event organisers for inviting me to read some material on hope and despair that ended up in my introduction at the event 'Free Alaa, Free them All' at McNeill's in Glasgow in March 2023. Free Alaa, free them all.

Ben Mabie initially reached out to me and provided useful comments on draft chapters. At Verso, thanks to Asher Dupuy-Spencer, Bruno George, Nick Walther, and everyone involved in the production, distribution and publicity processes.

When I write I always have my friends in mind. Most of the work that went into writing this book was undertaken in isolation; that it wasn't the product of loneliness is testament to all these people and more without whom I would have surely burnt out long before I was able to finish it.

Notes

Epigraph

1. Bertolt Brecht, 'To Those Born After', originally published in German in 1939 as 'An die Nachgeborenen', translated by Tom Kuhn. Copyright 1939, (c) 1961 by Bertolt-Brecht-Erben / Suhrkamp Verlag. Translation copyright (c) 2019, 2015 by Tom Kuhn and David Constantine, from *Collected Poems of Bertolt Brecht* by Bertolt Brecht, translated by Tom Kuhn and David Constantine. Used by permission of Liveright Publishing Corporation.

Introduction

1. Diane di Prima, *Revolutionary Letters* (San Francisco, CA: Last Gasp of San Francisco, 2005), p. 23.
2. Lisa Baraitser, *Enduring Time* (London: Bloomsbury, 2017), p. 50.
3. Masao Adachi and Kôji Wakamatsu (dirs.), *Red Army/PFLP: Declaration of World War*, Wakamatsu, Japan, 1971.
4. Leila Khaled, *My People Shall Live: Autobiography of a Revolutionary* (London: Hodder and Stoughton, 1973), p. 79.
5. Victor Serge, *Memoirs of a Revolutionary*, trans. by Peter Sedgwick (New York: NYRB, 2012), p. 305. See also p. 436.
6. Serge, *Memoirs of a Revolutionary*, pp. 206–7.
7. Huey P. Newton, *Revolutionary Suicide* (London: Penguin, 2009), p. 2.
8. Ibid., p. 359.
9. Lacy Banks, 'Black Suicide', *Ebony*, May 1970, pp. 76–84, p. 76. The article discusses the work of black psychiatrist Alvin Poussaint, author of works on the psychological dynamics associated with racial conflicts within the civil rights movement (discussed in Chapter 5).
10. Newton, 'On the defection of Eldridge Cleaver from the Black Panther Party and the defection of the Black Panther Party from the Black community: April 17, 1971' in *The Huey P. Newton Reader*, ed. by David Hilliard and Donald Weise (New York: Seven Stories Press, 2002), pp. 200–8.
11. Newton, *Revolutionary Suicide*, p. 175.

12. Ernesto Che Guevara, *Congo Diary: Episodes of the Revolutionary War in the Congo* (New York: Seven Stories, 2021) p. 249.
13. Guevara, *Congo Diary*, pp. 250, 252.
14. Ho Chi Minh, quoted in Newton, *Revolutionary Suicide*, p. 331; Khaled, *My People Shall Live*, p. 54.
15. Alaa Abd El-Fattah and Ahmed Douma, 'Graffiti for Two', in Alaa Abd El-Fattah, *You Have Not Yet Been Defeated*, translated by a collective (London: Fitzcarraldo Editions, 2022), pp. 187–208, p. 189. For a less despairing account of the aftermaths of the 'Arab Spring' see Walid el Houri, 'Beyond Failure and Success: Revolutions and the Politics of Endurance', *Radical Philosophy* 2: 2 (June 2018), pp. 72–8.
16. El-Fattah and Douma, 'Graffiti for Two', pp. 193, 200, 208.
17. Raymond Williams, *Border Country* (London: Readers Union, Chatto and Windus, 1962), p. 153.
18. Ibid., pp. 153–4.
19. Phil Brown, Michael Galan and Nancy Henley, 'Introduction', in *The Radical Therapist: The Radical Therapist Collective* (Harmondsworth: Penguin, 1974), pp. 7–10, p. 8.
20. I discuss how social movements during and in the aftermath of 1968 engaged with radical psychiatry (and radical psychiatry as a social movement in its own right) and survey some of the relevant literature, here: Hannah Proctor, 'Mad World: Radical Psychiatry and 1968', versobooks.com.
21. *Red Therapy* (London: Red Therapy, 1978), p. 2. Accessed in the East London Big Flame archives at May Day Rooms.
22. Ibid., p. 10.
23. Former Red Therapy member John Rowan recalls they were thrown out of Big Flame by therapy sceptics based in Liverpool (where Big Flame was founded) 'for being too interested in sexual politics and personal issues'. John Rowan, *The Horned God: Feminism and Men as Wounding and Healing* (London: Routledge, 1987), p. 21.
24. *Red Therapy*, p. 12. Co-written by two former members of Red Therapy and dedicated to the group, Sheila Ernst and Lucy Goodison's *In Our Own Hands: A Book of Self-Help Therapy* (London: Women's Press, 1981) expresses similar sentiments in its introduction: 'We hoped that if we could understand how certain attitudes were socially determined, we could, by a conscious act of will, choose to change or banish them. But even within a growing and effective movement active in the world, and with a radical restructuring of domestic life, our feelings and relationships did not change easily. Women were gaining new power but continued to feel depressed, inadequate and confused,' p. 3.
25. Gail Lewis interview in Brenna Bhandar and Rafeef Ziadah, eds, *Revolutionary Feminisms: Conversations on Collective Action and Radical Thought* (London: Verso, 2020, epub), pp. 142–89, p. 154. Lewis shared her memories of Red Therapy member Shelia Ernst at a memorial event at Birkbeck College, London in 2016.
26. Peter Sedgwick, *Psychopolitics* (London: Unkant, 2015), p. 251.
27. Paul Hoggett, Julian Lousada, Marie Maguire and Joanna Ryan, 'Battersea Action and Counselling Centre (BACC)', *Psychoanalysis and History* 24: 3, pp. 291–8. These commitments do not just belong in the past: Joanna Ryan, *Class and Psychoanalysis: Landscapes of Inequality* (London: Routledge, 2017).

28. Sheila Rowbotham, *The Past is Before Us: Feminism in Action Since the 1960s* (London: Penguin, 1989), pp. xv, 18. On the kinds of initiatives that arose from the movement see Sarah Crook, 'The women's liberation movement, activism and therapy at the grassroots, 1968–1985', *Women's History Review* 27: 7 (2018), pp. 1152–68. The introduction to a collection co-edited by former Red Therapy member Marie Maguire that also included essays by Red Therapy participants Sheila Ernst and Joanna Ryan, similarly described how hostility towards psychoanalysis in the women's movement shifted in response to women's psychological experiences and difficulties within it. See Marilyn Lawrence and Marie Maguire, eds, *Psychotherapy with Women: Feminist Perspectives* (London: Macmillan, 1997), p. 1.
29. Juliet Mitchell and Jacqueline Rose, 'Feminine Sexuality: Interview, 1982', *m/f* 8 (1983), pp. 3–16, p. 7.
30. Sheila Ernst and Marie Maguire, eds, *Living with the Sphinx: Papers from the Women's Therapy Centre* (London: Women's Press, 1981), pp. 1–29, p. 9.
31. Jacqueline Rose, 'Where does the Misery Come From? Psychoanalysis, Feminism and the Event', *Feminism and Psychoanalysis*, ed. by Richard Feldstein and Judith Roof (Ithaca, NY: Cornell University Press, 1989), pp. 25–39, p. 29.
32. Ibid., p. 28.
33. Fred Moten, 'The Case of Blackness', *Criticism* 50: 2 (2008), pp. 177–218, p. 208.
34. Ibid., p. 209.
35. Frantz Fanon and Jacques Azoulay 'Social therapy in a ward of Muslim men: Methodological difficulties', in *Alienation and Freedom*, ed. by Jean Khalfa and Robert J. C. Young, trans. by Steven Corcoran (London: Bloomsbury, 2018), pp. 353–71, p. 359, p. 363.
36. Lucie K. Mercier, 'The Translatability of Experience: On Fanon's Language Puzzle', *Critical Times* 6: 1 (2023), pp. 15–38, p. 26.
37. Frantz Fanon, 'Letter to the Resident Minister (1956)', in *Toward the African Revolution: Political Essays*, trans. by Haakon Chevalier (New York: Grove Press, 1964), pp. 52–4, p. 52, p. 53.
38. See Camille Robcis, *Disalienation: Politics, Philosophy and Radical Psychiatry in Postwar France* (Chicago: University of Chicago Press, 2021), pp. 68–9.
39. Jean-Paul Sartre, 'Preface', *The Wretched of the Earth*, trans. by Constance Farrington (New York: Grove Press, 1963), pp. 7–34, p. 30, p. 21.
40. Fanon, *Wretched of the Earth*, p. 309, p. 294.
41. Ibid., pp. 252–3. In his discussion of the case histories, David Marriott argues that Fanon suggests that some FLN fighters 'were often at greater risk from their own psyches than from their enemies', David Marriott, *Whither Fanon? Studies in the Blackness of Being* (Stanford: Stanford University Press, 2018), p. 190. See also Emily Kuby, '"Our Actions Never Cease to Haunt Us": Frantz Fanon, Jean-Paul Sartre, and the Violence of the Algerian War', *Historical Reflections* 41: 3 (2015), pp. 59–78.
42. The autobiography of former IRA member, 'Brighton bomber' Patrick Magee, expresses very similar sentiments. Patrick Magee, *Where Grieving Begins: Building Bridges after the Brighton Bomb: A Memoir* (London: Pluto Press, 2021).
43. See Nancy Luxon, 'Fanon's Psychiatric Hospital as a Waystation to Freedom', *Theory, Culture and Society* 38: 5 (2021), pp. 93–113, and Nica Siegel, 'Fanon's

Clinic: Revolutionary Therapeutics and the Politics of Exhaustion', *Polity* 55: 1 (2023), pp. 7–33.
44. Stuart Hall, 'Life and Times of the First New Left', *New Left Review* 61 (Jan–Feb 2010), pp. 177–96, p. 184. Hall, born in 1932, situated himself as part of a generation for whom 1956 marked a decisive turning point. Following the 'boundary-marking experiences' of the Soviet crushing of the Hungarian Revolution and the Suez Crisis, socialists lost faith in the Soviet project and came to realize that the independence of some former colonies would not signal the end of imperialism. While 1956 was also significant for people on the British left a generation older than Hall, more of whom were members of the Communist Party, this group had also been shaped by experiences of the Popular Front, the Spanish Civil War and anti-fascist organizing before and during the Second World War and represented a distinct tendency as a result.
45. On this context and historical moment see David Graeber, *Direct Action: An Ethnography* (Edinburgh: AK Press, 2009).
46. Reflections on the collective yet splintered disappointment of those dispersed aftermaths are discussed in existing texts sometimes directly, sometimes implicitly: see, for example, the collection *Bad Feelings* edited by Arts Against Cuts (London: Bookworks, 2015), the second issue of *LIES: A Journal of Materialist Feminism* (2015), the introduction to Jackie Wang's *Carceral Capitalism* (Los Angeles, CA: Semiotext(e), 2018), Luke Roberts, 'Fear of Retribution,' *Journal of British and Irish Innovative Poetry* 12(1): 26 (2020), pp. 1–23, or, in a context where the cost of loss was far more severe, an anonymous reflection written on the fifth anniversary of the Egyptian revolution: 'Fear the everyday state', *Libcom*, 11 February 2016. For a more formal oral history of the UK student movement see Matt Myers, *Student Revolt: Voices of the Austerity Generation* (London: Pluto, 2017). On corrosive interpersonal dynamics that can emerge in political groups by a group that emerged from that historical conjuncture see Endnotes, 'We Unhappy Few: The Communist Group', *Endnotes 5: The Passions and the Interests*, autumn 2019, pp. 16–113.
47. Yara Rodriguez Fowler captures the atmosphere of political scenes in London around this time in her novel, *There Are More Things* (London: Hachette, 2022).
48. Tobi Haslett discusses the divergences and interconnections between these two strands of struggle: 'the fights are fused and need each other. They form two spokes on a single wheel.' Tobi Haslett, 'Magic Actions', *n+1* 40, Summer 2020, nplusonemag.com. Addressing the UK context, Larne Abse Gogarty reflects on the passage of time between the 2010 student movement and Corbyn's defeat, noting that on the same day as the 2019 election police were found not guilty of hospitalising student movement activist Alfie Meadows after striking him violently during a 2010 demonstration: *What We Do Is Secret: Contemporary Art and the Antinomies of Conspiracy* (Berlin: Sternberg Press, 2023), pp. 137–62, p. 142.
49. Gargi Bhattacharyya, 'We, the heartbroken', Pluto, 2020, plutobooks.com.
50. Bobby London, 'Hurt People', *The New Inquiry*, March 29 2018, thenewinquiry.com.
51. Plan C's 'We Are All Very Anxious' responds to anxiety within social movements and proposes reviving and adapting consciousness-raising practices developed in the women's liberation movement in response to shared experiences of

precarity (Plan C, 'We Are All Very Anxious: Six Theses on Anxiety and Why It is Effectively Preventing Militancy, and One Possible Strategy for Overcoming It', 4 April 2014, weareplanc.org). For a recent example of a book addressing activist burnout that includes tips for self-care see Nicole Rose, *Overcoming Burnout* (Oakland, CA: PM Press, 2019).
52. See Micha Frazer-Carroll, *Mad World: The Politics of Mental Health* (London: Pluto Books, 2023).

1. Melancholia

1. Walter Benjamin, *The Arcades Project*, trans. and ed. by Rolf Tiedemann (Cambridge, MA: Belknap Press, 1999), p. 474.
2. Stuart Hall, *The Hard Road to Renewal: Thatcherism and the Crisis of the Left* (London: Verso, 1988), p. vii.
3. For a forceful criticism of some of Stuart Hall's analyses of Thatcherism, including an evisceration of his and Martin Jacques' celebratory essay about Live Aid, see A. Sivanandan, 'All that Melts into Air is Solid: the Hokum of New Times', *Race and Class* 31: 3 (1989), pp. 1–30.
4. Jacqueline Rose, 'Margaret Thatcher and Ruth Ellis', *New Formations* 6 (1988), pp. 1–29, p. 5, p. 7.
5. A version of her talk was published at newhumanist.org.uk.
6. Wendy Brown, 'Resisting Left Melancholy', *boundary 2* 26: 3 (1999), pp. 19–27, p. 20.
7. Walter Benjamin, 'Left-Wing Melancholy', *Screen*, 15: 2 (1974), pp. 28–32, p. 28, p. 29, p. 30, p. 31.
8. Brown, 'Resisting Left Melancholy', p. 22, p. 26.
9. Benjamin, 'Left-Wing Melancholy', p. 29, p. 30. This made me think of the liberal Corbyn-hating boomers described by David Graeber who professed to be on the left until a left-wing option actually presented itself: nybooks.com.
10. Jodi Dean, 'Communist Desire', in Slavoj Žižek, ed., *The Idea of Communism, volume 2* (London: Verso, 2013), pp. 77–102, p. 87. Rodrigo Nunes contrasts the two theories of melancholia offered by Brown and Dean in *Neither Vertical nor Horizontal: A Theory of Political Organisation* (London: Verso, 2021).
11. Enzo Traverso, *Left Wing Melancholia: Marxism, History, and Memory* (New York: Columbia University Press, 2016), p. 32.
12. RIP Sean Bonney. Sean Bonney, *Our Death* (Oakland, CA: Commune Editions, 2019), p. 34.
13. Stuart Hall, 'The Crisis of Labourism' (1984), in *Hard Road to Renewal*, pp. 196–210, p. 204, p. 205. For a historical account focused on support groups in London, see Diarmaid Kelliher, *Making Cultures of Solidarity: London and the 1984–5 Miners' Strike* (London: Routledge, 2021).
14. Vicky Seddon, ed., *The Cutting Edge: Women and the Pit Strike* (London: Lawrence and Wishart, 1986), p. 282. See also Anne Scargill and Betty Cook (with Ian Clayton), *Anne and Betty: United by the Struggle* (Pontefract: Route, 2020), p. 164. Thanks to Helen Charman for recommending these books to me.
15. Keith Harper, 'Miner's strike ends in bitter tears', *Guardian*, 4 March 1985.
16. Vicky Seddon, ed., *The Cutting Edge: Women and the Pit Strike* (London: Lawrence and Wishart, 1986), p. 121, p. 49.

17. Ibid., pp. 246–7.
18. Ibid., p. 247, p. 47.
19. Walter Benjamin, *The Arcades Project*, trans. and ed. by Rolf Tiedemann (Cambridge, MA: Belknap Press, 1999), p. 948.
20. Benjamin, 'Left-Wing Melancholy', p. 31.
21. Walter Benjamin, 'Experience and Poverty', *Walter Benjamin: Selected Writings, Volume 2: Part 2, 1931–1934*, ed. by Michael W. Jennings, Howard Eiland and Gary Smith, trans. by Rodney Livingstone and others (Cambridge, MA: Belknap Press, 1999), pp. 731–6, p. 733.
22. Benjamin, 'Left-Wing Melancholy', p. 29.
23. Bertolt Brecht, 'Dialectical Ode', *The Collected Poems of Bertolt Brecht*, trans. and ed. by Tom Kuhn and David Constantine with Charlotte Ryland (New York: Liveright, 2019, epub), p. 2015.

2. Nostalgia

1. Alaa Abd El-Fattah and Ahmed Douma, 'Graffiti for Two', in Alaa Abd El-Fattah, *You Have Not Yet Been Defeated*, translated by a collective (London: Fitzcarraldo Editions, 2022), pp. 187–208, p. 196.
2. Keston Sutherland, 'Revolution and Really Being Alive', Poetry and Revolution Conference, May 2012, Birkbeck, sro.sussex.ac.uk.
3. Alain Badiou, 'The Communist Hypothesis', *New Left Review* 49, Jan/Feb 2008, newleftreview.org.
4. Karl Marx, *The Civil War in France* (London: Lawrence and Wishart, 1933) p. 50.
5. Svetlana Boym, *The Future of Nostalgia* (New York: Basic Books, 2001).
6. Susan Stewart, *On Longing: Narratives of the Miniature, the Gigantic, the Souvenir, the Collection* (Durham, NC: Duke University Press, 1993), p. 23, p. 12.
7. For an argument emphasising the radical potential of political commemoration focused on commemorations of the Spanish Civil War in the US, with an emphasis on performance and in-person events, see Peter Glazer, *Radical Nostalgia: Spanish Civil War and Commemoration* (Rochester, NY: University of Rochester Press, 2005).
8. Jason E. Smith, 'The American Revolution', *Brooklyn Rail*, July 2021, brooklynrail.org.
9. On the enduring yet constantly metamorphosing significance of the Commune, see Quentin Deluermoz, 'The Commune, 1871: Present, Past, and Back Again', *Nineteenth-Century French Studies* 49: 3 & 4 (2021), pp. 348–57.
10. Georges Haupt, 'The Commune as Symbol and Example', *Aspects of International Socialism, 1871–1914*, trans. by Peter Fawcett (Cambridge: Cambridge University Press, 1986), pp. 23–47, p. 26.
11. Karine Varley, 'Reassessing the Paris Commune of 1871: A Response to Robert Tombs', 'How Bloody was the Semaine Sanglante? A Revision', *H-France Salon* 3 (2011): pp. 20–5, p. 20.
12. Laura C. Forster, 'The Paris Commune in the British socialist imagination, 1871–1914', *History of European Ideas* 46: 5 (2020), pp. 614–32, p. 617.
13. Colette E. Wilson, *Paris and the Commune, 1871–1878: The Politics of Forgetting* (Manchester: Manchester University Press, 2007), p. 2.

14. Franck Frégosi, 'The "Ascent" of the Communards' Wall at Père-Lachaise: A Secular Partisan Pilgrimage', *Archives de sciences sociales des religions* 155: 3 (2011), pp. 165–89.
15. Rosa Luxemburg, 'Order Prevails in Berlin (January 1919)', marxists.org.
16. C. L. R. James, 'They Showed the Way to Labor Emancipation: On Karl Marx and the 75th Anniversary of the Paris Commune' (1946) (originally published pseudonymously in *Labor Action*), marxists.org.
17. See Irina Shilova, 'Building the Bolshevik Calendar through Pravda and Izvestiia', *Toronto Slavic Quarterly* 14 (2007), and Jay Bergman, 'The Paris Commune in Bolshevik Mythology', *English Historical Review* 129: 541 (2014), pp. 1412–41. These passages on the Commune's significance in the Soviet Union are adapted from Hannah Proctor, 'Revolutionary Commemoration', *Radical Philosophy* 2: 1 (2018), pp. 47–57.
18. Andy Willimott, *Living the Revolution: Urban Communes and Soviet Socialism, 1917-1932* (Oxford: Oxford University Press, 2017), p. 42.
19. Richard Stites, *Revolutionary Dreams: Utopian Vision and Experimental Life in the Russian Revolution* (Oxford: Oxford University Press, 1989), p. 111.
20. Casey Harison, 'The Paris Commune of 1871, the Russian Revolution of 1905, and the Shifting of the Revolutionary Tradition', *History and Memory* 19: 2 (2007), pp. 5–42, p. 24.
21. Gavin Bowd, *The Last Communard: Adrien Lejeune, the Unexpected Life of a Revolutionary* (London: Verso, 2016), p. 56.
22. Patrick H. Hutton, *The Cult of the Revolutionary Tradition: The Blanquists in French Politics, 1864-1893* (Berkeley, CA: University of California Press, 1981), pp. 121–2.
23. Sébastien Fevry, 'The joyful power of activist memory: The radiant image of the Commune in the Invisible Committee's writings', *Memory Studies* 12: 1 (2019), pp. 46–60; Malia Wallen, 'Occupy Oakland Regroups, Calling for a Strike', *New York Times*, 1 November 2011; Jason Livingston, 'The Communards of Wall Street', *Brooklyn Rail*, May 2013, brooklynrail.org.
24. Kristin Ross, *Communal Luxury: The Political Imaginary of the Paris Commune* (London: Verso, 2015, epub), p. 25. (Ross cites the example of the Occupy Oakland activist who gives their name as 'Louise Michel' to the *New York Times*, p. 16).
25. Haupt, 'Commune as Symbol and Example', p. 47.
26. Robert Tombs, *The Paris Commune, 1871* (Harlow: Pearson Education, 1999), pp. 151–83.
27. Élie Reclus cited in John Merriman, *Massacre: The Life and Death of the Paris Commune of 1871* (New Haven, CT: Yale University Press, 2014), p. 177.
28. The exact figure remains contested, but Robert Tombs argues the actual number, though still very large, is likely far smaller than the figures cited in Communard accounts that became standard and which put it anywhere between 17,000 and 50,000. Most subsequent historians cite a number between 20,000 and 30,000. Robert Tombs, 'How bloody was la semaine sanglante of 1871? A revision', *The Historical Journal* 55: 3, pp. 679–704.
29. Tombs, *Paris Commune, 1871*, pp. 180–1.
30. Alisa Luxenberg, 'Creating Désastres: Andrieu's Photographs of Urban Ruins in the Paris of 1871', *The Art Bulletin* 80: 1 (1998), pp. 113–37.
31. Jeannene M. Przyblyski, 'Revolution at a Standstill: Photography and the Paris Commune of 1871', *Yale French Studies* 101 (2001), pp. 54–78.

32. Marx, *The Civil War in France*, p. 59.
33. Gay. L Gullickson, *Unruly Women of Paris: Images of the Commune* (Ithaca, NY: Cornell University Press, 1996).
34. On pathologising discourses and their entanglement with questions of morality, see Merriman, *Massacre*, p. 236.
35. On Lissagaray's *History of the Commune of 1871* as a work whose style and tropes are typical of works by exiled Communards, see Scott McCracken, 'The Commune in Exile: Urban Insurrection and the Production of International Space', in *Nineteenth-Century Radical Traditions*, ed. Joseph Bristow and Josephine McDonagh (London: Palgrave Macmillan, 2016), pp. 113–36.
36. Prosper-Olivier Lissagaray, *History of the Commune of 1871*, trans. by Eleanor Marx Aveling (London: Reeves and Turner, 1886), p. 459, p. 451, p. 400, p. 412.
37. Louise Michel, *The Red Virgin: Memoirs of Louise Michel*, ed. and trans. by Bullitt Lowry and Elizabeth Ellington Gunter (Tuscaloosa, AL: University of Alabama Press, 1981), p. 73.
38. Lissagaray, *History of the Commune of 1871*, p. 452, p. 465.
39. John Merriman, *Massacre: The Life and Death of the Paris Commune of 1871* (New Haven, CT: Yale University Press, 2014), p. 212.
40. Ibid., p. 207.
41. Alice Bullard, *Exile to Paradise: Savagery and Civilization in Paris and the South Pacific, 1790–1900* (Cambridge: Cambridge University Press, 2001), p. 97.
42. Matt K. Masuda, *The Memory of the Modern* (Oxford: Oxford University Press, 1996), p. 153. Regarding the 'virgin earth', Miranda Frances Spieler uses a legal lens to debunk the myth in the context of French Guiana (also a penal colony): 'To the extent that ex-citizens resembled colonial subjects, this arose not from living outside the law in vile nature but from living inside the law as inventions of human artifice.' Miranda Frances Spieler, *Empire and Underworld: Captivity in French Guinea* (Cambridge, MA: Harvard University Press, 2012), p. 8.
43. 'Fraternity, that hallmark of the Communard ethos, lost its allure in New Caledonia and was replaced only with solitude, inactivity, boredom, and despair.' Bullard, *Exile to Paradise*, p. 191.
44. Lissagaray, *History of the Commune of 1871*, p. 450.
45. Louise Michel, *The Red Virgin: Memoirs of Louise Michel*, ed. and trans. by Bullitt Lowry and Elizabeth Ellington Gunter (Tuscaloosa, AL: University of Alabama Press, 1981), p. 155.
46. Bullard, *Exile to Paradise*, pp. 183–5, pp. 192–3.
47. Johannes Hofer, 'Medical dissertation on nostalgia', trans. Carolyn Spiser Anspach, *Bulletin of the Institute of the History of Medicine* 2: 6 (1934), pp. 376–91, p. 386.
48. Lisa Gabrielle O'Sullivan, 'Dying For Home: The Medicine and Politics of Nostalgia in Nineteenth-Century France', PhD thesis, Queen Mary, University of London, 2006.
49. Michael S. Roth, 'Dying of the Past: Medical Studies of Nostalgia in Nineteenth-Century France', *History and Memory* 3: 1 (1991), pp. 5–29.
50. O'Sullivan, 'The Time and Place of Nostalgia: Re-situating a French Disease', *Journal of the History of Medicine and Allied Sciences* 67: 4 (2012), pp. 626–9, p. 642, p. 643.
51. Cited in Charles J. Stivale, 'Louise Michel's Poetry of Existence and Revolt', *Tulsa Studies in Women's Literature* 5: 1 (1986), pp. 41–61, p. 53.

52. O'Sullivan, 'Dying for Home', pp. 154–9; Roth, 'Dying of the Past', p. 15.
53. Peter Weiss, *The Aesthetics of Resistance, volume 1*, trans. by Joachim Neugroschel (Durham, NC: Duke University Press, 2005), p. 240.
54. Bullard, *Exile to Paradise*, p. 185, p. 194.
55. Niklas Plaetzer, 'Decolonizing the "Universal Republic": The Paris Commune and French Empire', *Nineteenth-Century French Studies* 49: 3/4 (2021), pp. 585–603, p. 587.
56. Massimiliano Tomba, *Insurgent Universality: An Alternative Legacy of Modernity* (Oxford: Oxford University Press, 2019), p. 72.
57. Edith Thomas, *Louise Michel* (Montreal: Black Rose Books, 1980), p. 148.
58. Ross, *Communal Luxury*, p. 81.
59. Plaetzer, 'Decolonizing the "Universal Republic"', p. 587.
60. Bullard, *Exile to Paradise*, pp. 46–7. See also Bronwen Douglas, *Across the Great Divide: Journeys in History and Anthropology* (Amsterdam: Harwood, 1998), pp. 150–2; Linda Latham, 'Revolt re-examined: The 1878 insurrection in New Caledonia', *The Journal of Pacific History* 10: 3 (1975), pp. 48–63; and Adrian Muckle, 'Killing the "Fantôme Canaque": Evoking and Invoking the Possibility of Revolt in New Caledonia (1853–1915)', *Journal of Pacific History* 37: 1 (2002), pp. 25–44, p. 26.
61. Michel, *The Red Virgin*, p. 111, p. 112.
62. Thomas, *Louise Michel*, p. 159.
63. Communards Victor Cosse and Simon Mayer cited in Masuda, *The Memory of the Modern*, p. 157.
64. Bullard, *Exile to Paradise*, pp. 203–9.
65. Carolyn J. Eichner, 'Civilization vs Savagery: Louise Michel and the Kanaks', *Salvage*, 22 May 2017.
66. Muckle, 'Killing the "Fantôme Canaque"', p. 26.
67. Ranajit Guha's *Elementary Aspects of Peasant Insurgency in Colonial India* (Durham, NC: Duke University Press, 1999), p. 15, p. 11.
68. Corinne David-Ives, 'Ataï's Return to New Caledonia: Reconciliation Politics and the Embarrassing Legacy of Colonial Anthropology', *Journal of New Zealand & Pacific Studies* 5: 2 (2017), pp. 175–88.
69. See Susan A. Ashley, *'Misfits' in Fin-de-Siecle France and Italy: Anatomies of Difference* (London: Bloomsbury, 2017), pp. 144–8.
70. Vincenzo Ruggiero, *Understanding Political Violence: A Criminological Analysis* (Maidenhead: Open University Press, 2006), pp. 40–2.
71. Hutton, *The Cult of the Revolutionary Tradition*, p. 123.
72. Walter Benjamin, 'Exposé of 1939', *The Arcades Project*, trans. and ed. by Rolf Tiedemann (Cambridge, MA: Belknap Press, 1999), pp. 14–26, p. 26, p. 25.
73. Benjamin, *Arcades*, 'Convolute D: Boredom, Eternal Return', p. 112.
74. Benjamin, 'Exposé of 1939', p. 25.
75. Benjamin, 'Convolute D', pp. 101–19, p. 111.
76. Peter Hallward, 'Blanqui's bifurcations', *Radical Philosophy* 185 (2014), pp. 36–44, p. 36, p. 39.
77. Louis-Auguste Blanqui, *Eternity by the Stars: An Astronomical Hypothesis*, trans. Frank Chouraqui (New York: Contra Mundum Press, 2013), p. 134.
78. Benjamin, 'Convolute J: Baudelaire, pp. 228–387, p. 339.

3. Depression

1. Kate Millett, *The Loony Bin Trip* (London: Virago, 1990), p. 283.
2. Depression, understood as a medical diagnosis rather than a mood, displaced melancholia in the middle of the twentieth century, with an emphasis on biological causes and psychopharmaceutical treatments taking hold in the 1970s and 1980s. 'Major depression' entered the *DSM-III* in 1980 (Jonathan Sadowsky, *The Empire of Depression: A New History* (Polity: Cambridge, 2021), p. 98.) On the growth of depression as a diagnosis, see Edward Shorter, *How Everyone Became Depressed: The Rise and Fall of the Nervous Breakdown* (Oxford: Oxford University Press, 2013).
3. Sianne Ngai, 'Shulamith Firestone's Airless Spaces', *Arcade Blog*, 21 August 2012, arcade.stanford.edu.
4. Ann Cvetkovich, *Depression: A Public Feeling* (Durham, NC: Duke University Press, 2012), p. 50. Cvetkovich was involved in the Public Feelings project and Feel Tank Chicago, out of which the concept 'political depression' emerged. Cvetkovich's fellow Public Feelings working group member Lauren Berlant also uses the term in *Cruel Optimism* (Durham, NC: Duke University Press, 2011), which I have excluded from my discussion here mostly because they say much less about the experience of actually being depressed but perhaps also because I didn't have the space – or do I mean courage? – to work through my ambivalent feelings towards their arguments.
5. Ibid., p. 18.
6. Ibid., p. 2, p. 14.
7. Ibid., p. 156, p. 32.
8. Ibid., p. 65, p. 12.
9. Ibid., p. 65, p. 194, p. 154, p. 194.
10. Fisher, 'Good for Nothing', theoccupiedtimes.org.
11. Johanna Hedva, 'Sick Woman Theory' (originally published in *Mask Magazine*, January 2016), johannahedva.com.
12. See, for example, Leah Lakshmi Piepzna-Samarasinha, *Care Work: Dreaming Disability Justice* (Vancouver: Arsenal Pulp Press, 2018).
13. Susan Faludi, 'Death of a Revolutionary', *The New Yorker*, 15 April 2013.
14. Kathi Weeks, 'The Vanishing Dialectic: Shulamith Firestone and the Future of the Feminist 1970s', *South Atlantic Quarterly* (October 2015), pp. 735–54, p. 745, p. 748.
15. Compare Weeks on Firestone to Victoria Hesford on Kate Millett. Victoria Hesford, *Feeling Women's Liberation* (Durham, NC: Duke University Press, 2013), p. 170.
16. Weeks, 'The Vanishing Dialectic', p. 747.
17. Ibid., p. 751. On these many problems, see Sophie Lewis's loving yet critical essay on *The Dialectic of Sex*, which extols Firestone's thrilling utopianism and humorous prose while expressing disappointment with aspects of her arguments. Sophie Lewis, 'Shulamith Firestone Wanted to Abolish Nature—We Should, Too', *The Nation*, 14 July 2021, thenation.com.
18. Luc Boltanski and Eve Chiapello, *The New Spirit of Capitalism*, trans. by Gregory Elliott (London: Verso, 2005), p. 4. I have chosen to focus on one text to

exemplify this narrative, but plenty of other examples could be found (though with varying political motivations and degrees of persuasiveness). See, for example, Régis Debray, 'A Modest Contribution to the Rites and Ceremonies of the Tenth Anniversary', *New Left Review* 1: 115, May/June 1979 or Christopher Lasch, *The Culture of Narcissism: American Life in An Age of Diminishing Expectations* (New York: W. W. Norton, 1979).
19. Boltanski and Chiapello, *The New Spirit of Capitalism*, p. 97, p. 424.
20. See also Sadowsky, *The Empire of Depression*, p. 99.
21. Benjamin Noys, *The Persistence of the Negative: A Critique of Contemporary Continental Theory* (Edinburgh: Edinburgh University Press, 2010), p. 2. I'm thinking particularly of Jean-François Lyotard, *The Postmodern Condition*, trans. by Geoff Bennington (Minneapolis, MN: University of Minnesota Press, 2010).
22. Alberto Toscano, 'Dreamworlds of Catastrophe', Sidecar, *New Left Review* blog, newleftreview.org.
23. Weeks, 'The Vanishing Dialectic', p. 752. See also Elizabeth Freeman, *Time Binds: Queer Temporalities, Queer Histories* (Durham, NC: Duke University Press), pp. 67–8.
24. Shulamith Firestone, *Airless Spaces* (New York: Semiotext(e), 1998), p. 57, p. 35, p. 71, p. 19, p. 33, p. 57, p. 58, p. 59.
25. Ibid., p. 5.
26. Ibid., p. 64, p. 160.
27. Millett, *Loony Bin Trip*, p. 226, p. 233, p. 164.
28. Ibid., p. 234.
29. Kate Millett, *Flying* (New York: Alfred A Knopf, 1974), p. 92.
30. Millett, *Loony Bin Trip*, p. 257, p. 262, p. 274, p. 275.
31. Ibid., p. 283.
32. Ibid., p. 314.
33. *The Loony Bin Trip* describes Millett's participation in political groups fighting the medical treatment and definitions of mental illness, attending Madness Network meetings in San Francisco and engaging with Network Against Psychiatric Assault. In her acknowledgments Millett thanks Judi Chamberlin and Sally Zinman, who were both involved in the mental patients liberation movement. See Linda J. Morrison, *Talking Back to Psychiatry: The Psychiatric Consumer/Survivor/Ex-Patient Movement* (London: Routledge, 2005).
34. Shulamith Firestone, *The Dialectic of Sex: The Case for Feminist Revolution* (New York: Bantam Books, 1970), p. 242, p. 9.
35. Stella Sandford, 'The Dialectic of *The Dialectic of Sex*' in *Further Adventures in the Dialectic of Sex: Critical Essays on Shulamith Firestone*, ed. by Stella Sandford and Mandy Merck (New York: Palgrave Macmillan, 2010), pp. 235–54, p. 241.
36. Firestone, *Dialectic of Sex*, p. 3.
37. Sandford, 'Dialectic of *The Dialectic of Sex*', p. 241.
38. I am unsure of the precise relationship between Cintron and Firestone, but a Lourdes Cintron in New York City has been involved in alternative mental health projects and activism (of the kind Millett also engaged in). See 'Citywide Mental Health Project blog', thecitywidementalhealthproject.wordpress.com.
39. Firestone, *Airless Spaces*, p. 38, p. 92.
40. Ibid., p. 56.
41. Ronald Fraser, ed., *1968: A Student Generation in Revolt* (London: Chatto and Windus, 1988), p. 296.

42. Luisa Passerini, *Autobiography of a Generation: Italy, 1968*, trans. by Lisa M. Erdberg (Middletown, CT: Wesleyan University Press, 1996), p. 2, p. 124, p. 4, p. 38.
43. Luisa Passerini, 'An Eclectic Ego-Histoire' in *History and Psyche: Culture, Psychoanalysis, and the Past*, ed. by Sally Alexander and Barbara Taylor (Basingstoke: Palgrave Macmillan, 2012), pp. 305–24, p. 317.
44. The original Italian title of Passerini's book is *Autoritratto di gruppo* and does not contain a reference to generations. On criticisms of 'generation' as a heuristic in post-'68 literature, see Kristin Ross, *May '68 and its Afterlives* (Chicago: University of Chicago Press, 2002), p. 203.
45. For a discussion of the formal qualities of the book that notes its use of montage technique and treats it as an 'explosion' of the genre of the case history, see Matt ffytche, 'Throwing the case open: The impossible subject of Luisa Passerini's Autobiography of a Generation', *History of the Human Sciences* 33: 3–4, pp. 33–46.
46. Passerini, *Autobiography of a Generation*, p, 3, p. 1, p. 10.
47. Ibid., p. 109, p. 76.
48. According to another interviewee: 'The individual had disappeared. I didn't have an individual life. I no longer did anything by myself. I didn't read a book, I lived in this herd.' Ibid., p. 89.
49. Ibid., p. 89, p. 96, p. 131.
50. Ibid., p. 155, p. 121, pp. 151–2.
51. Passerini, 'An Eclectic Ego-Histoire', p. 317
52. Passerini, *Autobiography of a Generation*, p. 7.
53. Ibid., p. 106, p. 160. The second quoted passage is also about the death of her father. For an illuminating discussion of this aspect of the book and the question of delay in relation to intergenerational trauma, see Lisa Baraitser, *Enduring Time* (London: Bloomsbury, 2017), pp. 93–114.
54. Ibid., p. 15.
55. Jean-François Vilar, *Nous cheminons entourés de fantômes aux fronts troués* (Paris: Seuil, 1993), pp. 100–2, cited in Kristin Ross, *May '68 and its Afterlives* (Chicago: University of Chicago Press, 2002), p. 196.
56. Vilar, cited in Ross, *May '68 and its Afterlives*, p. 196.
57. Ibid., p. 197.

4. Burnout

1. 'The Free Clinics: Ghetto Care Centers Struggle to Survive,' *American Medical News*, 21 February 1972, 12–14 cited in Alondra Nelson, *Body and Soul: The Black Panther Party and the Fight Against Medical Discrimination* (Minneapolis: University of Minnesota Press, 2011), p. 75.
2. Imogen Daal, *Burnout Survival Kit* (London: Bloomsbury, 2020).
3. Anne Helen Petersen, *Can't Even: How Millennials Became the Burnout Generation* (Boston, MA: Houghton Mifflin Harcourt, 2020, epub), p. 18, p. 25.
4. 'Burn-out refers specifically to phenomena in the occupational context and should not be applied to describe experiences in other areas of life.' World Health Organisation, 'Burn-out an "occupational phenomenon": International Classification of Diseases', 28 May 2019, who.int.

5. Pascal Chabot, *Global Burnout* (London: Bloomsbury, 2018). For my review of this book, see Hannah Proctor, 'Exhausting concepts', *Radical Philosophy* 2: 4 (2018).
6. Byung-Chul Han, *The Burnout Society* (Palo Alto, CA: Stanford University Press, 2015), p. 8.
7. Petersen, *Can't Even*, p. 22.
8. Sarah Jaffe, 'Emotions on Strike', *Dissent*, Winter 2021, dissentmagazine.org.
9. Herbert J. Freudenberger, 'Burnout: Past, Present and Future', *Loss, Grief and Care* 3: 1–2 (1989), pp. 1–10, p. 4, p. 7, p. 6, p. 3.
10. Freudenberger, 'Staff Burn-out', *Journal of Social Issues* 30: 1 (1974), pp. 159–65, p. 161.
11. Ibid., p. 165.
12. Gregory Weiss, *Grassroots Medicine: The Story of America's Free Health Clinics* (Lanham, ML: Rowan and Littlefield, 2006), p. 28.
13. David E. Smith, 'The Free Clinic Movement in the United States: A Ten Year Perspective', *Journal of Drug Issues* 6: 4 (1976), pp. 343–55, p. 346.
14. Weiss, *Grassroots Medicine*, p. 26.
15. 'Their predominant problems are urinary infections, venereal diseases, gynaecological cases, abscesses caused by dirty needles, and the consequences of heroin or barbiturate abuse. Quite a number are drug addicts and some are ambulatory psychotics. We have begun a methadone detoxification, a dental and a counseling program.' Herbert J. Freudenberger, 'The Free Clinic Concept', *International Journal of Offender Therapy* 15 (1971), pp. 121–33, p. 122.
16. Ibid., p. 121.
17. Herbert J. Freudenberger, 'The psychologist in a free clinic setting: An alternative model in health care', *Psychotherapy: Theory, Research & Practice* 10: 1 (1973), pp. 52–61, p. 57.
18. Ibid., p. 53.
19. Ibid., p. 53.
20. Freudenberger, 'Burnout', p. 6; Freudenberger, 'Staff Burn-out', p. 161.
21. Matthew J. Hoffarth, 'The making of burnout: From social change to self-awareness in the postwar United States, 1970–82', *History of the Human Sciences* (2017), pp. 1–16.
22. Ibid., p. 5.
23. Herbert J. Freudenberger, 'Treatment and Dynamics of the "Disrelated" Teenager and His Parents in the American Society', *Psychotherapy: Theory, Research and Practice* 6: 4 (1969), pp. 249–55, p. 249.
24. Matt ffytche, 'Psychoanalytic sociology and the traumas of history: Alexander Mitscherlich between the disciplines', *History of the Human Sciences* 20: 10 (2017), pp. 1–27. Writing in the late seventies, Christopher Lasch also discusses the significance of absent fathers in relation to youth revolt, Christopher Lasch, *The Culture of Narcissism: American Life in the Age of Diminishing Expectations* (New York: W. W. Norton, 1979), pp. 172–6.
25. Freudenberger, 'The Case of Missing Male Authority', *Journal of Religion and Health* 9 (1970), pp. 35–43, p. 42.
26. Ibid., p. 43.
27. Robert Liebert, *Radical and Militant Youth: A Psychoanalytic Inquiry* (New York: Praeger, 1971). I have written in more detail about this book here: hhnnc-cnnll.substack.com/p/militant-youth.
28. Jaffe, 'Emotions on Strike'. M. E. O'Brien, *Family Abolition: Capitalism and the Communizing of Care* (London: Pluto, 2023).

29. Bench Ansfield, 'Edifice Complex', *Jewish Currents*, 3 January 2023, jewishcurrents.org.
30. Mike Davis and Jon Wiener, *Set the Night on Fire: LA in the Sixties* (London: Verso, 2020), p. 597.
31. For a critical analysis of the US health care system published at that time, see Barbara Ehrenreich and John Ehrenreich, *The American Health Empire: Power, Profits, and Politics* (New York: Vintage Books, 1971).
32. Alondra Nelson, *Body and Soul: The Black Panther Party and the Fight Against Medical Discrimination* (Minneapolis: University of Minnesota Press, 2011), p. 18, p. 81. On the Young Lords' medical campaigns which also took inspiration from the Cuban example, see Johanna Fernandez, *The Young Lords: A Radical History* (Chapel Hill: University of North Carolina Press, 2020), pp. 135–54.
33. Callen Lorde homepage: callen-lorde.org.
34. Katie Batza, *Before AIDS: Gay Health Politics in the 1970s* (Philadelphia: University of Pennsylvania Press, 2018), p. 109.
35. ACT UP oral history project, Gregg Bordowitz Interview 17 December 2002, actuporalhistory.org.
36. See, for example, the distinction between solidarity and charity outlined in Dean Spade, *Mutual Aid: Building Solidarity During this Crisis (and the Next)* (London: Verso, 2020). These issues were outlined in the influential 1979 pamphlet by the London Edinburgh Weekend Return Group, see London Edinburgh Weekend Return Group, *In and Against the State: Discussion Notes for Socialists*, ed. by Seth Wheeler (London: Pluto Press, 2021).
37. Norma Armour cited in Nelson, *Body and Soul*, p. 94.
38. Jonathan Metzl, *The Protest Psychosis: How Schizophrenia Became a Black Disease* (Boston, MA: Beacon Books, 2009).
39. Terry Kupers, 'Radical Therapy Needs Revolutionary Therapy', *Radical Therapist* 2: 1 (1971), p. 16. On that broader context and 'radical psychiatry' in the US, see Michael Staub, *Madness is Civilization: When the Diagnosis was Social, 1948–1980* (Chicago: University of Chicago Press, 2011), and Lucas Richert, *Break on Through: Radical Psychiatry and the American Counterculture* (Cambridge, MA: MIT Press, 2019).
40. On campaigns against the Center for the Study and Reduction of Violence, see Nelson, *Body and Soul*, pp. 153–80.
41. On Rahim see ibid., p. 182. See also Rachel Judith Stern, 'Solidarity not Biomedicine: Common Ground's "New Model" of Providing Healthcare', mutualaiddisasterrelief.org.
42. Tim Shorrock, 'The Street Samaritans', *Mother Jones*, March/April 2006, motherjones.com.
43. See Kindred Southern Healing Justice Collective website: kindredsouthernhjcollective.org.
44. Leah Lakshmi Piepzna-Samarasinha, *Care Work: Dreaming Disability Justice* (Vancouver: Arsenal Pulp Press, 2018), p. 100.
45. Cassie Thornton, *The Hologram: Feminist, Peer-to-Peer Health for a Postpandemic Future* (London: Pluto Press, 2020), p. 2, p. 54. See also Kelly Hayes and Mariame Kaba, *Let This Radicalize You: Organizing and the Revolution of Reciprocal Care* (Chicago: Haymarket, 2023).
46. Peer Illner discusses the example of the Common Ground Health Clinic in New

Orleans and points to the dangers of romanticising small-scale activist initiatives. Peer Illner, *Disasters and Social Reproduction: Crisis Response Between the State and Community* (London: Pluto Press, 2021).
47. See Sean Brotherton, *Revolutionary Medicine: Health and the Body in Post-Soviet Cuba* (Durham: Duke University Press, 2012).

5. Exhaustion

1. Andrei Platonov, *Chevengur*, trans. by Anthony Olcott (Ann Arbor: Ardis, 1978), p. 166.
2. Jacques Rancière, *Proletarian Nights: The Workers' Dream in Nineteenth-Century France*, trans. John Drury (London: Verso, 2012).
3. Asad Haider, 'Emancipation and Exhaustion', *South Asian Avant-Garde (SAAG): A Dissident Literary Anthology*, March 2021, saaganthology.com.
4. Neel Mukherjee, *The Lives of Others* (London: Vintage Books, 2014), p. 173. In this fictional account Mukherjee's protagonist remains at a distance from 'the others'. On relations and class divisions between rural peasants and urban students in the Naxalite movement, see Sumanta Banerjee, *India's Simmering Revolution: The Naxalite Uprising* (London: Zed Books, 1980).
5. See David G. Schuster, *Neurasthenic Nation: America's Search for Health, Happiness, and Comfort, 1869–1920* (New Brunswick, NJ: Rutgers University Press, 2011) and Anna Katharina Schaffner, *Exhaustion: A History* (New York: Columbia University Press, 2016), pp. 85–110. On economies of energy and working bodies see Anson Rabinbach, *The Human Motor: Energy, Fatigue, and the Origins of Modernity* (Berkley: University of California Press, 1992).
6. Alexander Berkman, 'The Kronstadt Rebellion (1922)', in *The Russian Tragedy*, ed. by William G Nowlin (Sanday: Cienfuegos Press, 1977) pp. 69–108, p. 71.
7. Barbara Evans Clements, *Bolshevik Women* (Cambridge: Cambridge University Press, 1997), p. 220.
8. On Kislovodsk specifically and the development of Soviet sanatoria generally see Diane P. Koenker, *Club Red: Vacation Travel and the Soviet Dream* (Ithaca, NY: Cornell University Press, 2013), pp. 12–52.
9. Armand diary entry from the 1 September 1920 cited in Clements, *Bolshevik Women*, p. 220.
10. On neurasthenia and nervousness in late imperial Russia, see Laura Goering, '"Russian Nervousness": Neurasthenia and National Identity in Nineteenth-Century Russia', *Medical History* 47 (2003), pp. 23–46, and Susan K. Morrissey, 'The Economy of Nerves: Health, Commercial Culture, and the Self in Late Imperial Russia', *Slavic Review* 69: 3 (2010), pp. 645–75.
11. Frances Lee Bernstein, *Dictatorship of Sex: Lifestyle Advice for the Soviet Masses* (DeKalb: Northern Illinois University Press, 2011), p. 85. Indeed, these diagnoses were so widespread that psychiatrists expressed concern they were beginning to lose their meaning, see Kenneth M Pinnow, *Lost to the Collective: Suicide and the Promise of Soviet Socialism, 1921–1929* (Ithaca, NY: Cornell University Press, 2010), pp. 220–1.
12. On Red Army soldiers committing suicide in the aftermath of the Civil War, see Mark von Hagen, *Soldiers in the Proletarian Dictatorship: The Red Army and the*

Soviet Socialist State, 1917–1930 (Ithaca, NY: Cornell University Press, 1990), pp. 306–7.
13. In addition to Bernstein's account, see Sheila Fitzpatrick, 'Sex and Revolution: An Examination of Literary and Statistical Data on the Mores of Soviet Students in the 1920s', *Journal of Modern History* 50: 2 (1978), pp. 252–78.
14. I engage with some of these discussions about the revolution, sex and energy in Hannah Proctor, 'Reason Displaces All Love', *New Inquiry*, February 2014, thenewinquiry.com.
15. Bernstein, *Dictatorship of Sex*, p. 86.
16. Daniel Beer, *Renovating Russia: The Human Sciences and the Fate of Liberal Modernity, 1880–1930* (Ithaca, NY: Cornell University Press, 2008), pp. 176–8. The chapter 'Social Isolation and Treatment After the Revolution' provides a useful overview of the various debates (including within criminology), indicating how ideas from the tsarist era morphed without disappearing after the October Revolution (pp. 165–204).
17. Simon Pawley, 'Revolution in health: nervous weakness and visions of health in revolutionary Russia, c.1900–31', *Historical Research* 90: 247 (2017), pp. 191–209, p. 207; Koenker, *Club Red*, p. 13.
18. Beer cites the psychiatrist Lev G. Orshanskii discussing hooliganism: 'Not everyone was able to maintain their heroic behavior in the everyday life that followed [the revolution]. A new psychological stage arrived: nervous and physical exhaustion, insufficiency of strength, and through this exhaustion old ways began to reassert themselves.' Lev G. Orshanskii, 'Khuligan, Psikhologicheskii ocherk' (1927), in Beer, *Renovating Russia*, p. 175.
19. Beer, *Renovating Russia*, p. 187.
20. For a discussion of Aron Zalkind, *Revoliutsiia i molodezh'* [Revolution and Youth] (Moscow: Izdanie Kommunistich. un-ta im. Sverdlova, 1925), see Eric Naiman, *Sex in Public: The Incarnation of Early Soviet Ideology* (Princeton, NJ: Princeton University Press, 1997), pp. 170–3.
21. Aaron Soltz (Sol'ts) cited in Yuri Slezkine, *The House of Government: A Saga of the Russian Revolution* (Princeton, NJ: Princeton University Press, 2017), p. 224.
22. Victor Serge describes the exasperation and despair among his comrades in this period in *Memoirs of a Revolutionary*, trans. by Peter Sedgwick (New York: NYRB, 2012), pp. 135–82.
23. Leonard Schapiro, *The Communist Party of the Soviet Union* (London: Methuen, 1970, 2nd ed), p. 237.
24. Susan K. Morrissey points to some of the ambiguities of the discourses around exhaustion and mental illness in connection to suicides among revolutionaries, which were framed as legitimate responses to material hardships endured due to state repression, on the one hand, and as evidence of degeneracy, on the other. See Susan K. Morrissey, *Suicide and the Body Politic in Imperial Russia* (Cambridge: Cambridge University Press, 2006), pp. 285–6.
25. Pinnow, *Lost to the Collective*, p. 87.
26. Mark von Hagen, *Soldiers in the Proletarian Dictatorship: The Red Army and the Soviet Socialist State, 1917–1930* (Ithaca, NY: Cornell University, 1990), pp. 306–7.
27. Alexander Berkman, *The Bolshevik Myth: Diary 1920–22* (London: Hutchinson and Co, 1925), p. 303.

28. Emma Goldman, *Living My Life* (London: Penguin, 2006), p. 512, p. 510.
29. Leon Trotsky, *My Life: An Attempt at an Autobiography* (New York: Pathfinder Press, 1970), p. 507.
30. Pinnow, *Lost to the Collective*, p. 88.
31. Schapiro, *Communist Party of the Soviet Union*, p. 314.
32. Serge, *Memoirs of a Revolutionary*, p. 228 (on official responses to the suicide of 'left opposition' member Evgenia Bogdanovna Bosch); Adolf Joffe, 'Letter to Leon Trotsky', 16 November 1927, marxists.org. He also describes himself as suffering from 'inflammation of the nerves'.
33. Slezkine, *House of Government*, p. 220, p. 221, p. 222.
34. Schapiro, *Communist Party of the Soviet Union*, p. 314.
35. Serge, *Memoirs of a Revolutionary*, p. 234.
36. Robert Coles, 'Social Struggle and Weariness', *Psychiatry* 27: 4 (1964), pp. 305–15, p. 305.
37. Robert Coles, *Farewell to the South* (Boston: Little, Brown, 1972).
38. Anne C. Rose, *Psychology and Selfhood in the Segregated South* (Chapel Hill: University of North Carolina Press, 2009), pp. 159–60.
39. For more on Coles' work on desegregation and schools, see Robert Coles, *Children of Crisis* (Boston, MA: Little Brown, 1967), which also reflects on his subject position as a white northerner and the social/political assumptions he had before embarking on this work.
40. However, the black psychiatrist Kenneth Clark – famous for his experiments with Mamie Clark that investigated children's attitudes to black and white dolls – observed that 'only a white person could move freely in the South, speaking with members of both races, as Coles did' (Rose, *Psychology and Selfhood*, p. 160).
41. Coles, 'Social Struggle', p. 305.
42. Ibid., p. 308.
43. Erik H. Erikson, *Childhood and Society* (London: W. W. Norton, 1950).
44. Coles, 'Social Struggle, p. 314.
45. An argument that is closer to Erikson's is made in Jacob R. Fishman and Fredric Solomon, 'Youth and Social Action: Perspectives on the Student Sit-in Movement', *American Journal of Orthopsychiatry* 33 (1963), pp. 872–82.
46. Coles, 'Social Struggle', p. 309, p. 313, p. 309.
47. Ibid., p. 309, p. 314.
48. Ibid., p. 312.
49. Ibid., p. 310.
50. On the differences in experience Coles and Poussaint had in the South, see Rose, *Psychology and Selfhood*, p. 161.
51. Alvin Poussaint, 'The Stresses of the White Female Worker in the Civil Rights Movement in the South', *American Journal of Psychiatry* 123: 4 (1966), pp. 401–7.
52. Alvin F. Poussaint and Joyce Ladner, '"Black Power": A Failure for Racial Integration Within the Civil Rights Movement', *Archives of General Psychiatry* 18 (1968), pp. 385–91.
53. Ibid., p. 391.
54. Emma Jones Lapsansky, '"Black Power Is My Mental Health": Accomplishments of the Civil Rights Movement', in *Black America*, ed. by John F. Szwed (New York: Basic Books, 1970), p. 14, p. 13.

55. Toni Cade Bambara, 'The Apprentice', in *The Sea Birds are Still Alive* (London: Women's Press, 1984), pp. 24–42. p. 28, p. 27.
56. Bambara in a 1974 letter to Walter Burford cited in Linda Janet Holmes, *Joyous Revolt: Toni Cade Bambara, Writer and Activist* (Santa Barbara, CA: Praeger, 2014), p. 65.
57. Bambara, 'The Apprentice', p. 27, p. 32, p. 28.
58. Ibid., p. 33, p. 34, p. 36.
59. Ibid., p. 37, p. 38, p. 39, p. 34, p. 42.
60. Holmes, *Joyous Revolt*, p. 49, p. 57, pp. ix–x. On the political context in Atlanta in the preceding period, see Winston A. Grady-Willis, *Challenging U.S. Apartheid: Atlanta and Black Struggles for Human Rights, 1960–1977* (New Haven, NC: Duke University Press, 2006).
61. Toni Cade Bambara, *The Salt Eaters* (London: Women's Press, 1980), p. 3.
62. Avery Gordon, *The Hawthorne Archive: Letters from the Utopian Margins* (Bronx, NY: Fordham University Press, 2017), p. 40.
63. Ibid., p. 64. This phrase is uttered jokingly by another character.
64. Bambara, *The Salt Eaters*, p. 36, p. 5, p. 65.
65. Ibid., p. 39, pp. 30–1, p. 31, p. 34, p. 93.
66. Laura Whitehorn, who accompanied Bambara as part of the delegation, reflects on the experience and on 'The Sea Birds Are Still Alive', here: thefeministwire.com.
67. Holmes, *Joyous Revolt*, p. 84.
68. Bambara, *The Salt Eaters*, p. 98, p. 90, p. 91.
69. This shift is similar to the meta-narrative sketched in this book's chapter on depression. Susan Willis, *Specifying: Black Women Writing the American Experience* (London: Routledge, 1987), pp. 129–58.
70. Ishmael Reed, 'Reginald Martin, Toni Cade Bambara – Writers', *Airing Dirty Laundry* (Reading, MA: Addison Wesley Publishing, 1993), pp. 165–71, p. 168.
71. Holmes, *Joyous Revolt*, p. 103.
72. Bambara, *The Salt Eaters*, p. 35, p. 34, p. 39, p. 38.
73. Ibid., p. 98, p. 90.
74. Ibid., p. 10, p. 92.
75. Ibid., p. 100.
76. For a discussion of the spiritual healing processes that contextualises them within the cultural practices of South Carolina and Georgia Sea Islands where West African practices and cosmologies were adopted by enslaved Africans, see Gay Wilentz, 'A Laying on of Hands: African American Healing Strategies in Toni Cade Bambara's The Salt Eaters', in *Healing Narratives: Women Writers Curing Cultural Dis-ease* (New Brunswick, NJ: Rutgers University Press, 2000), pp. 53–78.
77. Bambara, *The Salt Eaters*, p. 104, p. 119.
78. Bambara, 'Going Critical', Toni Cade Bambara, *Deep Sightings and Rescue Missions: Fiction, Essays, and Conversations*, ed. by Toni Morrison (New York: Vintage 1996, epub), pp. 14–40, p. 26.
79. Bambara, *The Salt Eaters*, p, 234.
80. Donna Haraway, 'A Manifesto for Cyborgs: Science, Technology and Socialist Feminism in the 1980s', in *The Postmodern Turn: New Perspectives on Social Theory*, ed. by Steven Seidman (Cambridge: Cambridge University Press, 1994), pp. 82–115, p. 92.
81. Cited in Clements, *Bolshevik Women*, p. 221.

82. bell hooks, *Sisters of the Yam: Black Women and Self-Recovery* (London: Routledge, 2015), p. 21, p. 13, p. 24.
83. Avery Gordon, *The Hawthorne Archive: Letters from the Utopian Margins* (Bronx, NY: Fordham University Press, 2017) p. 37, p. 41.
84. Ruth Wilson Gilmore, foreword to Dan Berger, *The Struggle Within: Prisons, Political Prisoners, and Mass Movements in the United States* (Oakland, CA: PM Press, 2014, epub), pp. 11–20, p. 14, p. 13, p. 15.
85. See Derrick E White, *The Challenge of Blackness: The Institute of the Black World and Political Activism in the 1970s* (Gainesville: University Press of Florida, 2011).
86. C. L. R. James, Grace C. Lee, Pierre Chaulieu with the collaboration of Cornelius Castoriadis, *Facing Reality: The New Society, Where to Look for it and How to Bring it Closer* (Bewick, MI: Bewick Editions, 1974, originally published, 1958), p. 91 (my emphasis), p. 86.
87. Toni Cade Bambara (then Toni Cade), 'On the issue of roles', in *The Black Woman: An Anthology*, ed. by Toni Cade Bambara (New York: Signet, 1970), pp. 101–110, p. 110.
88. Akwugo Emejulu, 'George Floyd: why the sight of these brave, exhausted protesters gives me hope', *The Conversation*, 2 June 2020, theconversation.com.

6. Bitterness

1. Vivian Gornick, 'Rosa Luxemburg's Theory of Revolution', *Village Voice*, 1 March 1987.
2. Yoshikuni Igarashi, 'Dead Bodies and Living Guns: The United Red Army and Its Deadly Pursuit of Revolution, 1971–1972', *Japanese Studies* 27: 2 (2007), pp. 119–37, p. 131.
3. This summarises descriptions of a consciousness-raising group in Sue Bruley, 'Consciousness-Raising in Clapham; Women's Liberation as "Lived Experience" in South London in the 1970s', *Women's History Review* 22: 5 (2013), pp. 717–38. Bruley is a historian and conducted oral history interviews with members of this group but she had also been a member of the group so the account is partly autobiographical.
4. This account is based on a scene from the documentary *It Still Rotates* (1978), directed by Suliman Elnour, a member of the Sudanese Film Group.
5. John F. Levin and Earl Silbar, eds, *You Say You Want a Revolution: SDS, PL and Adventures in Building a Worker-Student Alliance* (San Francisco, CA: 1741, 2019), p. 88.
6. It should, however, be noted that self-criticism practices adopted by the Communist Party in China were preceded and influenced by Bolshevik practices and writings (though in the Soviet context the practice tended to be confined to Party members). Josef Stalin himself published works defending self-criticism in the late 1920s. See Martin King Whyte, *Small Groups and Political Rituals in China* (Berkeley: University of California Press, 1974). The Chinese Trotskyist Zheng Chaolin complained that when he was studying in Moscow in 1923 his cell's activities were taken up almost exclusively by 'individual criticism' sessions focused on 'abstract psychological attitudes' that 'sowed seeds of hatred' in people's hearts. Gregor Benton, ed., *Prophets Unarmed: Chinese Trotskyists in Revolution, War, Jail, and the*

Return from Limbo (Leiden: Brill, 2015), pp. 312–13. The broadly anti-Stalinist New Left's take up of criticism-self-criticism in the 1960s and 1970s did not tend to acknowledge any connection to Stalinist or Soviet practices.
7. An in-depth discussion of how groups have tried and/or failed to deal with instances of sexual abuse and bullying is beyond my consideration here. For a self-reflective consideration of how the political culture and sect-like 'revolutionary morality' within the British Trotskyist Workers Revolutionary Party participated in enabling prolific sexual abuse, physical violence and bullying by the leadership, see Simon Pirani, 'The Break-up of the WRP: From the Horses Mouth', *Libcom*, libcom.org. On the SWP in Britain, see Edward Platt, 'Comrades at War: the decline and fall of the Socialist Workers Party', *New Statesman*, 20 May 2014, newstatesman.com. There are also many examples of groups who have developed anti-carceral accountability practices and safer spaces policies in an attempt to address these kinds of issues; see, for example, feministactionsupportnetwork.tumblr.com.
8. William Hinton, *Fanshen: A Documentary of Revolution in a Chinese Village* (Berkeley: University of California Press, 1996), p. xii. The paragraph above glosses the opening of chapter 35, pp. 319–21.
9. Ibid., p. 184, p. 480.
10. Mao Zedong, 'Rectify the Party's Style of Work (1 February 1942)', in *Selected Works of Mao Tse-tung, vol. 3* (Oxford: Pergamon Press, 1965), pp. 35–51, p. 50.
11. Hinton, *Fanshen*, p. 350, p. 364, p. 383.
12. Ibid., p. 384, p. 388.
13. Ibid., p. 388.
14. Ibid., p. 395, p. 425. Later in the book another set of meetings is initiated but this time around most people stay in bed rather than attending. Rather than laying bare uncomfortable truths, rumours began to proliferate and along with them increasingly suspicious and 'sour' feelings (p. 524). Long after the initial purification meetings party members revealed that 'vindictive statements and unfair opinions voiced by the delegates before the gate had burned themselves into the consciousness of the Party members' (p. 567).
15. Ibid., p. 395, p. 568.
16. William Hinton, 'Background notes to Fanshen', *Monthly Review* 55: 5 (2003), monthlyreview.org.
17. Andrew Ross argues that 'Maoist precepts' including self-criticism and consciousness-raising have 'had a longer and more successful career run in the West than in China itself'. See Andrew Ross, 'Mao Zedong's Impact on Cultural Politics in the West' and he cites *Fanshen* as a major influence, *Cultural Politics* 1: 1 (2005), pp. 5–22, p. 12. For a discussion of how the function and form of criticism-self-criticism as a means of dealing with inner-party strife shifted with the onset of the Cultural Revolution in China, see Lowell Dittmer, 'The Structural Evolution of "Criticism and Self-Criticism"', *The China Quarterly* 56 (1973), pp. 708–29.
18. On the global significance of *Red Star Over China* including its translation into Chinese, see Julia Lovell, *Global Maoism* (London: Vintage, 2019), pp. 60–87.
19. Marcia Holmes provides a succinct overview here: bbk.ac.uk.
20. See, for example, Aminda M. Smith, *Thought Reform and China's Dangerous Classes: Reeducation, Resistance, and the People* (New York: Rowman and Littlefield, 2013).

21. Delegations from various political organisations in the US and Western Europe began to visit China from the early 1970s, though even those who visited China followed strict itineraries on tours overseen by the state. See Sally Taylor Lieberman, 'Visions and Lessons: "China" in Feminist theory-making, 1966–1977', *Michigan Feminist Studies* 6 (1991), pp. 91–108, p. 99.
22. On 'Third World Marxism', see Max Elbaum, *Revolution in the Air: Sixties Radicals Turn to Lenin, Mao and Che* (London: Verso, 2002).
23. Greg Calvert, 'In White America: Liberal Conscience vs. Radical Consciousness' in *Revolutionary Youth and the New Working Class: The Praxis Papers, the Port Authority Statement, the RYM Documents and Other Lost Writings of SDS*, ed. by Carl Davidson (Pittsburgh, PA: Changemaker Publications, 2011), pp. 11–20, pp. 11–12.
24. Mark Rudd, *Underground: My Life with SDS and the Weathermen* (New York: HarperCollins, 2009, epub) pp. 161–2.
25. See Mao Zedong, *Quotations from Mao Tse-tung*, marxists.org.
26. Cathy Wilkerson, *Flying Close to the Sun: My Life and Times as a Weatherman* (New York: Seven Stories Press, 2011), p. 238.
27. 'A Weatherman: You Do Need A Weatherman to Know Which Way the Wind Blows', *Leviathan*, December 1969, sds-1960s.org.
28. Bill Ayers, *Fugitive Days: Memoirs of an Antiwar Activist* (Boston, MA: Beacon Press, 2001), p. 160.
29. See Ron Jacobs, *The Way the Wind Blew: A History of the Weather Underground* (London: Verso, 1997), p. 94.
30. Susan Stern, *With the Weathermen: The Personal Journey of a Revolutionary Woman* (New Brunswick, NJ: Rutgers University Press, 2007), pp. 165–85.
31. Arthur M. Eckstein, *Bad Moon Rising: How the Weather Underground Beat the FBI and Lost the Revolution* (New Haven, CT: Yale University Press, 2016), p. 76.
32. Ayers, *Fugitive Days*, p. 147.
33. Ibid., p. 161; Jeremy Varon, *Bringing the War Home: The Weather Underground, the Red Army Faction, and Revolutionary Violence in the Sixties and Seventies* (Berkeley: University of California Press, 2004), p. 59.
34. Jonathan Lerner, *Swords in the Hands of Children: Reflections of an American Revolutionary* (New York: OR Books, 2017), p. 79.
35. On purging the group of informants, see Eckstein, p. 77. They did not succeed completely, however, as related in the memoirs of a former FBI informant: Larry Grathwohl, *Bringing Down America: An FBI Informer with the Weathermen* (New Rochelle, NY: Arlington House, 1976), p. 199.
36. Self-critical written reflections began to be produced soon after the townhouse explosion. In a communique from December 1970, Bernadine Dohrn claims that despite many having reservations about carrying out a bombing, the group had willed themselves into acting dangerously: 'Many had not slept for days. Personal relationships were full of guilt and fear.' 'New Morning, Changing Weather', 6 December 1970, rozsixties.unl.edu.
37. Ayers, *Fugitive Days*, p. 152, p. 161.
38. Varon, *Bringing the War Home*, p. 59. Dan Berger similarly claims that though intended to 'help people become better activists and human beings' the sessions functioned instead as 'a weapon of manipulation, of rigid discipline'. Dan Berger, *Outlaws of America: The Weather Underground and the Politics of Solidarity* (Oakland, CA: AK Press, 2006), p. 105.

39. David Gilbert, *Love and Struggle: My Life in SDS, the Weather Underground, and Beyond* (Oakland, CA: PM Press, 2012), p. 124.
40. William Hinton, *The Hundred Day War: The Cultural Revolution at Tsinghua University* (New York: Monthly Review Press, 1972), p. 7. For a first-hand account of the persecution of intellectuals at Peking University during the Cultural Revolution that includes vivid descriptions of brutal 'struggle sessions' (distinguished from self-criticism sessions, which tended to involve verbal rather than physical attacks), see Ji Xianlin, *The Cowshed: Memories of the Chinese Cultural Revolution*, trans. by Chenxin Jiang (New York: New York Review Books, 2016).
41. Berger, *Outlaws of America*, p. 130. Though Berger explains that later when the group was falling apart members attacked the leadership 'with an intensity that placed little value on treating comrades with respect and even surpassed the group's early criticism/self-criticism sessions', p. 234. On the retreat, see also Thai Jones, *A Radical Line: From the Labor Movement to the Weather Underground, One Family's Century of Conscience* (New York: Free Press, 2004), pp. 218–20.
42. The paper originated as a memo sent to the women's caucus of the Southern Conference Educational Fund (SCEF) in 1969 and its title was added by editors when the paper appeared in *Notes from the Second Year* in 1970.
43. Carol Hanisch, 'The Personal is Political', carolhanisch.org.
44. Alice Echols claims Sarachild was 'undoubtedly influenced by Mao' and that in 1988 Sarachild told Echols that she first read *Fanshen* in summer 1968, a few months after New York Radical Women first embarked on consciousness-raising. Echols, *Daring to be Bad: Radical Feminism in America, 1967–1975* (Minneapolis: University of Minnesota Press, 2019), p. 85, p. 320.
45. Ibid., p. 84. On this array of different influences, see also Sara Evans, *Personal Politics: The Roots of Women's Liberation in the Civil Rights Movement and the New Left* (New York: Vintage Books, 1980), p. 214.
46. Carol Hanisch, 'William Hinton and the Women of Long Bow', 3 April 1999, carolhanisch.org.
47. Irene Peskilis, 'Resistances to Consciousness', June 27 1969, redstockings.org.
48. Sally Taylor Lieberman, 'Visions and Lessons: "China" in Feminist theory-making, 1966-1977', *Michigan Feminist Studies* 6 (1991), pp. 91–108, p. 93.
49. See, for example, Quinn Slobodian, 'Guerrilla Mothers and Distant Doubles: West German Feminists Look at China and Vietnam, 1968–1982', *Zeithistorische Forschungen/Studies in Contemporary History* 12 (2015), pp. 39–65; Christina Van Houten, 'Simone de Beauvoir Abroad: Historicizing Maoism and the Women's Liberation Movement', *Comparative Literature Studies* 52: 1 (2015), pp. 112–29; and Richard Wolin, *The Wind from the East: French Intellectuals, the Cultural Revolution, and the Legacy of the 1960s* (Princeton, NJ: Princeton University Press, 2010).
50. Juliet Mitchell, *Women's Estate* (Harmondsworth: Penguin, 1971), p. 62. She cites *Fanshen* and discusses the influence of Hinton's descriptions of Long Bow on the New Left on pp. 22–3. Sheila Rowbotham cites *Fanshen* in her discussion of women's liberation in China and discusses the 'painful' yet transformative practice of 'speaking bitterness' among women that he relays in Sheila Rowbotham, *Women, Resistance and Revolution: A History of Women and Revolution in the Modern World* (New York: Vintage, 1972), pp. 184–7.
51. Hinton, *Fanshen*, p. 157.

52. For a summary of the movement's unravelling and its emotional fallout, see Ruth Rosen, *The World Split Open: How the Modern Women's Movement Changed America* (Harmondsworth: Penguin, 2001), p. 264.
53. Jo Freeman, 'Tyranny of Structurelessness' (1970), jofreeman.com.
54. Jo Freeman, 'Trashing', first published in *Ms*, April 1976, pp. 49–51, pp. 92–8, jofreeman.com.
55. In another example of tangled influences, Kate Millett described 'trashing' as a 'savage rite ... invented by Weathermen of the manly Left' that resulted from the purism, tyranny and dogmatism of the 'new and terrible orthodoxy with purge and heretic' that came to characterise the women's movement. Kate Millett, *Flying* (New York: Alfred A Knopf, 1974), p. 367, p. 160.
56. Freeman, 'Trashing', jofreeman.com.
57. She writes: 'Trying to change an entire society is a very slow, frustrating process in which gains are incremental, rewards diffuse, and setbacks frequent.' Ibid.
58. Rachel Blau DuPlessis and Ann Barr Snitow, eds, *Feminist Memoir Project: Voices from Women's Liberation* (New Brunswick, NJ: Rutgers University Press, 2007), p. 373.
59. Vivian Gornick, 'Women's Work: Two new books confront the legacy of the 1970s women's movement', *Book Forum*, Apr/May 2015, bookforum.com. See also her description of the movement's slow erosion around 1980 and her experience of falling into depression in *The Feminist Memoir Project*, pp. 372–3. Compare this with Kate Millett's reflections in 1974: 'I could not live the way I advocated, recommended to other people. That I was not free myself. We're all finding this out. A lot of my friends say the same thing, we recognize the gap between what we say and how we really live. It depresses us. We have discovered ambivalence.' Millett, *Flying*, p. 85.
60. Vivian Gornick, 'Introduction (2019)', in *The Romance of American Communism* (London: Verso, 2020), p. xviii. She also reflects on the women's liberation movement and the emergence of dogmatism in the book's conclusion, pp. 256–65.
61. Ibid., p. 22.
62. Ibid., p. 195, p. 233.
63. The loss experienced by party members who left after 1956 is the focus of an essay I co-wrote with Larne Abse Gogarty: 'Communist Feelings', *New Socialist*, 13 March 2019, newsocialist.org.uk.
64. Gornick, *Romance of American Communism*, p. 148, p. 153, p. 177.
65. Ayers, *Fugitive Days*, p. 160.
66. Gornick, *Romance of Ammerican Communism*, p. 178, p. xviii.
67. Ibid., p. 259, p. 19.
68. Arthur Koestler in Koestler et al., *The God that Failed: Six Studies in Communism* (London: Hamish Hamilton, 1950), pp. 25–82, p. 64.
69. Elbaum singles out Todd Gitlin's account of the sixties as exemplary of this tendency, Elbaum, *Revolution in the Air*, pp. 35–7.
70. For a crude example of this kind of pathologising approach focused on the Japanese movement, see William Regis Farrell, *Blood and Rage: The Story of the Japanese Red Army* (Washington, DC: Lexington Books, 1990). Pathologisation was also evident in reactions to the Red Army Faction (RAF) in West Germany. See Charity Scribner, *After the Red Army Faction: Gender, Culture and Militancy* (New York: Columbia University Press, 2015).

71. Elbaum, *Revolution in the Air*, p. 37.
72. Keeanga-Yamahtta Taylor, ed., 'The Combahee River Collective Statement', in *How We Get Free: Black Feminism and the Combahee River Collective* (Chicago: Haymarket Books, 2017, epub), pp. 28–45, p. 27.
73. Taylor, 'Barbara Smith Interview', in *How We Get Free*, pp. 46–100, p. 56, p. 66.
74. Asad Haider, *Mistaken Identity: Race and Class in the Age of Trump* (London: Verso, 2018).
75. Colleen Lye, 'Identity Politics, Criticism, and Self-Criticism', *The South Atlantic Quarterly* 119: 4 (2020), pp. 701–14, p. 706, p. 707.
76. Ibid., p. 701.
77. Mao Zedong, 'On Contradiction' (1937), marxists.org.
78. Taylor, ed., 'Combahee River Collective Statement', p. 44.
79. The many causes recall those invoked by Toni Cade Bambara in *The Salt Eaters*. Bambara and Barbara Smith were acquainted in New York in the 1960s, Linda Janet Holmes, *Toni Cade Bambara: A Joyous Revolt* (Santa Barbara, CA: Praeger, 2014), pp. 40–5.
80. Robin D. G. Kelley and Betsy Esch, 'Black like Mao: Red China and Black Revolution', in *Souls: Critical Journal of Black Politics and Culture* 1: 4 (1999), pp. 6–41, p. 39. See also Robeson Taj Frazier, *The East is Black: Cold War China in the Black Radical Imagination* (Durham, NC: Duke University Press, 2015).
81. Lye, 'Identity Politics, Criticism, and Self-Criticism', p. 709.
82. Kelley and Esch, 'Black like Mao', p. 37.
83. Slobodian, 'Guerrilla Mothers and Distant Doubles', p. 57. Though this was also the moment in which 'scar literature' reflecting on suffering during the Cultural Revolution began to be published in China.
84. Redstockings, 'Editors' Note to Nancy Milton's "Report on Separatism in China" in Redstockings', in *Feminist Revolution* (New York: Random House, 1978), p. 156.
85. Slobodian, 'Guerilla Mothers and Distant Doubles', p. 57.
86. Carol Hanisch, 'Paying the piper? Did I blow my life?', *Meeting Ground: A Project of the Women's Liberation Front* 12 (1990), pp. 1–3.
87. See Alyssa Battistoni, 'Bad Romance', *Dissent*, dissentmagazine.org, and Ari Brostoff, 'The Family Romance of American Communism', *n+1*, nplusonemag.com.
88. 'Bliss was it in that dawn to be alive' is a line Gornick takes from Wordsworth's *The Prelude* (published posthumously in 1850). I have stolen this insight from Danny Hayward who read an earlier draft of this chapter (though I possibly simplified his point in the process).
89. '"There's a Lot More That Needs to Be Done", An Interview with Barbara Smith', *The Drift* 9, 28 February 2023, thedriftmag.com.
90. Hinton, *Fanshen*, p. 609.

7. Trauma

1. Samah Jabr, 'A Deeper Pain', *The New Internationalist*, 1 November 2014, newint.org. This article is cited in the closing pages of Lara Sheehi and Stephen Sheehi, *Psychoanalysis under Occupation: Practicing Resistance in Palestine* (New York: Routledge, 2022), p. 206.

2. Dagmar Herzog, *Cold War Freud: Psychoanalysis in an Age of Catastrophes* (Cambridge: Cambridge University Press, 2018), p. 116. Ethan Watters claims that PTSD became 'the international lingua franca of human suffering' in this period. Watters, *Crazy Like Us: The Globalization of the American Psyche* (New York: Free Press, 2011), p. 71.
3. Didier Fassin and Richard Rechtman, *The Empire of Trauma: An Inquiry into the Condition of Victimhood*, trans. by Rachel Gomme (Princeton, NJ: Princeton University Press, 2009), p. 28, p. 5. On shifts in definition that occurred between *DSM-III* to *DSM-V*, see Anushka Pai, Alina M. Suris and Carol S. North, 'Posttraumatic Stress Disorder in the *DSM-5*: Controversy, Change, and Conceptual Considerations', *Behavioural Sciences* 7: 1 (2017), p. 7.
4. Though PTSD assumes that events in the outside world have psychological consequences, it does not necessarily recognise what roles people played in events. For example, in the aftermath of the uprisings in Ferguson in 2014 that followed the racist police murder of Michael Brown, both cops and members of the community were diagnosed with PTSD: Tara E. Galovski, Zoë D. Peterson, Marin C. Beagley, David R. Strasshofer, Philip Held, Thomas D. Fletcher, 'Exposure to Violence During Ferguson Protests: Mental Health Effects for Law Enforcement and Community Members', *Journal of Traumatic Stress* 29: 4 (2016), pp. 283–92.
5. Fassin and Rechtman, *Empire of Trauma*, p. 160.
6. Leslie Dwyer and Degung Santikarma, 'Posttraumatic Politics: Violence, Memory, and Biomedical Discourse in Bali', in *Understanding Trauma*, ed. by L. Kirmayer, R. Lemelson and M. Barad (Cambridge: Cambridge University Press, 2007), pp. 403–32, pp. 403–4. On the meaning of 'trauma' in the Indonesian context, see James T. Siegel, *A New Criminal Type in Jakarta: Counter-Revolution Today* (Durham, NC: Duke University Press, 1998), pp. 134–5 and Wulan Dirgantoro, 'Aesthetics of Silence: Exploring Trauma and Indonesian Paintings After 1965', *Ambitious Alignments: New Histories of Southeast Asian Art, 1945–1990*, ed. by Stephen H. Whiteman, Sarena Abdullah, Yvonne Low and Phoebe Scott (Singapore: Power Publications and National Gallery Singapore, 2018), pp. 199–224, p. 218 (with thanks to her for sharing this publication with me).
7. Adrian Vickers, 'Where are the bodies: The haunting of Indonesia', *The Public Historian* 32: 1 (2010), pp. 45–58, which also provides a useful overview of the existing literature on the massacres of 1965–1966.
8. Ibid., p. 46. See also Ariel Heryato, 'Where Communism Never Dies: Violence, Trauma and Narration in the Last Cold War Capitalist Authoritarian State', *International Journal of Cultural Studies* 2: 2, pp. 147–77, p. 151.
9. See Mary S. Zurbuchen, 'History, Memory, and the "1965 Incident" in Indonesia', *Asian Survey* 42: 4 (2002), pp. 564–81.
10. Crocodile Hole, the place from which the corpses of the generals were exhumed, is still the site of a giant monument and accompanying museum memorializing their deaths, and it was the site for the Suharto regime's significant state rituals. John Roosa, *Pretext for Mass Murder: The September 30th Movement and Suharto's Coup d'état in Indonesia* (Madison: University of Wisconsin Press, 2006), p. 10.
11. Dwyer and Santikarma, 'Posttraumatic Politics', p. 407.

12. On how perceptions of the monument to victims of the bombing diverged from the designers' intentions, see Jeff Lewis, Belinda Lewis and I Nyoman Darma Putra, 'The Bali Bombings Monument: Ceremonial Cosmopolis', *The Journal of Asian Studies* 72: 1 (2013), pp. 21–43.
13. Between December 1965 and March 1966 Dwyer and Santikarma estimate 80,000 to 100,000 Balinese people were killed ('Posttraumatic Politics', p. 415). On the massacres in Bali, see also Geoffrey Robinson, *The Dark Side of Paradise: Political Violence in Bali* (Ithaca, NY: Cornell University Press, 1995) and Adrian Vickers, 'Reopening Old Wounds: Bali and the Indonesian Killings', *The Journal of Asian Studies* 57: 3 (1998), pp. 774–85. For a collection of essays discussing 1965–66 massacres in Indonesia that also assesses the reexamination of the events that occurred after the fall of the Suharto regime, see the special issue on 'The Legacy of Violence in Indonesia' in *Asian Survey* 42: 4 (2002).
14. Dwyer and Santikarma, 'Posttraumatic Politics', p. 405.
15. Ibid., p. 423, p. 428. They also stress that some clinicians were attentive to these tensions and caution against characterising Balinese culture as static and monolithic. Discussions of PTSD that raised concerns about cultural relativism were published in the period in which the trauma industry was expanding. See Patrick Bracken and Celia Petty, eds, *Rethinking the Trauma of War* (London: Save the Children/Free Association Books, 1998), Joshua Breslau, 'Introduction: Cultures of Trauma: Anthropological Views of Posttraumatic Stress Disorder in International Health', *Culture, Medicine and Psychiatry* 28 (2004), pp. 113–26, and Derek Summerfield, 'The Invention of Post-Traumatic Stress Disorder and the Social Usefulness of a Psychiatric Category', *British Medical Journal* 322 (2001), pp. 95–8. Fassin and Rechtman discuss the furore generated by the publication of the latter article, pp. 25–8.
16. Dwyer and Santikarma, 'Posttraumatic Politics', p. 416.
17. Samah Jabr, 'A Deeper Pain', *The New Internationalist*, 1 November 2014. See also Amani M. Abusoboh, 'Post-Traumatic Stress Disorder Scale and Palestinian Trauma', *Pangaea Journal*, sites.stedwards.edu. Fassin and Rechtman discuss how psychiatrists and humanitarians working for Médecins Sans Frontières and Médecins du Monde in Palestine during the Second Intifada (2000–5) were often individually motivated by indignation at the Israeli occupation but the language of trauma adopted by the organisations allowed them to 'give an account of the violence of war, not of its causes but of its consequences, not of politics but of suffering.' Fassin and Rechtman, *Empire of Trauma*, p. 197. On the use of PTSD in Indigenous political campaigns in North America in the 1990s, see Melanie K. Yazzie, 'Traumatic Monologues', *The Baffler* 59, September 2021.
18. David Becker cited in Ben Shepherd, 'After a Fight', *Times Literary Supplement*, the-tls.co.uk.
19. Herzog, *Cold War Freud*, pp. 113–22.
20. Allan Young, *The Harmony of Illusions: Inventing Post Traumatic Stress Disorder* (Princeton: Princeton University Press, 1995), p. 94; Hannah Decker, *The Making of DSM-III: a Diagnostic Manual's Conquest* (Oxford: Oxford University Press, 2013), p. 309. Young also emphasises how dramatic a 'revolutionary' turn the *DSM-III* represented, p. 100.

21. Young, *Harmony of Illusions*, pp. 95–6.
22. Rick Mayes and Allan V. Horowitz, 'DSM-III and the Revolution in Classification of Mental Illness', *Journal of the History of the Behavioral Sciences* 41: 3 (2005), pp. 249–67, p. 252.
23. Ibid., p. 263, p. 264.
24. Young, *Harmony of Illusions*, p. 113. Wilbur J. Scott, 'PTSD in DSM-III: A Case in the Politics of Diagnosis and Disease', *Social Problems* 37: 3 (1990), pp. 294–310, p. 307, p. 117.
25. Herzog, *Cold War Freud*, pp. 89–122, p. 122.
26. Roger Luckhurst, *The Trauma Question* (London: Routledge, 2008), p. 59. See also, Ben Shepherd, *A War of Nerves: Soldiers and Psychiatrists, 1914–1994* (London: Pimlico, 2002), pp. 355–68.
27. Joseph Darda, *How White Men Won the Culture Wars: A History of Veteran America* (Berkeley: University of California Press, 2021), p. 44.
28. Nadia Abu El-Haj, *Combat Trauma: Imaginaries of War and Citizenship in post-9/11 America* (London: Verso, 2022), p. 40, p. 37, p. 155. She also argues that in practice clinicians have often operated with more nuanced understandings of trauma than those in the *DSM*.
29. Robert Jay Lifton, *Home from the War: Vietnam Veterans: Neither Victims nor Executioners* (New York: Simon and Schuster, 1973), p. 414.
30. Ibid., p. 128, p. 281, p. 132, p. 287.
31. Ibid., pp. 17–18.
32. Bussarawan Teerawichitchainan and Kim Korinek, 'The long-term impact of war on health and wellbeing in Northern Vietnam: Some glimpses from a recent survey', *Social Science & Medicine* 74 (2012), pp. 1995–2004.
33. Heonik Kwon, 'Rethinking the Traumas of War', *South East Asia Research* 20: 2, pp. 227–37, p. 228.
34. On the commemoration of war deaths in Vietnam, see Shaun Kingsley Malarney, *Culture, Ritual and Revolution in Vietnam* (London: Routledge, 2002). On the publicly disavowed psychological and physical impact of the war and its aftermath on women who joined the shock brigades that includes some speculative diagnoses, see François Guillemot, 'Death and Suffering at First Hand: Youth Shock Brigades during the Vietnam War (1950–1975)', *Journal of Vietnamese Studies* 4: 3 (2009), pp. 17–60.
35. It is interesting to compare Kwon's work to anthropologist James Siegel's discussion of the prevalence of communist ghosts in Indonesia after the fall of the Suharto in Indonesia. Siegel, *Naming the Witch* (Palo Alto, CA: Stanford University Press, 2006).
36. Kwon, 'Rethinking', p. 231.
37. Heonik Kwon, *After the Massacre: Commemoration and Consolation in Ha My and My Lai* (Berkeley: University of California Press, 2006), p. 125.
38. Kwon, 'Rethinking', p. 233, p. 234.
39. Heonik Kwon, *Ghosts of War in Vietnam* (Cambridge: Cambridge University Press, 2008), pp. 25–6.
40. Avery F. Gordon, 'Some Thoughts on Haunting and Futurity', *borderlands* 10: 2 (2011), pp. 1–21, p. 2, p. 4.
41. For a useful discussion of the relatively late turn to historical trauma within psychoanalysis, see Matt ffytche, 'Psychoanalytic Sociology and the Traumas of

History: Alexander Mitscherlich between the Disciplines', *History of the Human Sciences* 20: 10 (2017), pp. 1–27, p. 10.
42. Carla Fischer Canessa, 'Psychoanalysis and Dictatorship in Chile: A Non-Existing Relationship', *Psychoanalytic Dialogues* 26: 4 (2016), pp. 476–85, p. 477. See also Susan Mailer, 'Out of Sight Out of Mind? An Uneasy Compromise: Commentary on Dr. Carla Fischer's Paper "Psychoanalysis and Dictatorship in Chile: A Non-Existing Relationship"', *Psychoanalytic Dialogues* 26: 4 (2016), pp. 486–90. Similarly, in Argentina and Brazil during the dictatorships of the late twentieth century official Psychoanalytic Associations continued to operate. On Brazil see Aline Rubin, Belinda Mandelbaum and Stephen Frosh, '"No Memory, No Desire": Psychoanalysis in Brazil During Repressive Times', *Psychoanalysis and History* 18: 1 (2016), pp. 93–118. On Argentina, see Nancy Caro Hollander, 'Psychoanalysis Confronts the Politics of Repression: The Case of Argentina', *Social Science and Medicine* 28: 7 (1989), p. 757, and Mariano Ben Plotkin, *Freud in the Pampas: The Emergence and Development of a Psychoanalytic Culture in Argentina* (Stanford, CA: Stanford University Press, 2001).
43. Canessa, 'Psychoanalysis and Dictatorship in Chile', p. 478.
44. David Becker, 'The Deficiency of the Concept of Posttraumatic Stress Disorder When Dealing with Victims of Human Rights Violations', in *Beyond Trauma: Cultural and Societal Dynamics*, ed. by Robert J. Kleber, Charles R. Figley and Berthold P.R. Gersons (New York: Springer Science, 1995), pp. 99–114, p. 100.
45. See Herzog, *Cold War Freud*, pp. 113–22.
46. Becker, 'Deficiency', p. 101, p. 105.
47. Ibid., p. 104, p. 107.
48. Herzog, *Cold War Freud*, p. 118.
49. See David Becker and Margarita Diaz, 'The Social Process and the Transgenerational Transmission of Trauma in Chile', in *International Handbook of Multigenerational Legacies of Trauma*, ed. by Y. E. Danielli (Berlin: Plenum Press, 1998), pp. 435–45, p. 438. In this essay they identify three traumatic sequences – the coup and beginning of repression, repression under the dictatorship, the aftermath of the dictatorship – analogous to the sequences identified by Keilson.
50. David Becker, Elizabeth Lira, Maria Isabel Castillo, Elena Gomez, and Juana Kovalskys, 'Therapy with Victims of Political Repression in Chile: The Challenge of Social Reparation', *Journal of Social Issues* 46: 3 (1990), pp. 133–49, p. 142. According to Herzog, Becker later came to view this approach as overly idealistic (Herzog, *Cold War Freud*, p. 120).
51. Nancy Caro Hollander, 'Buenos Aires: Latin Mecca of Psychoanalysis', *Social Research* 57: 4 (1990), pp. 889–919, p. 907.
52. David Becker, Maria Isabel Castillo, Elena Gomez, Juana Kovalskys and Elizabeth Lira, 'Subjectivity and Politics: The Psychotherapy of Extreme Traumatization in Chile', *International Journal in Mental Health* 18: 2 (1989), pp. 80–97, p. 94.
53. Becker et al., 'Subjectivity', p. 83.
54. Becker and Díaz, 'Social Process and the Transgenerational Transmission', p. 436.
55. Becker and Díaz, 'Social Process and the Transgenerational Transmission', p. 444.

56. Margarita Díaz Cordal, 'Traumatic effects of political repression in Chile: A clinical experience', *The International Journal of Psychoanalysis* 86: 5 (2005), pp. 1317–28, p. 1312.
57. Ruth Leys, *Trauma: A Genealogy* (Chicago: University of Chicago Press, 2000), p. 7.
58. Ibid., p. 37.
59. Díaz Cordal, 'Traumatic effects of political repression in Chile', p. 1325.
60. Dominick LaCapra, 'Absence, Loss', *Critical Inquiry* 25: 4 (1999), pp. 696–727, p. 712. LaCapra also distinguishes between structural and historical trauma, the former being a universal part of individual subject formation whereas the latter is tied to specific circumstances.
61. Díaz Cordal, 'Traumatic effects of political repression in Chile', p. 1325, p. 1326.
62. Rob White, 'After Effects', *Film Quarterly*, 12 July 2012, filmquarterly.org.
63. Roger Luckhurst gives a helpful synoptic overview of this body of work and its influences in *The Trauma Question*, pp. 4–13. On this intellectual history, the broader historical context and the connection between trauma studies and Holocaust studies in the 1990s, see also, Karyn Ball, 'Trauma and Memory Studies', *Oxford Encyclopedia of Literary Theory* (Oxford: Oxford University Press, 2021).
64. See Leys, *Trauma*, particularly the book's closing two chapters, pp. 229–97. Leys's book devotes a chapter to Bessel van der Kolk, though it was published before the publication of *The Body Keeps the Score* in 2014 and predates the more pervasive, popular reception of his work. On van der Kolk, see Danielle Carr, 'Tell Me Why It Hurts', *New York Magazine*, 31 July 2023, nymag.com.
65. Roger Luckhurst cites Shoshana Felman's writings on Claude Lanzmann's nine-hour film *Shoah* (1985) as the paradigmatic example of this approach for writing about film (and also notes that Lanzmann vehemently rejected the notion of a 'trauma aesthetic'). For a searing attack on 'Holocaust piety' and theorists (including Felman) who argue that the horrors of Nazism cannot be represented, see Gillian Rose, 'Beginnings of the day – Fascism and representation', *Mourning Becomes the Law: Philosophy and Representation* (Cambridge: Cambridge University Press, 1996), pp. 41–62.
66. Rebecca Comay, *Mourning Sickness: Hegel and the French Revolution* (Stanford: Stanford University Press, 2011), p. 4, p. 148.
67. Becker et al., 'Subjectivity', p. 140.
68. Raúl Zurita, *INRI*, trans. by William Rowe (New York: New York Review Books, 2018), p. 13. Thanks to Ed Luker for sending me his copy of this book in the post during lockdown.
69. Becker and Díaz, 'Social Process and the Transgenerational Transmission', p. 439.
70. Tomás Moulian, 'A Time of Forgetting: The Myths of the Chilean Transition', NACLA Report on the Americas 32: 2 (1998), pp. 16–22, p. 22.
71. Sergio Villalobos-Ruminott, 'Chilean Revolts and the Crisis of Neoliberal Governance', *Radical Philosophy* 2: 7 (2020), pp. 9–16, p. 10.
72. William Rowe, 'Translator's Afterword', in Zurita, *INRI*, pp. 133–37, p. 133.

8. Mourning

1. Peter Apps, *Show Me the Bodies: How We Let Grenfell Happen* (London: Oneworld, 2021).

2. Brenna Bhandar, 'Organised State Abandonment: The Meaning of Grenfell', *Critical Legal Thinking*, 21 September 2018.
3. Nadine El-Enany, 'The Colonial Logic of Grenfell', *Verso Blog*, 3 July 2017.
4. Joe Hill, 'Don't mourn, organize!', *Jacobin*, 19 November 2015.
5. George Hardy, *These Stormy Years: Memories of the Fight for Freedom on Five Continents* (London: Lawrence and Wishart, 1956), p. 161.
6. For example, Franklin Rosemont mentions that the front page of the New York Times on 11 July 1985 featured a photograph of a black South African wearing a t-shirt with the slogan printed on it. Franklin Rosemont, *Joe Hill: The IWW & the Making of a Revolutionary Working Class Counterculture* (Oakland, CA: PM Press, 2015).
7. David Wojnarowicz, *Close to the Knives: A Memoir of Disintegration* (New York: Vintage Books, 1991), p. 203.
8. Jacqueline Rose, 'Virginia Woolf and the Death of Modernism', in *On Not Being Able to Sleep: Psychoanalysis and the Modern World* (London: Vintage, 2004), pp. 72–88, p. 73.
9. Ibid., p, 73, p. 88.
10. Eve Kosofsky Sedgwick, 'Paranoid Reading and Reparative Reading, or, You're so Paranoid you probably Think this Essay is about You', in *Touching Feeling: Affect, Pedagogy, Performativity* (Durham, NC: Duke University Press, 2003), pp. 123–151.
11. Douglas Crimp, 'Mourning and Militancy', *October* 51 (1989), pp. 3–18, p. 16.
12. Ibid., pp. 4–5, p. 5, p. 10.
13. Sigmund Freud, 'Mourning and Melancholia', *Standard Edition of the Complete Psychological Works of Sigmund Freud*, Vol. 14 (1914–1916), ed. and trans. by James Strachey et al. (London: Hogarth Press), pp. 243–58, p. 244.
14. Here Crimp contrasts his approach to that taken by Michael Moon in 'Memorial Rags', which proposes to read mourning through the lens of fetishism. See Michael Moon, 'Memorial Rags' in *Professions of Desire: Lesbian and Gay Studies in Literature*, ed. by George E. Haggerty and Bonnie Zimmerman (New York: Modern Language Association of America, 1995), pp. 233–40.
15. Crimp, 'Mourning and Militancy', p. 7, pp. 8–9, p. 10, p. 9.
16. Freud, 'Mourning and Melancholia', p. 245; Crimp, 'Mourning and Militancy', p. 12.
17. Sarah Schulman, *The Gentrification of the Mind: Witness to a Lost Imagination* (Berkeley: University of California Press, 2012), p. 45, p. 46, p. 48. On the 'state-condoned violence and murder' enabled by politicians like Reagan and Helms, see also David Wojnarowicz, 'Do Not Doubt the Dangerousness of the 12-Inch Politician', in *Close to the Knives*, pp. 138–64, p. 148.
18. Crimp, 'Mourning and Militancy', p. 15.
19. Ibid., p. 16.
20. Jacqueline Rose, *Sexuality in the Field of Vision* (London: Verso, 1986), p. 10.
21. Crimp, 'Mourning and Militancy', p. 17, p. 16.
22. Sarah Schulman, *Let the Record Show: A Political History of ACT UP New York, 1987–1993* (New York: Farrar, Straus and Giroux, 2021), p. 406. Though she also acknowledges it was not always possible to bear the loss, 'In some cases, we went insane with grief' (p. 575).
23. Crimp, 'Mourning and Militancy', p. 18.

24. Tamar Garb, 'Painting/Politics/Photography: Marlene Dumas, Mme Lumumba and the Image of the African Woman', *Art History* (2020), pp. 1–25, p. 20.
25. Schulman, *Let the Record Show*, pp. 611–31.
26. Freud, 'Mourning and Melancholia', p. 249.
27. Sean Purdy, 'Brazil's June Days of 2013: Mass Protest, Class, and the Left', *Latin American Perspectives* 227: 46 (4 July 2019), pp. 15–36, p. 16.
28. Soreanu is critical of the orthodox left's sometimes dismissive accounts of this spontaneous movement and its diverse demands. I am more interested in her theorisations of protest as a site for collectively working through the past than I am in her political assessments of the protests. The Sean Purdy article cited above provides a useful class analysis of the movement that is critical of accounts that emphasised the significance of social media over the class composition of the crowds and the shifts in Brazilian capitalism to which they were responding. Brazil's 'June Days' are central to Vincent Bevin's discussion of the global mass uprisings between 2010–20. He explicitly analyses them in relation to the subsequent election of Bolsonaro and activist concerns about horizontality, leaderlessness and political plurality that Soreanu broadly ignores. Vincent Bevins, *If We Burn: The Mass Protest Decade and the Missing Revolution* (London: Wildfire, 2023).
29. Raluca Soreanu, *Working-through Collective Wounds: Trauma, Denial, Recognition in the Brazilian Uprising* (London: Palgrave Macmillan, 2018), p. 3, p. 98.
30. Ibid., p. 7, p. 196, p. 128.
31. Ibid., p. 18.
32. Sigmund Freud, 'Group Psychology and the Analysis of the Ego', in *Standard Edition of the Complete Psychological Works of Sigmund Freud, vol XVIII (1920–21)*, ed. and trans. by James Strachey (London: Hogarth Press, 1955), pp. 69–143, p. 77, p. 79.
33. The most prominent example is Wilhelm Reich, *The Mass Psychology of Fascism* (first published in German in 1933).
34. Soreanu, *Working-through Collective Wounds*, p. 29.
35. Ibid., p. 102.
36. Stephen Frosh, *Hauntings: Psychoanalysis and Ghostly Transmissions* (Houndsmills: Palgrave Macmillan, 2013), p. 4.
37. Soreanu, *Working-through Collective Wounds*, p. 121, p. 54, p. 46, p. 118, p. 22.
38. Ibid., p. 26, p. 27, p. 165.
39. See Nadine El-Enany, 'The Colonial Logic of Grenfell', Verso Blog, July 2017, versobooks.com, and Barnaby Raine, 'What Burns?', June 2017, medium.com.
40. I owe this observation to a tweet by Rees Arnott Davis.
41. Soreanu, *Working-through Collective Wounds*, p. 22, p. 94. Soreanu does not claim that the 2013 protests can be reducible to this but argues that the unresolved traumas of the dictatorship are one aspect of the movement whose meanings are contested and overdetermined. For a discussion of how Soreanu's account diverges from existing narratives of the events, see Felipe Massao Kuzuhara, 'Review: Working Through Collective Wounds', *Psychoanalysis and History* 21: 3.
42. For a discussion of the failures of Dilma Rousseff and the PT at this moment, see Rodrigo Nunes, 'Brazil's perfect storm of dissent', *Al Jazeera*, 20 June 2013.
43. See Ludmila Abilio et al., 'The Long Brazilian Crisis: A Forum', ed. and introduced by Juan Grigera and Jeffery R. Webber, *Historical Materialism*, historicalmaterialism.org.

44. Rodrigo Nunes, 'Brazil Transformed', *New Left Review* (Sidecar), 10 November 2022.
45. Soreanu, *Working-through Collective Wounds*, p. 192.
46. 'Burning Issues: Hannah Black interviewed by Larne Abse Gogarty', *Art Monthly* 441 (November 2020), pp. 1–6, p. 4. On riots as joyous and exuberant experiences that are also often simultaneously acts of mourning, see Vicky Osterweil, *In Defense of Looting: A Riotous History of Uncivil Action* (New York: Bold Type Books, 2020).
47. Tobi Haslett, 'Magic Actions: Looking back on the George Floyd Rebellion', *n+1*, Summer 2021, nplusonemag.com.
48. Angela Y. Davis, *Freedom is a Constant Struggle: Ferguson, Palestine and the Foundations of a Movement* (Chicago: Haymarket Books, 2016), p. 15.
49. On rejecting the 'normal' or the notion of a hoped for 'return to normal' after the pandemic, see Dionne Brand, 'On narrative, reckoning and the calculus of living and dying', *Toronto Star*, 4 July 2020.
50. This invokes Walter Benjamin's line from his 1940 *Theses 'On the Concept of History'*: 'Even the dead will not be safe from the enemy when he is victorious.'
51. This statement responds to observations made in Jacqueline Rose's essay, 'To Die One's Own Death', *London Review of Books*, 19 November 2020.
52. Saree Makdisi, 'No Human Being Can Exist', 25 October 2023, nplusone.com.
53. Abdaljawad Omar, 'Can the Palestinian Mourn?', Rusted Radishes, Nov 2023, rustedradishes.com.

Afterword

1. Muriel Rukeyser, 'Tenth Elegy, Elegy in Joy', in *Elegies* (New York: New Direction, 2013), p. 59.
2. Sean Bonney, '21/What if the summer never ends', in *Our Death* (Oakland: Commune Editions, 2019), p. 92.
3. Gillian Rose, *Love's Work* (London: Vintage, 1997), p. i.
4. Cited in Sara Crangle, 'The agonies of ambivalence: Anna Mendelssohn, La poétesse maudite,' *Modernism/Modernity* 25: 3, pp. 461–97, p. 468.
5. Muriel Rukeyser, '1/26/39', in *The Collected Poems of Muriel Rukeyser*, ed. by Janet Kaufman and Anne Herzog (Pittsburgh: University of Pittsburgh, 2005), p. 165.
6. Hannah Black, *Tuesday or September or the End* (New York: Capricious, 2021), p. 33, p. 123.
7. Ibid., p. 131.
8. Ibid., p. 131.
9. Jackie Wang, *Carceral Capitalism* (South Pasadena: Semiotext(e), 2018), p. 304.
10. Muriel Rukeyser, *Savage Coast* (New York: Feminist Press, 2014), p. 37.
11. Audre Lorde, *Sister Outsider: Essays and Speeches* (Berkeley: Crossing Press, 1984, 2007), p. 18.
12. Agnes Smedley, *Daughter of Earth* (New York: Feminist Press, CUNY, 2019).
13. Victor Serge, *Notebooks: 1936–1947* (New York: NYRB, 2019), p. 413.
14. North Yorkshire Women Against Pit Closures, *Strike 84-85* (Leeds: North Yorkshire Women Against Pit Closures, 1985), pp. 61–2.

15. Jeannene M. Przyblyski, 'Courbet, the Commune, and the Meanings of Still Life in 1871', *Art Journal* 55 (1996), pp. 28–37, p. 37.
16. Bruno Jasieński, *I Burn Paris*, trans. by Soren A. Gauger and Marcin Piekoszewski (Prague: Twisted Spoon Press, 2012), p. 300.
17. Jalal Movaghary-Pour, 'Interview: "Fight with hope, fight without hope, but fight absolutely" with Mike Davis', *LSE Blog*, 1 March 2016, blogs.lse.ac.uk.

Index

A

Abdelhadi, Eman, 207
absent fathers, impacts of, 95–7
Abu El-Haj, Nadia, 167
The Act of Killing (documentary), 183
ACT UP, 67, 189, 192
Adorno, Theodor, 33
The Aesthetics of Resistance (Weiss), 55
Airless Spaces (Firestone), 65, 70, 72, 73–4, 76, 77, 78
Allemane, Jean, 56
Allende, Salvador, 171, 176, 180, 184
al-Mokrani, Muhammad, 56
Alprentice 'Bunchy' Carter Free Clinic, 98
Amini, Mahsa, 200
Ansfield, Bench, 98
anti-adaptive healing, 16, 76, 205
'Apocalyptic Populism' (Brown), 34
'The Apprentice' (Bambara), 106, 118–20, 121, 122, 127, 128
'Arab Spring', 219n14
The Arcades Project (Benjamin), 60
Argentinian Psychoanalytic Association (APA), 174
Armand, Inessa, 107–8, 110, 126
Authoritarian Personality (Adorno et al.), 33
Autobiography of a Generation: Italy, 1968 (Passerini), 80–4
Ayers, Bill, 140–1, 150
Azoulay, Jacques, 17

B

Badiou, Alain, 43, 46
Baku Commune of 1918, 47
Bali, Kuta bombings, 161, 163
Balzac, Honoré de, 53
Bambara, Toni Cade, 106, 118–26, 127, 128
Banks, Lacy, 4, 5
Baraitser, Lisa, 2
Battersea Action and Counselling Centre, 14
Battistoni, Alyssa, 156
The Battle of Chile (film), 176, 177
Batza, Katie, 99
Baudrillard, Jean, 180
Beauvoir, Simone de, 77
Becker, David, 164, 172–3, 174–5, 181, 183
Beer, Daniel, 109
Benjamin, Walter, 31, 34, 35, 39, 41, 60, 61

Berger, Dan, 239–40n41, 239n38
Berkman, Alexander, 107, 111
Bernstein, Frances Lee, 108
Bettelheim, Bruno, 174
Bevins, Vincent, 171
Beyond the Pleasure Principle (Freud), 177, 196–7
Bhattacharyya, Gargi, 23
Big Flame, 220n22
Bion, Wilfred, 26–7
bitterness, 130–57
Black, Hannah, 200, 206, 212
Black Arts Movement, 118
'A Black Feminist Statement' (CRC), 152
black liberation movement, 127, 139
Black Lives Matter, 97, 117
Black Panther Party, 4, 5, 72, 99, 100
Black Power, 117–8
The Black Woman (Bambara), 128
Blanqui, Louis Auguste, 59–61
Blanquists, 49, 59–60
Blida-Joinville psychiatric hospital (Algeria), 17
Bloody Week of 21 to 28 May (*semaine sanglante)*, 49, 51
Boggs, Grace Lee, 128
Bolsonaro, Jair, 199
Boltanski, Luc, 71
Bonney, Sean, 203
Border Country (Williams), 9–10
Bordowitz, Gregg, 67, 99
Boric, Gabriel, 184
Boym, Svetlana, 43
brainwashing, 138
Brazil, 248–9n28
Brecht, Bertolt, v, 41, 48, 141
Briet, Pierre Urbain, 54
British Black Panthers, 198
Brixton Black Women's Group, 13

Brostoff, Ari, 156
Brown, Michael, 22, 200, 201
Brown, Wendy, 34, 35, 40
Buckow Elegies (Brecht), 41
Bullard, Alice, 51, 55–6
burnout. *See also* burnout society; movement burnout
  according to Freudenberger, 91–2
  according to WHO, 90
  origins of term, 91
  use of term, 89
Burn-Out: How to Beat the High Cost of Success (Freudenberger), 98
burnout society, 90–1
Burnout Survival Kit (Daal), 90
Byung-Chul Han, 90

C

Callen-Lorde Community Health Project (originally Community Health Project), 99
Calvert, Greg, 139
Canessa, Carla Fischer, 172
Can't Even: How Millennials Became the Burnout Generation (Petersen), 90
Can't Get You Out of My Head (Curtis), 72
capitalist realism, 68, 72
'The Case of Missing Male Authority' (Freudenberger), 95–7
Central Executive Committee Rest Home (Tetkovo), 111
Chabot, Pascale, 90
Chiapello, Eve, 71
Chicago Westside Group, 146
Chile, Obstinate Memory (film), 177
Chilean Psychoanalytic Association, 171, 172

Cintron, Lourdes, 77, 229n38
Civil Action group, 152
civil rights movement, 106, 112, 113, 117, 144
Clark, Kenneth, 235n40
Cleaver, Eldridge, 5
Clements, Barbara Evans, 108
Coles, Robert, 112–7, 124, 126, 128
colonial nostalgia, 57–8
Comay, Rebecca, 177
Combahee River Collective (CRC), 152, 153, 155, 156
Common Ground Health Clinic, 101, 232n46
Commune, 224n8
Communist Party of Indonesia (PKI), 162–3, 164
community care, structures of, 97
Community Health Project (later Callen-Lorde Community Health Center), 99
Condition of the English Working Class (Engels), 108–9
Congo Diary (Guevara), 5
consciousness-raising, 130, 138, 143, 144, 145, 146, 152, 237n3
Corbyn, Jeremy, 23, 31, 156
The Cordillera of Dreams (film), 177–8, 184, 185
Courbet, Gustave, 211
CRC (Combahee River Collective), 152, 153, 155, 156
Crenshaw, Kimberlé, 152–3, 155
Crimp, Douglas, 188–90, 191, 192–3, 195, 196, 198–9, 202
criticism-self-criticism, 131, 138, 139, 140–1, 142, 143, 147
'Criticism-Self-Criticism' (Mao), 139
Crocodile Hole, 243n10
Cultural Revolution, 239n40
Cunningham, Cath, 39
Curtis, Adam, 72
The Cutting-Edge: Women and the Pit Strike (Seddon), 37–8
Cvetkovich, Ann, 65–9, 75, 76, 78, 81, 84

D

Daal, Imogen, 90
Darda, Joseph, 166–7
Daughter of Earth (Smedley), 208–9
Davis, Angela Y., 127, 201
Davis, Mike, 98, 99, 212–3
The Days of the Commune (Brecht), 48
Dean, Jodi, 35–6, 40
depression, 62–86, 114, 227–8n2. *See also* political depression
Depression: A Public Feeling (Cvetkovich), 65–9
Derrida, Jacques, 177
Diagnostic and Statistical Manual of Mental Disorders
 DSM-III, 165–6
 DSM-IIIR, 166
 DSM-V, 27, 167
The Dialectic of Sex: The Case for Feminist Revolution (Firestone), 65, 70, 71, 73, 76–9, 83, 228n17
Díaz, Margarita, 174–6, 183
Di Prima, Diane, 1
disrelation, 95
Dohrn, Bernadine, 239n36
dolls, 235n40
Douma, Ahmed, 7–8, 10
Drabble, Barbara, 38
Durkheim, Emile, 4
Dwyer, Leslie, 163–4

E

Eagleton, Terry, 15
East London Big Flame, 11
Ebony (magazine), 4
Echols, Alice, 240n44
El Barrio Free Clinic (originally East LA Clinic), 98
Elbaum, Max, 151
Elementary Aspects of Peasant Insurgency in Colonial India (Guha), 58–9
El-Fattah, Alaa Abd, 7–9, 10
'Emancipation and Exhaustion' (Haider), 104
Emejulu, Akwugo, 129
Enduring Time (Baraitser), 2
Engels, Friedrich, 35, 77, 108–9
Erikson, Erik, 96, 113
Ernst, Sheila, 15, 220n27
  In Our Own Hands: A Book of Self-Help Therapy, 220n23
Esch, Betsy, 154
Eternity by the Stars (Blanqui), 60
Everything for Everyone: An Oral History of the New York Commune, 2052–2072 (O'Brien and Abdelhadi), 207
exhaustion, 103–29. *See also* nervous exhaustion; political exhaustion
Exhaustion: A History (Schaffner), 107
'Experience and Poverty' (Benjamin), 41

F

Facing Reality (James), 128
Fanon, Frantz, 16, 17–20, 28, 99
Fanshen (Hinton), 133–8, 139, 144–5, 157
Fanshen Women, 144

Fassin, Didier, 161–2
Felman, Shoshana, 177
Ferenczi, Sándor, 197
Ferrari, Joe, 192
Ferré, Théophile, 47
Firestone, Shulamith, 64, 65, 70–1, 72, 73–4, 76–9, 81, 83, 84, 143, 147, 229n38
Fisher, Mark, 68, 69, 72, 81, 84
Floyd, George, 7, 23, 44, 129, 200, 201
Flying (Millet), 70, 75, 79, 83
Forster, Laura C., 45
Foucault, Michel, 90
free clinic movement, 91, 92–5, 97, 98–9, 100, 102
Freeman, Jo, 146–7
FRELIMO (Mozambique Liberation Front), 122
Freud, Sigmund, 15, 27, 28, 40, 168, 174, 177, 187–8, 189–90, 191, 194, 195–7, 198, 200, 201, 208
Freudenberger, Herbert J., 89, 91–2, 93–8, 99, 100, 102
Fromm, Erich, 96
Front de Libération Nationale (FLN), 18

G

Garb, Tamar, 193
Garner, Eric, 201
Gay Men's Health Project Clinic, 99
Gaza War
  2014, 164
  2023, 202
Geldof, Bob, 32
Gentrification of the Mind (Schulman), 190–1
Gilbert, David, 142
Gilmore, Ruth Wilson, 101, 127–8

The God that Failed: Six Studies in Communism (Koestler), 151
Gogarty, Larne Abse, 222n47
'Going Critical' (Bambara), 125
Goldman, Emma, 111
'Good for Nothing' (Fisher), 68
Goodison, Lucy, 220n23
Gordon, Avery, 127, 128, 171
Gordon, Eric A., 131, 133
Gornick, Vivian, 130, 147–51, 154, 155–6
Gorz, André, 127
Grandier, Albert, 52
Grenfell, Francis, 198
Grenfell Tower fire (14 June 2017), 186–7, 198
'Griffiti for Two' (El-Fattah and Douma), 7–8
'Group Psychology and the Analysis of the Ego' (Freud), 195–6
Guangzhou Commune, 48
Guardian, report on miners' strike (UK 1984–85), 37
Guevara, Ernesto ('Che'), 5–6, 99
Guha, Ranajit, 58–9
Guzmán, Patricio, 164, 176–8, 179–82, 183, 184–5, 197

H

Habit (Bordowitz), 67
Haider, Asad, 104
Hall, Stuart, 20, 31–2, 34, 37, 39, 221–2n43, 223n3
Hallward, Peter, 60, 61
Handsworth Songs (Black Audio Film Collective), 186
Hanisch, Carol, 143–4, 155
The Hard Road to Renewal: Thatcherism and the Crisis of the Left (Hall), 31–2

Haslett, Tobi, 7, 201, 222n47
Haupt, Georges, 45, 48
Haywood, Bill, 187
Hedva, Johanna, 69
Hendin, Herbert, 4
Herzog, Dagmar, 166
Hill, Joe, 187
Hinton, William, 133–8, 139, 141, 143, 144, 145, 156, 157
History of the Commune of 1871 (Lissagaray), 50
Ho Chi Minh, 6
Hofer, Johannes, 53
Hoffarth, Matthew J., 94
Holloway Prison, 23, 205
Holmes, Linda Janet, 120
Holocaust piety, 247n65
Home from the War: Vietnam Veterans: Neither Victims nor Executioners (Lifton), 167–8
hooks, bell, 126–7
hooliganism, 234n18
Hughes, Langston, 42
The Hundred Day War: The Cultural Revolution at Tsinghua University (Hinton), 142
Hunter, Edward, 138
'Hurt People' (London), 23–4
Hutton, Patrick, 60

I

I Burn Paris (Jasieński), 212
identity politics, 152–3
ILAS (Latin American Institute of Mental Health and Human Rights), 172, 173, 174, 181, 184
Illner, Peer, 232n46
Indonesia, New Order regime, 162–3
Indonesian massacres, 243–4n13

In Our Own Hands: A Book of Self-Help Therapy (Ernst and Goodison), 220n23
INRI (Zurita), 182, 183, 184–5
Institute of the Black World, 128
insurgent social reproduction, 97
interpersonal dynamics, 222n45
Ioffe, Adolf, 111

J

Jabr, Samah, 161, 164
Jackson, George, 6
Jacobs, John, 143
Jacques, Martin, 32
Jaffe, Sarah, 91, 97, 98
The Jakarta Method (Bevins), 171
James, C. L. R., 47, 128, 209
Jasieński, Bruno, 212
Jemaah Islamiyah, 161
jikohihan (self-criticism), 130. *See also* self-criticism
July, Serge, 85
June Journeys (June Days), 194

K

Kanak people, 51, 57–9
Kästner, Erich, 34, 41
Keilson, Hans, 173
Kelley, Robin D. G., 154
Keniston, Kenneth, 96
Khaled, Leila, 2–3, 5, 6
Khrushchev, Nikita, 128, 149
Kindred Southern Healing Justice Collective, 101, 102
Klein, Naomi, 21
Koedt, Anne, 143
Koestler, Arthur, 150–1
Kraeplin, Emil, 165
Kronstadt naval base uprising (March 1921), 110, 111
Kunanbayev, Abai, 22
Kupers, Terry, 100–1
Kuta bombings, 161, 163
Kwon, Heonik, 169, 170, 245n35

L

LaCapra, Dominick, 176
Ladner, Joyce, 117
Lagos, Ricardo, 182
Lapsansky, Emma Jones, 117–8
Lasch, Christopher, 231n24
Latin American Institute of Mental Health and Human Rights (ILAS), 172, 173, 174, 181, 184
Laub, Dori, 177
left melancholy, 33, 34–6, 37, 38, 41, 44, 210
'Left-Wing Melancholy' (Benjamin), 34
Lenin, V. I., 46, 47, 108, 110, 111, 207
Lenin Rest Home (Maryino), 111
Lerne, Jonathan, 141
Lesbians and Gays Support the Miners, 38
Let the Record Show (Schulman), 192
Lewis, Gail, 13, 220n24
Leys, Ruth, 175, 177
Liebert, Robert, 97
Lierop, Robert van, 122
Lifton, Robert Jay, 167–8, 176
Lissagaray, Prosper Olivier, 50–1, 52
Little Red Book (Mao), 139
Live Aid, 32
The Lives of Others (Mukherjee), 105–6, 107
Lombroso, Césare, 59
London, Bobby, 23–4
Long Beach Free Clinic, 98

Long Bow cadre, 133, 134, 135, 138, 139, 141, 144, 145
The Look of Silence (documentary), 182, 183
The Loony Bin Trip (Millett), 70, 74–6, 77, 229n33
Lorde, Audre, 208
Love's Work (Rose), 203
Luckhurst, Roger, 247n63, 247n65
Lula da Silva, Luiz Inácio, 199
Lumumba, Patrice, 5, 193
Lumumba, Pauline Opango, 193
A Luta Continua (documentary), 122
Luxemburg, Rosa, 46–7, 209
Lye, Colleen, 152–4, 155

M

Maguire, Marie, 14, 15, 220n27
Makdisi, Saree, 202
Mangrove (film), 198
Maoist precepts, 238n17
Mao Zedong, 134, 136, 138, 139, 142, 153, 154
Marcuse, Herbert, 96
'Margaret Thatcher and Ruth Ellis' (Rose), 32
Marriott, David, 221n40
Martin, Trayvon, 201
Marx, Eleanor, 50
Marx, Karl, 35, 43, 49, 51, 77, 174
Maslach, Christina, 94
Mass Psychology of Fascism (Reich), 33
May '68 and its Afterlives (Ross), 84–6
McClain, Elijah, 200
Meadows, Alfie, 222n47
melancholia, 31–41. *See also* left melancholy

Memoirs of a Revolutionary (Serge), 3, 118
'Memorial Rags' (Moon), 248n14
Mendelssohn, Anna, 204–5
Mercier, Lucie K., 17
m/f (journal), 15
Michel, Louise, 48, 50, 52, 54, 56, 57
Millett, Kate, 62, 64, 70, 74–6, 79, 83, 84, 147, 229n33, 240n55, 241n59
miners' strike (UK 1984û85), 37–9, 209–10
Mitchell, Juliet, 145
Mitscherlich, Alexander, 96
Moon, Michael, 248n14
Mori, Tsuneo, 130
Morrissey, Susan K., 234n24
Moten, Fred, 16, 17
Moulian, Tomás, 183–4
mournful militancy, 41, 193, 194, 200, 202
mourning, 186–202
Mourning and Melancholia (Freud), 40, 187–8, 189–90
'Mourning and Militancy' (Crimp), 188–9
movement burnout, 97
Mozambique Liberation Front (FRELIMO), 122
Mubenga, Jimmy, 201
Muckle, Adrian, 58
Mukherjee, Neel, 105–6, 107
My Imaginary Country (film), 184
My Lai, 167, 168, 169–70, 171

N

Nelson, Alondra, 99
nervous exhaustion, 27, 107, 108, 110, 111, 112

nervousness, 108, 233n10
Network Against Psychiatric Assault, 229n33
neurasthenia, 107, 108, 111, 233n10
New Economic Policy (NEP, 1921–28), 108, 109, 112
The New Inquiry, 'Hurt People' article, 23–4
New Left, 10, 20, 139, 149, 237n6, 240n50
New Soviet Person, 112
The New Spirit of Capitalism (Boltanski and Chiapello), 71
Newton, Huey P., 4–5
New York Radical Women, 144, 147
Ngai, Sianne, 65
Nietzsche, Friedrich, 61
1968: A Student Generation in Revolt, 79–80
No Logo (Klein), 21
non-reformist reform, 127, 128
nostalgia, 42–61
Nostalgia for the Light (film), 177, 180, 181–2, 185
Notes from the Second Year: Women's Liberation (Firestone and Koedt), 143
Nunes, Rodrigo, 199

O

O'Brien, M. E., 97, 207
October Revolution (1917), 3, 27, 46, 47, 106, 107, 110, 151
Ono, Shin'ya, 140
'On the Issue of Roles' (Bambara), 129
Oppenheimer, Joshua, 182, 183
Orshanskii, Lev G., 234n18
orthodox left, 248–9n28
O'Sullivan, Lisa, 53, 54

P

Page, Cara, 101
'Paranoid Reading and Reparative Reading' (Sedgwick), 188
Paris Commune of 1871, 43, 45–8, 54, 56, 58, 211
Passerini, Luisa, 64, 80–4
The Pearl Button (film), 177, 180, 183, 184, 197
'The Personal Is Political' (Hanisch), 143
Peslikis, Irene, 144
Petersen, Anne Helen, 90, 91, 97
Phillips, Dorothy, 38–9
Piepzna-Samarasinha, Leah Lakshmi, 101
Pinochet, Augusto, 164, 171–2, 184
PKI (Communist Party of Indonesia), 162–3, 164
Plaetzer, Niklas, 57
Plan C, 222n50
Platonov, Andrei, 103
political commemoration, 224n6
political delegations, 238n21
political depression, 66, 67, 68, 70
political exhaustion, 64, 104
political funerals, 193
political nostalgia, 43, 44, 54–5
'Posttraumatic Politics: Violence, Memory, and Biomedical Discourse in Bali' (Dwyer and Santikarma), 163
post-traumatic stress disorder (PTSD), 161, 162, 163–73, 175, 177, 243n4, 244n15, 244n17
post-Vietnam syndrome, 167
Poussaint, Alvin, 116–7, 219n8
Preston, George, 182
Proletarian Nights (Rancière), 104
Przyblyski, Jeannene M., 211

psychological manipulation, 138, 146
Psychopolitics (Sedgwick), 13
'Public Feelings', 66
Pyne, Anne Forer, 144

R

Radical and Militant Youth: A Psychoanalytic Inquiry (Liebert), 97
radical psychiatry, 220n19
Radical Therapist collective, 10–1
Rahim, Malik, 101
Rancière, Jacques, 104
Rechtman, Richard, 161–2
Reclus, Élie, 49
Red Army/PLFP: Declaration of World War (documentary), 2–3
Red Star Over China (Snow), 138
Redstockings, 144, 154
Red Therapy, 11–3, 14, 15, 16, 220n22, 220n23, 220n24, 220n27
Reed, Ishmael, 123
Reich, Wilhelm, 15, 16, 28, 33, 191
'Resisting Left Melancholy' (Brown), 34, 40
Revolution and Youth (Zalkind), 109
revolutionary subjective universality, 42
Revolutionary Suicide (Newton), 4
Revolution in the Air (Elbaum), 151
Riesman, David, 96
Roe v. Wade, 155
The Romance of American Communism (Gornick), 148, 155–6
Rose, Gillian, 203
Rose, Jacqueline, 15–6, 28, 32–3, 34, 187–8, 191–2, 194
Rosemont, Franklin, 247n6

Ross, Andrew, 238n17
Ross, Kristin, 48, 56, 84–6
Rousseff, Dilma, 199
Rowan, John, 220n22
Rowbotham, Sheila, 14–5
Rowe, William, 184–5
Rudd, Mark, 139, 152
Rukeyser, Muriel, 203, 205, 208
Russakova, Liuba, 3
Ryan, Joanna, 14, 220n27

S

Saban Community Clinic, 99
Sadowsky, Jonathan, 71, 72
The Salt Eaters (Bambara), 106–7, 119, 120–2, 123–6, 128, 156
Sanders, Bernie, 23, 33, 156
Santikarma, Degung, 163–4
Sarachild, Kathie, 144
Sartre, Jean-Paul, 18
Savage Coast (Rukeyser), 208
Schaffner, Anna Katharina, 107
Schulman, Sarah, 190–1, 192, 193
SDS (Students for a Democratic Society), 131, 139, 140, 152
'The Sea Birds are Still Alive' (Bambara), 122, 125
Second Intifada, 244n17
Seddon, Vicky, 37–8
Sedgwick, Eve Kosofsky, 188, 189
Sedgwick, Peter, 13
self-criticism, 130, 131, 132, 139, 140, 141, 149, 153, 154, 155, 237n6, 238n17, 239n36. *See also* criticism-self-criticism
semaine sanglante (Bloody Week of 21 to 28 May), 49, 51
Serge, Victor, 3, 112, 118, 209
Sexuality in the field of Vision (Rose), 191–2

Sexual Politics (Millett), 70
Shakur, Afeni, 72
Shanghai People's Commune of 1967, 48
'Sick Woman Theory' (Hedva), 69
Siegel, James, 245n35
Silouan, Staretz, 203
Sisters of the Yam: Black Women and Self-Recovery (hooks), 126–7
Slezkine, Yuri, 111
Slobodian, Quinn, 154–5
Smedley, Agnes, 208–9
Smith, Barbara, 152, 156–7
Smith, David E., 92
Smith, Jason E., 44
SNCC (Student Non-Violent Coordinating Committee), 113, 117
Snow, Edgar, 138
social movements, 220n19
Social Solidarity Health Centre, 101–2
'Social Struggle and Weariness' (Coles), 112–7
socialthérapie, 17
Society for Old Bolsheviks, 111
sôkatsu (collective examination of organisational problems), 130
Soltz, Aron, 109
'Song of the Captives' (Michel), 54
Soreanu, Raluca, 194–5, 196, 197, 198, 199, 200, 249n41
Southern Conference Educational Fund (SCEF), 240n42
Souza, Amarildo de, 199–200
Spanish Civil War, 224n6
Spieler, Miranda Frances, 226n41
spiritual healing processes, 236n76
Spitzer, Robert, 165
Stalin, Joseph, 48, 237n6
Stewart, Susan, 44

St Marks Clinic, 99, 100, 101
Student Non-Violent Coordinating Committee (SNCC), 113, 117
Students for a Democratic Society (SDS), 131, 139, 140, 152
Suharto, 162–3
suicide, 3–5, 50, 71, 73, 74, 76, 77, 79, 85, 110, 111, 112
Sutherland, Keston, 42–3, 46

T

Tahrir Square, 8, 9, 48
Thatcher, Margaret, 31, 32–3, 34
Thatcherism, 223n3
Thiers, Adolphe, 49
Thorburn, Margo, 38
Thornton, Cassie, 101
thought reform, 138
The Thousand Year War (Hinton), 156
Tomba, Massimiliano, 56
Tombs, Robert, 225n27
Toscano, Alberto, 72
Tosquelles, François, 17
Totem and Taboo (Freud), 168
trashing, 240n55
'TRASHING: The Dark Side of Sisterhood' (Freeman), 146–7
trauma, 161–85, 243n6, 246n49, 246n60, 247n63, 247n64
Trauma: A Genealogy (Leys), 175
'Trauma: Care and Cure' conference (2002), 162
trauma industry, 161, 166
Traverso, Enzo, 36
Troops Out, 11, 12
Trotsky, Leon, 47, 111
Truth Commission (Brazil), 171
Tuesday or September or The End (Black), 206

'Tyranny of Structurelessness' (Freeman), 146

U
United Red Army, 140
US health care system, 231n31

V
van der Kolk, Bessel, 177
Varon, Jeremy, 142
Verdure, Augustin, 52
Vietnam, 245n34
Vietnam Veterans Against the War (VVAW), 167
Vilar, Jean-François, 85
Villalobos-Ruminott, Sergio, 184
'virgin earth', 226n41

W
Weathermen (later Weather Underground), 139, 140, 143, 152
Weather Underground (formerly Weathermen), 138, 139–40, 141, 143, 147, 150, 153
Weeks, Kathi, 70–1, 72, 76, 81
Weiss, Gregory L., 93
Weiss, Peter, 55
What Is to Be Done? (Lenin), 207–8
'Where Does the Misery Come From?' (Rose), 15
Whitehorn, Laura, 122
WHO (World Health Organization), on burnout, 90
Widodo, Joko, 183
Wiener, Jon, 98, 99
Wilkerson, Cathy, 139

Williams, Raymond, 9–10, 212
Willis, Susan, 123
Wilson, Darren, 22, 201
Wojnarowicz, David, 187, 193
Women's Estate (Mitchell), 145
Women's Liberation Conference (1978), 13
women's liberation movement, 11, 13, 14, 64, 65, 70, 75, 77, 121, 138, 143, 145, 148, 150, 152, 154, 220n27, 241n59
Women's Therapy Centre (North London), 15
Worker's Opposition's 'New Course', 111
Workers Revolutionary Party (WRP), 237–8n7
Working-through Collective Wounds: Trauma, Denial, Recognition in the Brazilian Uprising (Soreanu), 194
World Health Organization (WHO), on burnout, 90
The Wretched of the Earth (Fanon), 16, 18, 19

Y
Young Lords' medical campaigns, 231n32

Z
Zalkind, Aron, 109
Zhenotdel, 107
Zimmerman, George, 201
Zurita, Raúl, 182–3, 184–5